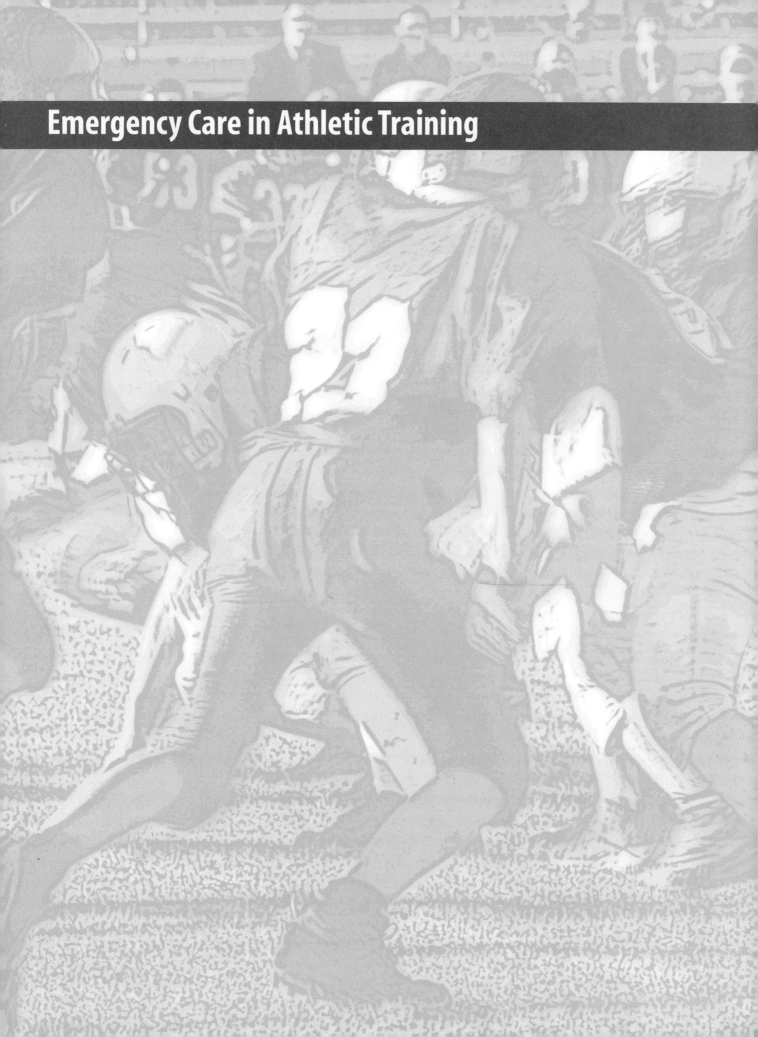

Emergency Care in Athletic Training

Emergency Care in Athletic Training

Keith M. Gorse, MEd, ATC

Instructor and Clinical Coordinator
Department of Athletic Training
Duquesne University
Pittsburgh, Pennsylvania

Robert O. Blanc, MS, ATC, EMT-P

Director of Athletic Performance
University of Pittsburgh
Pittsburgh, Pennsylvania

Francis Feld, MS, MEd, CRNA, ATC, NREMT-P

Certified Registered Nurse Anesthetist, UPMC-Mercy Hospital, Pittsburgh, Pennsylvania
Prehospital RN Ross West View EMSA, Pittsburgh, Pennsylvania
Prehospital RN University Ambulance Service, State College, Pennsylvania
Deputy Chief, Allegheny County Hazardous Materials Medical Team,
  Pittsburgh, Pennsylvania
Supervisory Nurse Specialist, PA-1 Disaster Medical Assistance Team,
  Pittsburgh, Pennsylvania
Formerly Athletic Trainer for the University of Pittsburgh and Pittsburgh Steelers Football
  Teams

Matthew Radelet, MS, ATC, CSCS

Current Student Physician Assistant Program
A.T. Still University
Arizona School of Health Sciences
Mesa, Arizona

Formerly Associate Athletic Trainer
The University of Arizona
Tucson, Arizona

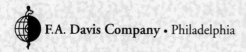
F.A. Davis Company • Philadelphia

F. A. Davis Company
1915 Arch Street
Philadelphia, PA 19103
www.fadavis.com

Printed in the United States of America

Last digit indicates print number: 10 9 8 7 6 5 4 3 2 1

Publisher, Health Professions and Medicine: Margaret M. Biblis
Senior Acquisition Editors: Christa Fratantoro and Quincy McDonald
Manager of Content Development: George W. Lang
Senior Developmental Editor: Jennifer A. Pine
Art and Illustration Manager: Carolyn O'Brien

As new scientific information becomes available through basic and clinical research, recommended treatments and drug therapies undergo changes. The author(s) and publisher have done everything possible to make this book accurate, up to date, and in accord with accepted standards at the time of publication. The author(s), editors, and publisher are not responsible for errors or omissions or for consequences from application of the book, and make no warranty, expressed or implied, in regard to the contents of the book. Any practice described in this book should be applied by the reader in accordance with professional standards of care used in regard to the unique circumstances that may apply in each situation. The reader is advised always to check product information (package inserts) for changes and new information regarding dose and contraindications before administering any drug. Caution is especially urged when using new or infrequently ordered drugs.

Library of Congress Cataloging-in-Publication Data

Emergency care in athletic training/Keith M. Gorse ... [et al.].
   p. ; cm.
Includes bibliographical references.
ISBN-13: 978-0-8036-1496-3
ISBN-10: 0-8036-1496-9
1. Sports emergencies. 2. Sports injuries. I. Gorse, Keith M.
[DNLM: 1. Athletic Injuries—therapy. 2. Emergencies—psychology. 3. Emergency Treatment—methods.
4. Sports Medicine—methods. QT 261 E53 2010]
RD97.E46 2010
617. 1'027–dc22

2009023704

Certified athletic trainers are health care professionals who are experts in injury prevention, assessment, treatment, and rehabilitation, particularly in the orthopedic and musculoskeletal disciplines. Athletic trainers have been recognized by the American Medical Association as allied health care professionals since the early 1990s. To be eligible for board certification, athletic training students must graduate from an accredited undergraduate or graduate athletic training curriculum, which consists of course work and clinical experience in several areas, including assessment and evaluation, acute care, general medical conditions, and pathology of injury and illness. Athletic trainers must hold a minimum of a bachelor's degree from an accredited program. In addition to board certification, many states regulate the athletic training profession through licensure, registration, or certification.

One of the most critical components of being an athletic trainer is the ability to provide appropriate care to a suddenly injured or ill athlete. *Emergency Care in Athletic Training* is a specialized textbook that addresses the specific educational needs of athletic training students and certified athletic trainers who are preparing to handle emergency medical situations in all areas of athletics.

Until recently, many athletic training educators have had to rely on general first aid materials that do not adequately address the needs of their programs. The authors of this textbook have stepped up to fulfill the growing need for more dynamic material that focuses on providing immediate medical care in athletics. *Emergency Care in Athletic Training* is written specifically for athletic trainers, athletic training students, and other sports medicine professionals focusing on the skills, knowledge, practice, and preparation needed to handle athletic emergency situations. Special features, such as the "Emergency Situations" that begin every chapter, help students use critical thinking skills by providing them with real-world examples. Students can see how well they responded by checking the resolution in the "Emergency Action" section at the end of the chapter. Additional case studies at the end of each chapter help students work through emergency care problems. Students can readily review the chapter material with the "Chapter Highlights" and test themselves on their comprehension with end-of-chapter quizzes.

Emergency Care in Athletic Training is a textbook that will help instruct athletic training students and athletic trainers about the emergency situations they will inevitably face throughout their careers. Athletic training educators and certified athletic trainers will now have access to the essential resource they need to address all athletic emergencies.

Contributors

Kevin M. Guskiewicz, PhD, ATC
Professor and Chair
Director, Sports Medicine Research Laboratory
University of North Carolina
Chapel Hill, North Carolina

Vincent N. Mosesso, Jr, MD, FACEP
Department of Emergency Medicine
UPMC Presbyterian Emergency Department
Pittsburgh, Pennsylvania

Johna Register-Mihalik, MA, ATC
Department of Exercise and Sport Science
University of North Carolina
Chapel Hill, North Carolina

Stephen Russo, PhD
Licensed Clinical and Sport Psychologist
Nova Southern University
Fort Lauderdale, Florida

David Stone, MD
Assistant Professor and Team Physician
Division of Sports Medicine
UPMC Center for Sports Medicine
Pittsburgh, Pennsylvania

Giampietro Vairo, MS, ATC
Assistant Athletic Trainer
Penn State University
State College, Pennsylvania

Scott Wissink, MD
Family Practice Medicine
UPMC Monroeville
Monroeville, Pennsylvania

Reviewers

Joel W. Beam, EdD, ATC, LAT
Program Director, Assistant Professor
Department of Athletics and Physical Therapy
University of North Florida
Jacksonville, Florida

Debbie I. Craig, PhD, ATC, LAT
Program Director, Assistant Professor, Athletic Training Education Program
Department of Rehabilitation Sciences
Northern Arizona University
Flagstaff, Arizona

Eric J. Fuchs, DA, ATC, EMT
Assistant Professor and Clinical Coordinator of Athletic Training Education Program
Department of Exercise and Sports Science
Eastern Kentucky University
Richmond, Kentucky

Bonnie M. Goodwin, MESS, ATC
Director, Athletic Training Education Program
Department of Health and Sport Sciences
Capital University
Columbus, Ohio

Brian M. Hatzel, PhD, ATC
Assistant Professor
Department of Movement Science
Grand Valley State University
Allendale, Michigan

Michelle M. Lesperance, MS, ATC, LAT
Program Director of Athletic Training Education Program, Assistant Professor of Kinesiology
Department of Kinesiology
Greensboro College
Greensboro, North Carolina

Joseph S. Lueken, MS, LAT, ATC
Athletic Trainer/Instructor
Department of Athletics
Indiana University
Bloomington, Indiana

Brendon P. McDermott, MS, ATC
Laboratory Instructor/Research Assistant
Department of Kinesiology
University of Connecticut
Storrs, Connecticut

Gary E. McIlvain, MS, ATC
Assistant Professor/ATEP Clinical Coordinator
Division of Exercise Science, Sport and Recreation
Marshall University
Huntington, West Virginia

Joseph B. Myers, PhD, ATC
Associate Professor
Department of Exercise and Sport Science
University of North Carolina
Chapel Hill, North Carolina

Matthew Rothbard, MS, ATC
Clinical Assistant Professor
Department of Kinesiology
Towson University
Towson, Maryland

Susan Saliba, PhD, ATC, MPT
Senior Associate Athletic Trainer, Associate Professor, Curry School of Education, School of Medicine
Department of Athletics
University of Virginia
Charlottesville, Virginia

Stacy Walker, PhD, ATC
Assistant Professor
Department of School of Physical Education, Sport, and Exercise Science
Ball State University
Muncie, Indiana

Sharon West, PhD, ATC
Associate Professor, ATEP Director
Department of Sport Sciences
University of the Pacific
Stockton, California

Acknowledgments

Keith would like to bestow his sincere love and appreciation to his wife, Betsy, and his children, Erin and Tyler. They were a main source of encouragement and support through the entire research and writing process. Keith would also like to thank the entire faculty, staff, and students in the Athletic Training Department at Duquesne University for their support over the last 8 years.

Rob would like to thank his mother; his wife, Peggy; his children, Jason, Jordan, and Shannon; and his entire family for the support they have given him. Rob would also like to thank the staff and volunteers at Tri-Community South, EMS for the education and mentoring they provided to him over his 17 years there.

Francis would like to thank Christine and Zoe for their love and support. He would also like to thank the paramedics and EMTs of Ross West View and Penn State EMS who are not only colleagues but also friends. We've been through tough situations and they only made us stronger.

Matt would like to gratefully acknowledge Susie Kenney for her support and assistance throughout the most difficult parts of this long project. Her many hours of work helped make this book possible. He would also like to thank Melanie Weiser and Doug Cantaoi for their assistance arranging for and being part of the photographs in Chapter 12.

Contents

Chapter 1

Organization and Administration of Emergency Care

Keith M. Gorse, MEd, ATC

KEY TERMS

Bloodborne
    pathogens
Documentation
Emergency action plan

Emergency medical services
First responder
Legal need
Patient assessment

Sports medicine staff
    and emergency team

 EMERGENCY SITUATION

During the second half of a boy's high school basketball game a player collapses on the court. Play is immediately stopped by the referee, and he goes to check on the player. The referee then yells for assistance from the athletic trainer covering the event. The athletic trainer runs onto the court to check on the unresponsive player. He checks all vitals and finds that the player is not breathing and has no pulse. At this point, what should the athletic trainer do to help the stricken player?

Call 911
AED - Ambo Bag
CPR 30:2

Emergency medical situations can occur in athletics at any time. When they do occur, it is important to have the proper **emergency action plan** (EAP) in place to provide the best possible care to the athletes with potentially life-threatening injuries or illness. The development and implementation of the EAP will help ensure that the quality of care provided to the athletes is the best possible. The goal of the sports medicine staff of any athletic organization is to have an EAP that will minimize the time needed to provide an immediate response to a potentially life-threatening situation or medical emergency.

Because medical emergencies can occur during any activity, the sports medicine staff must be prepared for any type of situation. Emergency care preparation includes the formation of an EAP, proper coverage of athletic events and practices, maintenance of emergency equipment and supplies, utilization of appropriate personnel involved with the sports medicine team, and the continuing education of the sports medicine team in emergency medical care (Box 1-1). Although every precaution may be taken by the athletic organization and its sports medicine staff, it is important to understand that medical emergencies may still occur. With proper organization and administration, however, these situations can be handled in a timely, effective, and professional manner.

Factors to consider in the proper organization and administration of emergency care in athletic activity include the following:

1. Development and implementation of an EAP
2. The **sports medicine staff and emergency team**
3. Initial **patient assessment** and care
4. Emergency communication
5. Emergency equipment and supplies
6. Venue locations
7. Emergency transportation
8. Emergency care facilities
9. **Legal need** and **documentation**

Box 1-1 Components of Emergency Care Preparation

- **Development of an EAP**
- **Proper coverage of athletic events and practices**
- **Maintenance and upkeep of emergency equipment and supplies**
- **Selection of appropriate personnel as part of the sports medicine team**
- **Continuing education of the sports medicine team in emergency medical care**

This chapter provides a framework for emergency care involving athletic trainers from an organizational and administrative perspective. The major chapter topic will concern issues relating to the development of the EAP and its contents. The chapter ends with an explanation of the legal need for emergency management for athletic organizations and their facilities and the proper documentation needed to reduce the liability factor and therefore the chances of a lawsuit.

Develop and Implement an EAP

Significant research regarding athletic injuries has been collected over the past decade, and it has been found that almost one third of athletes are injured in some way during their careers.[1–3] In a National Athletic Trainers' Association Position Statement it was recommended that each organization or institution that sponsors athletic activities or events develop and implement a written EAP.[4] Emergency action plans should be developed by organizational or institutional personnel in consultation with local **emergency medical services.**

✪ *STAT Point 1-1. Emergency action plans should be developed by organizational or institutional personnel in consultation with local emergency medical services.*

The EAP needs to be implemented for the safety of all athletic personnel, including athletes. It should be concise yet detailed enough to facilitate prompt and appropriate action. The development of an EAP and proper use of this plan often can make the difference in the outcome of an injury. All components of an EAP are connected, and they all must be considered to ensure a complete and favorable outcome in a potentially dangerous situation (Fig. 1-1). Once the importance of the EAP is realized and the plan has been developed, the EAP must be implemented. This is done through documentation of the plan, education of those involved, and frequent rehearsal of the plan itself.[4]

✪ *STAT Point 1-2. Once developed, the EAP is implemented through documentation of the plan, education of those involved, and frequent rehearsal of the plan itself.*

The EAP must provide a clear explanation of how it is going to work, allowing continuity among all members of the sports medicine staff and emergency team members. It is important to have a separate plan for different athletic venues and for practices versus games. Emergency team members, such as team physicians, may not necessarily be present at all athletic events, and this should be taken into account during development of the various EAPs. Also, the location and type of equipment required may be different among the

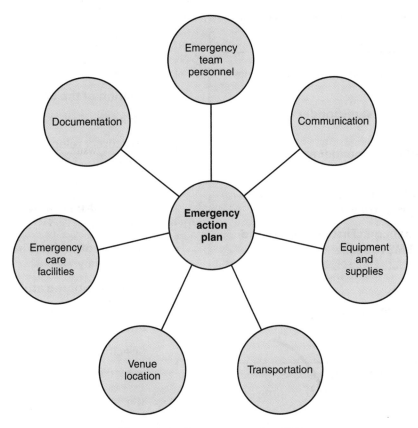

Figure 1-1. Components of an EAP.

sports teams and venues. For example, outdoor sports with a high risk of heat illness may require a large tub or wading pool to be used for emergency cooling of athletes at risk of heat stroke. This equipment would not be required for indoor sports.

It is important to properly educate all members of the emergency team regarding the EAP and its contents. All members of the team should be familiar with the emergency medical services (EMS) that will provide coverage to the venues. Each emergency team member, in addition to the athletic organization administrators, should have a written copy of the EAP that provides complete documentation of their roles and responsibilities in all emergency situations. A copy of the EAP specific to each venue should be posted by an available phone or some other prominent marked position at that site.

✪ *STAT Point 1-3. A copy of the EAP specific to the venue should be posted by an available phone or some other prominent marked position at that site.*

The emergency team must rehearse the EAP. This provides the team members with a chance to maintain their emergency skills at a high level of competency. It also provides the opportunity for athletic trainers and other emergency medical personnel to communicate regarding specific procedures in their respective areas. The EAP rehearsal can be accomplished through meetings held several times

throughout the year. One suggestion is to rehearse prior to the preseason for the high-risk sports, such as football in the fall, ice hockey in the winter, and lacrosse in the spring. Updates should be addressed as needed throughout the year because venues, emergency medical procedures, and emergency team members may change at any time.

Sports Medicine Staff and Emergency Team

The implementation of an EAP cannot take place without the formation of an emergency team. The primary members of this team consist of the sports medicine staff, which includes the athletic trainer and the team physician.[5] During an emergency the makeup of the emergency team can vary depending on who is at the scene at the time of the emergency. The emergency team can include athletic trainers, team physicians, athletic training students, team coaches, and equipment managers (Box 1-2). Any member of the emergency team can act as a **first responder.** A first responder is defined as a person who has been trained to provide emergency care before EMS arrives on the scene.[6] For this reason, all members of the emergency team should be trained and certified in first aid, cardiopulmonary resuscitation (CPR), automatic external defibrillation (AED), and prevention of disease

---

Box 1-2   The Emergency Team and Roles

- **Athletic trainer: First responder and immediate care**

- **Team physician: First responder and immediate care**

- **Team coach: First responder and activate emergency medical system**

- **Athletic training student: First responder and equipment retrieval**

- **Equipment manager: First responder and direction of EMS to scene**

---

transmission (**bloodborne pathogens**). Frequent EAP review and practice should be required for all members of the emergency team.

✪ *STAT Point 1-4. During an emergency, the makeup of the emergency team can vary depending on who is at the scene at the time of the emergency.*

In any emergency situation the roles of the members of the emergency team will vary depending on how many people are on the team, the venue that is being used, and the preferences of the athletic trainer (who is usually in charge of executing the EAP). The four roles within the emergency team are as follows:[5]

1. Immediate care of the athlete
2. Emergency equipment retrieval
3. Activation of the EMS system
4. Direction of EMS to the scene of the emergency

The first and most important role involves the immediate care of the injured athlete. The most qualified individual on the scene is usually the athletic trainer or team physician, either or both of whom should provide acute care in an emergency situation. This person should be trained in patient care and have good knowledge of the organization's EAP. Individuals who are less qualified, such as coaches or equipment managers, should yield to those who have more appropriate medical care training.[7]

Emergency equipment retrieval may be performed by a person on the emergency team who is familiar with the names and locations of the specific equipment that is required. Athletic training students would fit this role nicely. All necessary emergency equipment should be on site, in good condition, and easily accessible. Examples of emergency equipment include splints, spine board, bag valve mask, an AED device, first aid kit, and cell phone.

Activation of the EMS system is a priority where emergency transportation is not already present at the location of

---

Box 1-3   Activation of the Emergency Medical Service System

Activation of the EMS System:

1. **Make the Call—911 (if available) OR:**
2. **Use direct telephone numbers to local police, fire, and/or ambulance departments**

Provide Information to the EMS System:

1. **Name, address, and telephone number of the caller**
2. **Number of athletes involved in the emergency**
3. **Condition of the athlete(s)**
4. **Treatment initiated by members of the emergency team**
5. **Specific directions to the emergency scene**

---

the emergency.[8] If EMS is not at the scene, the system should be activated as soon as the situation is deemed to be an emergency. The person chosen for this role, such as a team coach, should be someone who is calm under pressure and who can communicate well over the telephone. This person should be able to communicate the nature of the emergency and the location of the emergency with specific directions to the venue (Box 1-3).

The emergency team should designate an individual to be in charge of opening any locked gates or doors and directing the local EMS to the scene of the emergency. An appropriate person for this responsibility would be an equipment manager because he or she typically is responsible for keys to locked gates or doors around the playing areas.

When assembling the emergency team, it is important to prepare each member of the team to adopt any of the emergency role situations. It may be a good idea to have more than one individual assigned to each of the four roles. This allows the emergency team to function without delay in the event that some members are not present.

Initial Patient Assessment and Care

Immediate care of any injured person needs to be the main concern for the emergency team. A CHECK—CALL—CARE system should be put into place for every member of the emergency team to follow when an emergency occurs (Box 1-4).[9]

The emergency team must CHECK the scene and the athlete. Team members first should make sure that it is safe to enter the area to help the injured person and, if there

---

Box 1-4 CHECK—CALL—CARE System

CHECK

- The scene to make sure it is safe to aid the athlete
- The scene to find evidence on what happened to the athlete
- The victim for airway, breathing, circulation, fractures, and bleeding

CALL

- 911 or the local emergency management service
- Give proper directions to the injury site
- Meet ambulance at scene and direct to injured athlete

CARE

- Calm and reassure the injured athlete
- Reassess and monitor all vital signs
- Control any bleeding
- Immobilize any injured body part
- Provide CPR/AED and appropriate first aid as needed

---

were no witnesses, check the area around the athlete to see what may have caused the injury. The emergency team should then check the injured person and see if he or she is conscious or unconscious. A team member should then check all vital signs: airway, breathing, and circulation. As the vital signs are being assessed, another emergency team member checks for bleeding and physical deformity on the athlete. While the CHECK mode is in progress an emergency team member should be stabilizing the injured person to ensure his or her safety. The injured party should not be permitted to move around because movement may cause further injury.

The emergency team must CALL 911 or the local emergency medical service and ensure the condition of the injured athlete is communicated to the EMS so the team arrives on the scene prepared for appropriate action. Proper directions to the site venue must be given to local EMS for quick and efficient travel time. An emergency team member should meet the ambulance as it arrives on the scene. This person should then direct the ambulance to the site of the injured athlete.

The emergency team must CARE for the injured athlete until the local EMS arrives at the accident site. Care should include the calming and reassuring of the injured person, assessing the injury, and monitoring all vital signs. The injured

athlete should be kept from moving injured body parts with immobilization techniques such as splints and spine boards. A properly stocked first aid kit with a working AED should always be available on site in case of an emergency.

All emergency team members need to have appropriate protection from bloodborne pathogens while taking care of any injured person.[10] Such articles of protection might include latex gloves and protective eyewear. Proper clean up of bodily fluids, such as blood or vomitus, and disposal of contaminated articles in biohazard containers or bags must be done as part of the proper management of any emergency situation.

The entire emergency team should stay at the site of the accident and help with the CHECK—CALL—CARE system. The team members should assist local EMS as needed with the transport of the injured person to the nearest emergency medical facility. This includes placing the athlete on a spine board or gurney and then assisting as necessary with placement into the ambulance. If necessary, EMS should then be escorted away from the emergency site; in some cases, such as on large college campuses with many roads that are either closed to vehicles or one-way only, EMS personnel may require some direction.[9] Only when the injured person is released to appropriate emergency medical personnel for transport can any member of the emergency team leave the site of the accident.

Emergency Communication

Communication is the key to quick and effective delivery of emergency care in any athletic trauma situation. Athletic trainers, other emergency team members, and EMS personnel must work together to provide the best possible care for injured athletes. Communication prior to an event is a good way to establish a positive working relationship between all groups of professionals.[11] If emergency medical transportation is not available on site during a particular event, then direct communication with the emergency medical system at the time of injury or illness is necessary.

Access to a working telephone or other telecommunications device, whether fixed or mobile, should be assured. The communications system should be checked prior to each practice or competition to ensure it is in proper working order.[12,13] A backup communications plan should be in effect should there be failure of the primary communication system. Currently the most common method of communication is a cellular telephone. However, at any athletic venue it is important to know the location of a working telephone other than a cellular phone because cellular service may not always be reliable or batteries may fail (Fig. 1-2).

✪ *STAT Point 1-5. A backup communications plan should be in effect should there be failure of the primary communication system.*

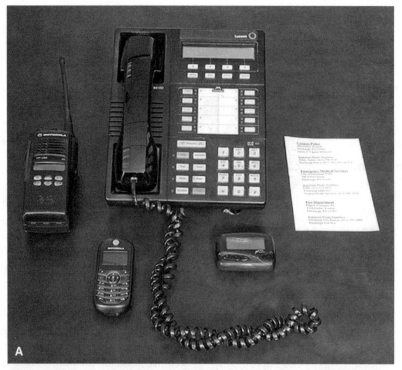

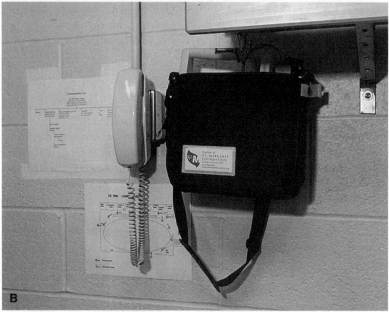

Figure 1-2. Emergency communication system: **(A)** common modes of communication; **(B)** communication tree posted beside landline phone.

A list of all appropriate emergency numbers, such as local emergency medical services, should be posted by the communication system most used by the athletic trainers and should be readily available to all emergency team members. Specific directions to on-site venues should also be included and posted with the emergency numbers. Such directions should include the actual street address of the venue, main road, secondary road, and other landmark information that will assist EMS personnel in arriving at the scene as soon as possible.[4]

Emergency Equipment and Supplies

All appropriate emergency equipment and supplies must be on hand at all athletic practices and events (Figs. 1-3 and 1-4). All assigned emergency team members should be aware of the location and function of all emergency equipment and supplies. Ensure that emergency equipment and supplies are properly inventoried annually and stored in a secure storage area for safekeeping by the athletic training staff.[9,14]

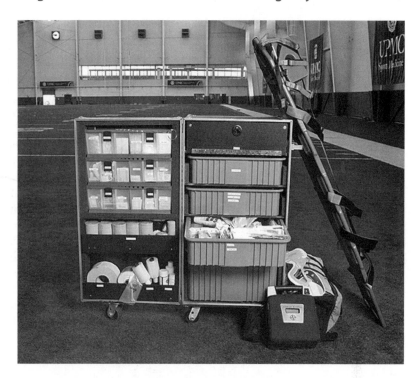

Figure 1-3. Emergency equipment (AED) on the sideline.

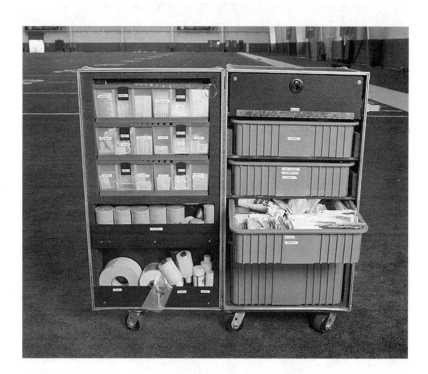

Figure 1-4. First aid kit with contents clearly labeled for easy access.

All athletic personnel and administrators must recognize the importance of the availability of AEDs as stated by guidelines set forth by the American Heart Association.[15] These guidelines state that early defibrillation is considered a critical component of basic life support *(see Chapter 4 for more detailed information)*. It is also important to utilize proper airway techniques for resuscitation when necessary *(see Chapter 3 for more detailed information)*. Emergency team members should be educated in the proper use of AEDs and airway adjuncts before being allowed to use them.[16]

All emergency equipment and supplies must be in good operating condition and should be checked regularly (Box 1-5). The middle of an emergency situation is not the time to find out that a piece of emergency equipment is missing or is not working. Each emergency team member must be trained in advance in how to use all first aid equipment and

Box 1-5   Emergency Equipment and Supply List

- **Equipment**
- **AED unit**
- **Immobilization splints**
- **Stretcher/spine board**
- **Airway bag—valve mask**

- **Supplies**
- **First aid kit**
- **Sterile bandages**
- **Tape and elastic wraps**
- **Bloodborne pathogen kits**

supplies. Also, the use of equipment and supplies should be regularly practiced by all emergency team members so that there is no delay in the effective use of the equipment during an actual emergency.

Venue Locations

The EAP should be specific to venue locations and any unique features that might be found as part of that facility (Fig. 1-5). The EAP for each venue should include information concerning the accessibility to emergency personnel, communications systems, emergency equipment, and emergency vehicle transportation.[4]

At all home venues, the host athletic trainer should communicate the EAP for the venue to the visiting team and its medical personnel. Specific areas reviewed should include all available emergency personnel, location of communication systems, and available emergency equipment (Box 1-6).

At neutral or away venues, the athletic trainer or any other member of the emergency team should identify the availability of communication with emergency medical services for that location.[4] It is also important that the name and location of the nearest emergency care facility and the availability of emergency transportation at the venue be identified prior to the event.

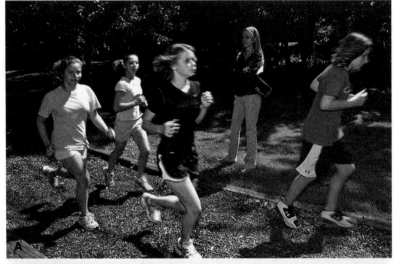

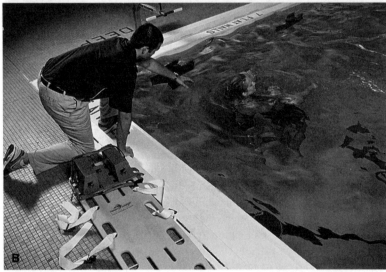

Figure 1-5. Venues with unusual requirements or needing a venue-specific EAP: **(A)** cross-country course, **(B)** swimming pool, **(C)** narrow stairs, **(D)** ice-hockey rink.

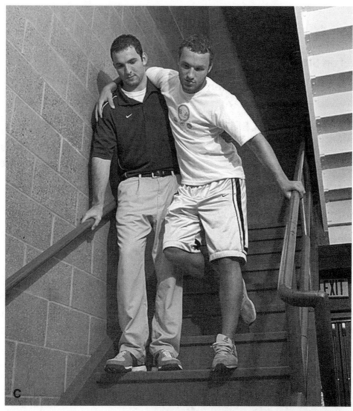

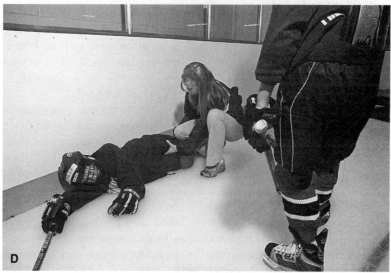

Figure 1-5. cont'd

Emergency Transportation

The EAP should include a policy for transportation of the sick and injured for all athletic events. By definition, an emergency dictates that transport should be via EMS vehicles (ambulance). The policy on transportation should explain in detail when and where an ambulance will be during all athletic events.[17] Emphasis should be placed on having an ambulance on site for all high-risk or collision sporting events, such as football, lacrosse, and ice hockey.[18] In some cases, the number of spectators who are expected to attend an event may warrant the presence of one or more ambulances on site, even if the sport is not considered collision or high risk in nature. Although spectators typically are not the responsibility of the sports medicine team, this point should be clear with administrators. If the team's medical staff is also responsible for the care of spectators, staffing for the event and the EAP itself must reflect this fact.

Box 1-6   Specific Venue Location EAP

---

1. **Emergency Personnel on Site**

   Practices, games, tournaments, and all other activities

   Athletic trainers, physicians, coaches, EMS personnel

2. **Emergency Communication**

   Phones and handheld radios

   Emergency phone numbers

3. **Emergency Equipment**

   AED, first aid kits, splints, spine boards

   Ambulance on site

4. **Emergency Procedures**

   Includes all venue drawings, maps, and directions

   Instructions on all CHECK—CALL—CARE items

   Directions to nearest emergency care facility

Box 1-7   Basic Life Support (BLS) Versus Advanced Life Support (ALS)

BLS: Emergency medical technician (EMT); basic airway support, AED, splinting, spine boarding

ALS: Paramedic; advanced airway support, invasive procedures such as IVs, use of medications as directed by physician

---

✪ *STAT Point 1-6. If the team's medical staff is also responsible for the care of spectators, staffing for the event and the EAP itself must reflect this fact.*

EMS response time to an accident should also be considered when developing a transportation policy. Consideration should also be given to the level of transportation service and equipment that is available. An example of this would be that of Basic Life Support (BLS) versus Advanced Life Support (ALS) availability (Box 1-7). Another issue that must be reviewed is the level of training of all emergency personnel who staff the attending ambulance service.[11]

It is critical that working emergency communication systems are in place between the on-site sports medicine staff and the emergency medical service that would be dispatching an ambulance in an emergency.[5] In the event that an ambulance is on site, a location should be designated for the ambulance with clear, direct access to the competition area and a clear route for entering and exiting the athletic venue (Fig. 1-6).

During an emergency evaluation, the emergency medical service assists the sports medicine staff in identifying emergencies that require critical care intervention and in determining transportation decisions.[18] In any emergency situation, the injured athlete should be transported by ambulance, where the necessary staff and equipment are available to deliver appropriate emergent care. For this reason, the sports medicine staff should not transport athletes in personal or institution vehicles. It is also very important that a plan is in place for supervision of activity areas if the emergency medical service and/or the sports medicine staff leave the site to accompany the injured athlete to a nearby emergency care facility.[4]

Emergency Care Facilities

The EAP should include information regarding the transportation directions to an emergency medical facility from all athletic venues. When selecting an appropriate emergency care facility, consider the proximity of the emergency facility to the venues and the level of care available at the facility.[4]

Notify the emergency care facility and local emergency medical services that are used by the athletic organization in advance of all athletic events that are scheduled at any of the organization's venues.[2] It is also recommended that the EAP be reviewed and practiced with both the emergency care facility administrators and medical staff in regard to important information concerning athlete care. An example of the information that must be reviewed is the proper removal of athletic equipment, such as football helmets and shoulder pads, in the emergency care facility.[18,19]

Legal Need and Documentation

The development of EAPs by athletic trainers, team physicians, and administrators is a legal need and duty to ensure the highest quality of care provided to all physically active participants. Allied health professionals, which include athletic trainers, are measured in part by the standards of care provided to athletes in emergency situations, which is one reason why it is important to have a written document in place.[20,21] The National Athletic Trainers' Association has stated that a well-organized and well-written EAP document that is regularly rehearsed is absolutely essential for all athletic organizations and sports medicine programs.[12,22]

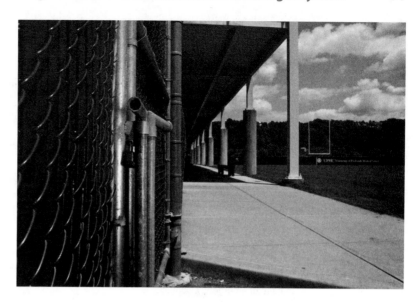

Figure 1-6. In the event of an emergency, a locked gate could pose a problem.

The athletic organization administrators and sports medicine team members must anticipate that a possible emergency situation may occur during any athletic activity.[5] Injuries to the head, spine, and limbs are possible in both practice and competition. It is clear that a duty exists on the part of the athletic organization and the sports medicine team to provide proper care for any medical conditions that result from athletic participation. Although it is not common in athletic activity, the athletic trainers and the rest of the sports medicine team must always be prepared for any type of life- or limb-threatening injury.[4] Failure to have an EAP in place, and to rehearse it regularly, may result in inefficient or inadequate care, which could lead to charges of negligence against the athletic organization administration and sports medicine team members.[4]

Several legal cases have supported the need for written EAPs, the most prominent of which is *Kleinknecht vs. Gettysburg College*.[12] As part of the 1993 decision, the court stated that Gettysburg College owed a duty to all its recruited athletes and that the college must provide "prompt and adequate emergency services while athletes were engaged in school-sponsored intercollegiate athletic activities."[12] The same court also ruled that reasonable measures must be ensured and in place to provide adequate and prompt treatment in any emergency situation. It can be concluded from this ruling that planning is critical to ensure that athletes get proper emergency care, which further reinforces the need for a written EAP as a requirement for all athletic organizations.[4]

The following are important pieces of documentation needed as part of the EAP:

1. Athlete Emergency Information Card, used to describe current medical conditions and medications being used by the athlete. This card should only be used when there is written approval from the athlete in accordance with patient confidentiality considerations (Fig. 1-7).

2. Individual Injury Evaluation Form, used for the documentation of the athlete's injuries (Fig. 1-8).

3. Delineation of the person or group responsible for documenting the events of the emergency situation.[4]

4. Follow-up documentation on the evaluation of response to emergency situation.[4]

5. Documentation on personnel training and regular rehearsal of the emergency action plan.[4]

6. Documentation of purchase, inventory, and maintenance of all emergency equipment and supplies.[4]

7. School/athletic organization coaches' Emergency Information Palm Card, provided to members of the sports medicine team and coaching staff for easy EAP reference (Fig. 1-9).

It is important to involve athletic organization administrators, coaches, and sports medicine staff in the development process of the EAP. The EAP should be reviewed and updated annually by all involved personnel.[4] All revisions to the EAP should be approved by all members at all levels of the athletic organization, sports medicine staff, emergency team members, and local emergency medical services. Finally, it is most important that all parts of the EAP are practiced and rehearsed by all members involved before each given athletic season begins.

Middle Road Athletic Association
Baseball and Softball

Medical Release

NOTE: To be carried by any Regular Season or Tournament Team Manager together with team roster or eligibility affidavit.

Player: _____ Date of Birth: _____

League Name: _____ I.D. Number: _____

Parent or Guardian Authorization:
In case of emergency, if family physician cannot be reached, I hereby authorize my child to be treated by Certified Emergency Personnel (i.e. EMT, First Responder, E.R. Physician).

Family Physician: _____ Phone: _____

Address: _____

Hospital Preference: _____

In case of emergency, contact:

_____
Name   Phone   Relationship to Player

_____
Name   Phone   Relationship to Player

Please list any allergies/medical problems, including those requiring maintenance medication (i.e. Diabetic, Asthma, Seizure Disorder).

The purpose of the above listed information is to ensure that medical personnel have details of any medical problem that may interfere with or alter treatment.

Medical Diagnosis: _____

Medication Dosage: _____

Frequency of Dosage: _____

Date of last Tetanus Toxoid Booster: _____

Mr./Mrs./Ms. _____
                    Authorized Parent/Guardian Signature

Figure 1-7. Athlete Emergency Medical Information Card.

**MIDDLE ROAD ATHLETIC ASSOCIATION
ACCIDENT/INJURY EVALUATION FORM**

Report all incidents that require assistance. Turn completed form in to the Middle Road Athletic Association Board within 24 hours of the incident.

Name of injured: _____

Address: _____

Date of birth: _____ Sex: _____ Phone (H) _____ (C) _____

Location of incident: _____ Date: _____ Time: _____

Sport involved: _____

Age level: _____

Position playing at time of injury: _____

How did injury occur? _____

_____

_____

Describe the nature of the injury and the body parts affected: _____

_____

_____

What care was provided? _____

Attended by: _____

Was the family notified?   Yes _____ No _____ Who was notified? _____

Physician called?   Yes _____ No _____ Name and phone # _____

Shaler EMS called?   Yes _____ No _____ Ambulance _____ Police _____ Fire _____ Other _____

Where taken? Name of hospital: _____ Other: _____

Witnesses: Name _____ Address _____

           Name _____ Address _____

Report prepared by: _____ Title: _____ Date: _____

Figure 1-8. Individual Injury Evaluation Form.

SHALER – Middle Road – Coaches

Emergency Card

Shaler EMS:	911 or 555-XXX-XXXX	St. Margaret Hospital E.R.: 555-XXX-XXXX
Shaler Fire:	911 or 555-XXX-XXXX	Children's Hospital: 555-XXX-XXXX
Shaler Police:	911 or 555-XXX-XXXX	Allegheny County Poison Control: 555-XXX-XXXX

MRAA President:
Bill Fragapane: 555-XXX-XXXX

Softball REP
Tom Sorce: 555-XXX-XXXX

Baseball REP:
Keith Gorse: 555-XXX-XXXX

MRAA Vice President:
Mark Dobson: 555-XXX-XXXX

Coach's Role in Emergency: CHECK – CALL – CARE

1. Immediate **CHECK** of athlete or spectator (Airway – Breathing – Circulation – Bleeding)

2. Do not move injured person – Stabilize

3. **CALL** emergency phone number & give proper directions to site* (Police – EMS – Fire)

4. **CARE** for injured person (Control bleeding – CPR / AED – Rescue Breathing – Choking – Immobilize)

5. NEEDS: First aid kit – Phone – Blankets – Ice packs – AED

* Make sure you have someone in charge of directing emergency vehicles to field (from road)

Figure 1-9. Emergency Information Palm Card.

 # EMERGENCY ACTION

The athletic trainer should have an EAP in place. The emergency team, which includes the athletic trainer, coach, and referee, should activate this plan immediately and check the basketball player's vitals, call for emergency personnel, and then care for the player until help arrives. The athletic trainer should have emergency equipment at the scene to start immediate care. This includes CPR supplies and an AED unit. Contact with local emergency services should be initiated by the basketball coach right away. Proper directions should be given to the sports facility. Emergency care should be started by the athletic trainer and assisted by the referee until emergency services arrive. The athletic trainer, referee, and coach should then aid the emergency service personnel as needed until the player is transported to the nearest hospital emergency room. The emergency team should then document everything done for the player from the time he was stricken to the point that he was transported to the hospital.

CHAPTER HIGHLIGHTS

- Organizations that sponsor athletic activities must have a written EAP. This plan should be able to adapt to any emergency situation.

- EAPs must be written documents and should be distributed to all members of the sports medicine staff and emergency team. This includes athletic trainers, team physicians, athletic training students, equipment managers, coaches, and school nurses.

- The EAP for the athletic organizations identifies the personnel involved in carrying out the plan and outlines their qualifications. All emergency team members should be trained and certified in CPR, AED, first aid, and bloodborne pathogen prevention.

- The EAP should include a section that provides the personnel of the emergency team with information on initial patient assessment and care that includes the Check—Call—Care criteria.

- The EAP should specify all equipment and supplies needed to help carry out the tasks required in case of an emergency. The plan should also outline the location of all emergency equipment.

- The EAP should establish a clear mechanism for communication with the appropriate emergency medical service in the area.

- Identification of the type of transportation for the injured individual(s) should also be part of the plan.

- The EAP should be specific to each activity site and venue. Each site and venue used should have a separate plan that is derived from the overall organizational policies on emergency planning.

- The EAP should incorporate the emergency care facilities being used for the care of the injured individuals. These emergency care facilities, such as local hospital emergency rooms, should be included in the development of the EAP for the organization.

- The EAP should be reviewed and rehearsed annually, although it is recommended to review and rehearse more than once a year. The EAP should also be revised whenever appropriate and it should be documented that the revision took place.

- All personnel involved with the organization and involved with the EAP share a professional and legal duty to provide the best emergency care to an injured individual. This includes the responsibility of developing and implementing an EAP.

- The EAP should be reviewed and approved by the administration and legal counsel of the involved athletic organization.

Chapter Questions

1. What is the purpose of your initial CHECK of the injured athlete?

   A. To check for minor injuries

   B. To ask for information about injury

   C. To check for life-threatening injuries

   D. To obtain consent for treatment

2. Which of these conditions warrants calling EMS personnel?

   A. Suspected fracture

   B. Injury to the head or spine

   C. Possible abdominal injury

   D. All of the above

3. Once the EAP has been developed, it is implemented through:

   A. Documentation

   B. Education

   C. Rehearsal

   D. All of the above

4. One of the roles of the emergency team is to:

   A. Check only for breathing and pulse

   B. Wait until EMS arrives to care

   C. Direct EMS to the scene

   D. None of the above

5. What information should the athlete's medical information card include?

    A. Family contact information

    B. Directions to sports venue

    C. Primary injury evaluation

    D. Long-term treatment goals

6. The EAP should be reviewed and rehearsed by the emergency team:

    A. Only once a year

    B. As many times as possible

    C. No more than twice a year

    D. Three or four times a year

7. Professional responsibilities for emergency team members include:

    A. CPR training

    B. First aid training

    C. Bloodborne pathogen training

    D. All of the above

8. The EAP should be specific to:

    A. Each activity

    B. Each venue location

    C. One specific site

    D. A and C only

9. Documentation needed for an EAP includes:

    A. Potential athlete medical conditions

    B. Inventory of emergency supplies

    C. Coaches' pocket information card

    D. All of the above

10. Consideration for an appropriate emergency care facility includes:

    A. Connection with team physician

    B. Size of emergency room

    C. Proximity to venue location

    D. None of the above

■ *Case Study 1*

Paul, the head athletic trainer for the local high school, was working a football game when the team quarterback ran headfirst into an opposing team linebacker, fell to the ground, and was motionless. Paul ran onto the field with his team physician and began a primary evaluation. The athlete appeared to have a head injury but was not unconscious. The athlete was able to answer questions but complained of a headache, blurred vision, tingling in his right hand, and slight neck pain. Paul had the athlete sit up, look at the scoreboard, and read the score and time of the game. The athlete was able to read the score and time of game, but he could not turn his head to see the scoreboard without discomfort. The team physician checked the injured athlete's eyes and ears, looking for abnormalities, while Paul took the athlete's helmet off and asked questions about the mechanism of injury. After a few minutes it was decided to have the athlete stand and try to walk off the field with aid from his teammates.

Once on the sidelines Paul and the team physician began to perform a secondary evaluation on the athlete. During this time the athlete complained of more head and neck pain. He felt nauseated and could not stand in one place.

The team physician told Paul that the athlete should go to the hospital for further examination and tests. Paul called over to the attending school district police crew to transport the athlete to the hospital via police van. At the hospital, it was found that he had a mild concussion and a nondisplaced compression fracture of the 5th cervical vertebrae.

Case Study 1 Questions

1. What are your concerns regarding the evaluation and care of this football player's injury?

2. What would you have done differently, if anything, if you had been in Paul's position?

3. Who, if anyone, is at fault in this case? If more than one person, how would that be determined by a judge or jury if there would be legal action taken by the injured athlete?

■ *Case Study 2*

Lisa is an athletic trainer for a local high school. A female soccer player has just collapsed on the soccer field during a game. Lisa runs out onto the field and begins a primary evaluation and determines that the athlete is not breathing and does not have a pulse; she begins CPR. During this time, other members of the emergency team, which include an athletic training student and a coach, are unsure of what to do to assist Lisa and the athlete. They also do not know where the emergency supplies are located. The only instruction the athletic training student was given by Lisa was to call the local emergency medical services.

Case Study 2 Questions

1. How would an EAP help alleviate the problems in this situation?
2. What would you have done differently, if anything, if you had been in Lisa's position?
3. What legal ramifications could occur as a result of this situation?

References

1. Arnheim DD, Prentice WE. Principles of Athletic Training. 9th ed. Madison, WI: WCB/McGraw-Hill Inc; 1997.

2. Dolan MG. Emergency care: Planning for the worst. Athl Ther Today. 1998;3(1):12–13.

3. Kleiner DM, Glickman SE. Considerations for the athletic trainer in planning medical coverage for short distance road races. J Athl Train. 1994;29:145–151.

4. Anderson C, Kleiner M. National Athletic Trainers' Association Position Statement: Emergency planning in athletics. J Athl Train. 2002;37(1):99–104

5. Kleiner DM. Emergency management of athletic trauma: Roles and responsibilities. Emerg Med Serv. 1998;10:33–36.

6. National Safety Council. First aid and CPR. 4th ed. Sudbury, MA: Jones and Bartlett; 2001.

7. Courson RW, Duncan K. The emergency plan in athletic training emergency care. Boston: Jones & Bartlett Publishers; 2000.

8. National Athletic Trainers' Association. Establishing communication with EMTs. NATA News. June 1994:4–9.

9. American Red Cross. Sports injury: Emergency first aid care and prevention. Washington, DC: American Red Cross; 1988.

10. Benson MT, ed. Guidelines 2H: Blood-borne pathogens and intercollegiate athletics. NCAA Sports Medicine Handbook. Overland, KS: National Collegiate Athletic Association; 1993:24–28.

11. Feld F. Technology and emergency care. Athl Ther Today. 1997;2(5):28.

12. *Kleinknecht v. Gettysburg College*, 989 F2d 1360 (3rd Cir 1993).

13. Ray R. Management strategies in athletic training. Champaign, IL: Human Kinetics; 2000.

14. Rubin A. Emergency equipment: What to keep on the sidelines. Phys Sportsmed. 1993;21(9):47–54.

15. American Heart Association. Guidelines 2000 for cardiopulmonary resuscitation and emergency cardiovascular care: International consensus on science. Curr Emerg Cardiovasc Care. 2000;11:3–15.

16. Marenco JP, Wang PJ, Link MS, et al. Improving survival from sudden cardiac arrest: The role of the automated external defibrillator. JAMA. 2000;285: 1193–1200.

17. Fincher AL. Managing medical emergencies, Part I. Athl Ther Today. 2001;6(3):44.

18. Feld F. Management of the critically injured football player. J Athl Train. 1993;28(3):206.

19. Kleiner DM, Almquist JL, Bailes J, et al. Prehospital care of the spine-injured athlete. Dallas: Inter-Association Task Force for Appropriate Care of the Spine-Injured Athlete; 2001.

20. Rankin JM, Ingersoll C. Athletic training management: Concepts and applications. St. Louis: Mosby–Year Book Inc; 1995:175–183.

21. Herbert DL. Legal aspects of sports medicine. Canton, OH: Professional Reports Corp; 1990:160–167.

22. Herbert DL. Do you need a written emergency response plan? Sports Med Stand Malpract Rep. 1999;11:S17–S24.

Suggested Readings

1. National Athletic Trainers Association: www.nata.org
2. National Collegiate Athletic Association: www.ncaa.org
3. American Sports Medicine Institute: www.asmi.org
4. American Red Cross: www.redcross.org
5. American Heart Association: www.amhrt.org
6. National Safety Council: www.nsc.org
7. National Center for Sports Safety: www.sportssafety.org
8. American College of Sports Medicine: www.acsm.org
9. American Academy of Orthopaedic Surgeons: www.aaos.org

Chapter 2

Physical Examination of the Critically Injured Athlete

Francis Feld, MEd, MS, CRNA, ATC, NREMT-P

KEY TERMS

[handwritten: test]

[handwritten: BP cuff]

Aneroid sphygmo-
  manometer
Auscultation
Bradycardia
Bradypnea *[handwritten: <12 per min]*
Capillary refill
Cheyne-Stokes
  respirations
Crepitus
Cyanosis
Diastolic blood
  pressure

Golden hour
Hypertension
Hypotension
Hypoxia
Korotkoff sounds
Mucosa
Patent
Perfuse
Primary survey
Pulse oximetry
Secondary survey
Shock

Stridor
Supraventricular
  tachycardia
Systolic blood pressure
Tachycardia
Tachypnea *[handwritten: high]*
Tympanic
Ventilation
Vital signs

[handwritten: 200 systolic- Dyastolic-]

EMERGENCY SITUATION

During warm-ups for a varsity football game, the athletic trainer is suddenly summoned to the far corner of the field where she is told a cheerleader has been injured. The athletic trainer runs to the area where she sees a large group of cheerleaders and spectators crowded around an individual on the ground. A quick glance shows the cheerleader is not moving and is not responding to shouts from his fellow cheerleaders.

The athletic trainer quickly notes that the athlete's right ankle and elbow are deformed but have no obvious signs of bleeding. The cheerleader does not respond to the athletic trainer's voice commands.

Imagine you are the athletic trainer. What are your priorities in managing this athlete? How would you proceed?

Evaluation of the injured or ill athlete consists of conducting a physical examination and obtaining a complete set of **vital signs**. Physical examination can be either a focused body systems approach or a global head-to-toe approach. Each chapter in this text will concentrate on emergency care of a body system, but because most injuries in athletics are traumatic, a head-to-toe approach is best suited for the global examination and will be used here. A head-to-toe approach is also the most commonly used method for physical examination by emergency medical services (EMS). Because EMS will almost always be summoned for a critically injured or ill athlete, it is best to utilize the same type of system to facilitate a smooth transition of care and get the athlete to the hospital quickly.

A physical examination has four components: inspection, palpation, percussion, and **auscultation** (Fig. 2-1). Inspection involves a close examination of the injured area looking for deformity, contusions, abrasions, swelling, and bleeding. Palpation involves touching the injured area to note abnormal findings such as deformity or **crepitus**. Percussion consists of tapping the injured area to elicit **tympanic** sounds. Percussion is used for thoracic and abdominal injuries and is difficult to perform in the athletic arena. Auscultation refers to listening to lung sounds with a stethoscope and, although difficult in a noisy environment, it is a crucial skill for any seriously injured athlete, especially when the athlete is short of breath. In this chapter we will first look at the procedures involved with a physical examination and then describe how to obtain vital signs.

The **golden hour** is the time between onset of injury and definitive surgical treatment. This universally accepted concept for the management of trauma patients means that

paramedics concentrate on a rapid assessment and packaging of the patient to keep their on-scene time to less than 10 minutes. If the response time was 10 minutes and the transport time is also 10 minutes, you can readily see that half of the golden hour is gone before the patient even arrives at a hospital, preferably a trauma center. Therefore, it is important that no time is lost by the athletic trainer in deciding to summon EMS after the injury occurs. Although not all athletic injury emergencies are related to trauma, it is reasonable to extend the trauma management concept to medical patients to avoid delays in getting the athlete to definitive care.

Scene Assessment and Safety

When approaching an athlete who is down, avoid tunnel vision; instead, get a global picture of the scene. Is the scene safe? How many athletes are injured? Are there hazards in the area such as electrical cords, water, or blood? Is the athlete moving? Are bystanders or teammates trying to move the athlete? Do you have sufficient resources and equipment to manage the injured athlete? If the athlete is an assault victim, where are the assailant and the weapon? All of these questions must be answered as you approach so that you do not become injured yourself. Failure to see the big picture is often called tunnel vision and can lead to significant dangers being missed (Fig 2-2).

Body Substance Isolation Precautions

Protection against the transmission of infectious diseases such as hepatitis or HIV is an important consideration when treating any patient. The degree of protection depends on the procedure performed and the body fluids you might come in contact with. Hand washing is the single most effective way to prevent the transmission of diseases, and the provider should always wash his or her hands before and after each patient contact. Use warm water and thoroughly spread the lathered soap over the entire hand and wrist areas for at least 15 seconds. Rinse completely with a strong stream of water and dry completely. If soap and water are not available, waterless alcohol-based soap can be used until soap and water become available. Repeated use of these waterless soaps will lead to dry and cracked skin, which increases the likelihood of disease transmission because the skin is no longer intact.

Wearing disposable latex or vinyl gloves is mandatory when there is any chance of coming into contact with blood or bodily fluids. With the increasing concerns over latex allergies, the use of vinyl gloves is preferred. The use of eye goggles, gowns, and masks is frequently indicated for many invasive procedures performed by advanced providers, but their use in the athletic environment is rare. Box 2-1 provides a listing of the level of protection indicated for various procedures.

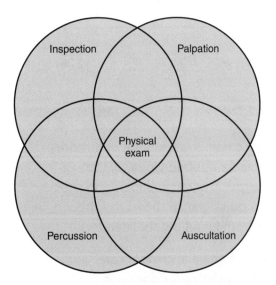

Figure 2-1. A good physical examination involves four components: inspection, palpation, percussion, and auscultation. Percussion is difficult to impossible to perform in the athletic environment.

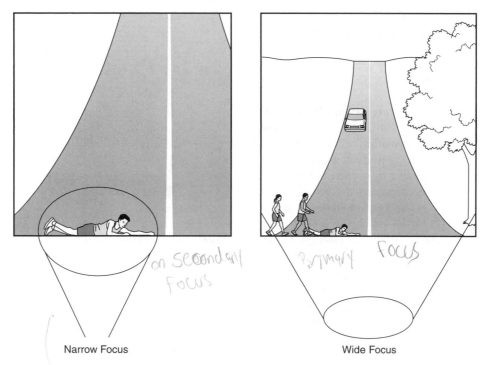

Narrow Focus

Wide Focus

on secondary Focus *Primary Focus*

Figure 2-2. Tunnel vision can miss significant dangers and must be avoided. The light at the end of the tunnel may be an oncoming truck.

Box 2-1   Level of Protection for Various Procedures

Procedure	Gloves	Mask	Gown	Eye Protection
Control minor bleeding	Yes	No	No	No
Control major bleeding	Yes	Yes	Yes	Yes
IV starts	Yes	No	No	No
Vital signs	No	No	No	No
IM injection	Yes	No	No	No
Advanced airway procedures	Yes	Yes	No	Yes

Primary Survey

The **primary survey** is a rapid head-to-toe assessment designed to identify and immediately correct life- and limb-threatening injuries. Within the first minute, you must determine if the athlete is critically injured and activate the emergency action plan (EAP). The primary survey consists of five parts, each described in the following text. A common mnemonic used to help remember these parts of the primary survey is simply the first five letters of the alphabet: *ABCDE* (Box 2-2).

Remember that the primary survey must be completed quickly. If the injury is serious, the situation is classified as a

Box 2-2   Parts of the Primary Survey

A: Stabilize cervical spine and check the *airway*.

B: Check for *breathing*.

C: Check for *circulation*.

D: Check for neurological *disability* (or apply *defibrillator*).

E: Check level of *exposure*.

"load and go," which means EMS is summoned immediately and all interventions within the scope of the providers are accomplished quickly and efficiently.

Airway and Cervical Spine

One should always assume the injured athlete has a cervical spine injury until it is proved otherwise. Stabilize the head and keep it in a neutral position with reference to the neck. Now evaluate the airway and determine responsiveness. It the athlete speaks in a clear and normal voice, you are assured the airway is **patent.** If the athlete is unconscious, look and listen for signs of airway compromise such as snoring. Either lifting the chin or using a modified jaw thrust maneuver with the cervical spine neutral can relieve an airway obstruction. *(See Chapter 3 for more information about airway management procedures.)* Abnormal airway sounds such as gurgling or **stridor** indicate the presence of a possible foreign body that must be removed. Always remove an athlete's mouth guard during any evaluation.

Breathing

Look and feel for the chest to rise, indicating the athlete is breathing. Look to see that the chest rises in a symmetrical fashion. Asymmetry may indicate significant chest trauma. Evaluate the rate and quality of breathing. If the athlete is not breathing, begin rescue breathing with either a pocket mask or bag valve mask. *(See Chapter 3 for more information about airway management procedures.)* A respiratory rate less than 8 or greater than 30 is significant and cause for concern. Note the color of the oral **mucosa** and nailbeds to look for **cyanosis,** which is a bluish color indicating **hypoxia.** Breathing must be adequate to ensure oxygenation of tissues (**ventilation**).

Circulation

Quickly feel the radial pulse and note if it is fast or slow, regular or irregular, and strong or weak. If the radial pulse is absent, check the carotid pulse. A weak or absent radial pulse is a strong indication that the athlete is in critical condition and mortality and morbidity are increased (Fig. 2-3).[1] Now check **capillary refill.** Press on the nailbed of any finger and quickly release, noting how quickly color returns. Color should return within 3 seconds or as quickly as you can say the words "capillary refill." If capillary refill is delayed, the athlete's circulation is not sufficient to **perfuse** the vital organs.

Disability/Defibrillation

Disability refers to a brief neurological examination. It is time consuming to perform a focused neurological examination, and merely asking the athlete to move his or her arms and legs is sufficient for a primary survey. If the athlete

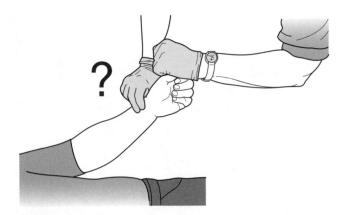

Figure 2-3. A weak or absent radial pulse indicates inadequate perfusion and shock.

is in cardiac arrest, the automatic external defibrillator should be used immediately.

Exposure

Clothing or equipment may need to be removed to examine the injured athlete. Modesty or environmental concerns should be taken into account but should never inhibit the examination.

Secondary Survey

After the primary survey is complete and life-threatening conditions are managed, a **secondary survey** is performed. This consists of a complete head-to-toe examination to rule out other injuries that may not be apparent on the primary examination. All components of the primary survey are continuously monitored so that any deterioration in the athlete's condition is immediately recognized and corrected. Findings will need to be clearly communicated to EMS personnel once they arrive on the scene.

Secondary Survey Examination

Starting at the head use a look, listen, and palpate approach. Look for contusions, abrasions, lacerations, and deformity. Listen to breath sounds in the chest. Palpate body parts for crepitus, pain, and rigidity or masses. Listen for abnormal sounds while palpating.

✪ *STAT Point 2-1. During a secondary survey examination, use a look, listen, and palpate method.*

Head-to-Toe Examination

Look at the pupils while examining the head. Pupils should be midline, equal, and round, and they should react to light and accommodation; the acronym PERRLA is frequently

Box 2-3	Pupil Examination: PERRLA

P Pupils

E Equal

R Round

R Reactive

L Light

A Accommodation (The pupils move in conjunction with each other and in the proper direction based on stimulation—for instance: "Follow my finger as it moves in different directions." The pupils should move simultaneously and smoothly as they follow the finger.)

used (Box 2-3). Palpate for deformity or pain in the cervical spine and ensure the trachea is in a midline position. Palpate the chest for pain or asymmetrical motion. Auscultate lung sounds high in the axilla bilaterally to determine the presence of equal breath sounds (Fig. 2-4). Palpate each quadrant of the abdomen for pain or rigidity. Compression of the iliac crests evaluates stability of the pelvis. Carefully but quickly palpate each leg and arm for deformity or pain. Check pulses in each extremity to ensure they are present and equal. For the lower extremities, use of the posterior tibial or dorsal pedal pulse is recommended. This entire examination should be accomplished in 1 minute or less. Once the primary and secondary surveys are completed, a complete set of vital signs should be obtained and recorded.

Vital Signs

Vital signs are appropriately named—they provide crucial information necessary to manage a seriously injured athlete. There are six easily measured vital signs: pulse, blood pressure, respiratory rate, temperature, **pulse oximetry,** and pain assessment (Box 2-4). Vital signs should be repeated as often as the patient's condition warrants. The athlete who is critically ill or injured should have vital signs measured at least every 3 minutes, whereas the less seriously injured may have vital sign intervals of 5 to 15 minutes. Box 2-5 lists normal values for vital signs. It is important to remember that normal is a relative term and there may be wide variations. As a general rule, well-conditioned athletes will have pulse rates, blood pressures, and respiratory rates on the low side of the ranges listed. The values for children are for ages 6 years to puberty. At puberty, vital sign values tend to mimic those for adults.

Pulse Rate

Count the pulse rate by palpating the radial artery at the wrist. An accurate pulse rate requires counting the rate for at least 30 seconds. Very slow or fast rates may require a full minute to obtain an accurate pulse rate. Note whether the pulse is strong or weak and regular or irregular. A weak pulse is considered thready and may indicate inadequate tissue perfusion, one form of **shock.** *(For more information on shock, see the appendix at the end of this chapter.)* An irregular rate requires careful evaluation and could indicate anything from sinus arrhythmia (a benign rhythm common in athletes) to premature beats to atrial fibrillation. An irregular rate should be further evaluated with an electrocardiogram (EKG) monitor to make a definitive diagnosis.

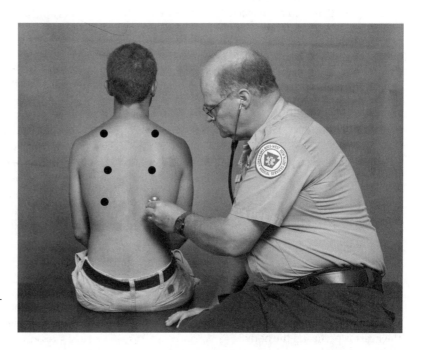

Figure 2-4. Listen to breath sounds on the posterior thorax in six places and compare each side bilaterally.

Box 2-4   The Six Vital Signs

- Pulse
- Blood pressure
- Respiratory rate
- Temperature
- Pulse oximetry
- Pain assessment

Box 2-5   Normal Vital Signs

	Adult	Child
Pulse	60-100	>20
Blood pressure	120/80	70 + 2 × age
Respiratory rate	10–20	>20
Temperature	98.6°F	98.6°F
	(37.0°C)	(37.0°C)
Pulse oximetry	>95%	>95%
Pain	0	0

A normal pulse rate is 60 to 100 beats per minute. Rates higher than 100 are called **tachycardia,** whereas rates lower than 60 are called **bradycardia** and rates higher than 150 are called **supraventricular tachycardia.** The young athletic population is different than the general population, and resting pulse rates less than 60 are common and are no cause for alarm as long as the athlete is alert and oriented. Rates higher than 100 are expected during physical activity and are cause for alarm only if they do not quickly return to a normal level when activity ceases.

✪ *STAT Point 2-2. Pulse rates higher than 100 are to be expected in athletes during activity and are cause for alarm only if they do not quickly return to a normal level when activity ceases.*

The radial artery is used most often only because it is readily accessible. Pulse rates may be determined by palpating any artery. Other arteries used include the femoral, carotid, brachial, temporal, posterior tibial, and dorsal pedal. The brachial artery is most commonly used in children younger than age 6. Direct pressure to the brachial and femoral pulse sites will slow or stop arterial bleeding distally. These are referred to as pressure points (Fig. 2-5). If the athlete is monitored with a pulse oximeter or EKG monitor, it is important to correlate the heart rate displayed on the monitor with a manual pulse rate. This ensures that every beat of the heart is perfusing the body.

Blood Pressure

Blood pressure is most commonly measured using a stethoscope and a device called an **aneroid sphygmomanometer** (blood pressure cuff). This device consists of a cuff with an inflatable bladder, a bulb to inflate the bladder, a valve to release the air from the bladder, and a pressure dial that displays cuff pressure in millimeters of mercury (mm Hg). Blood pressure is most often measured using the upper arm, although the forearm and thigh may also be used (Fig. 2-6). The cuff must be an appropriate size for the athlete and it must be applied snugly. Cuffs that are too small will give falsely high readings, whereas cuffs that are too large will give falsely low readings. The cuff width should cover at least 80% of the arm or be 20% to 50% greater than the diameter of the arm. Many cuffs have proper sizing guides easily visible on the cuff itself; it is important to follow manufacturer's instructions for use of these sizing guides. Pediatric cuffs and large adult and thigh cuffs should be available so that proper-sized cuffs are used when appropriate.

The cuff is placed on the upper arm directly on the skin, and the brachial artery is palpated at the elbow. The cuff should never be applied over clothing, and the arm should be at the level of the heart. Once the artery is located, the stethoscope is placed over the artery and the cuff is inflated. **Korotkoff sounds** are the noises heard through the stethoscope and are the result of the cuff collapsing the artery and producing turbulent blood flow. The cuff should be inflated 15 to 20 mm Hg beyond the point that the Korotkoff sounds disappear. The valve is then slowly opened and air is allowed to escape from the bladder. **Systolic blood pressure** (SBP) is when the Korotkoff sounds are heard again and the **diastolic blood pressure** (DBP) is when the sounds are absent. Systolic blood pressure is the pressure during ventricular contraction, whereas diastolic pressure is the pressure during ventricular rest. The gradient between the two is referred to as pulse pressure. The **mean arterial pressure** (MAP) is as follows:

$$MAP = \frac{SBP + 2(DBP)}{3}$$

Automatic blood pressure cuffs are available, but they may not be cost effective for the athletic training room. These are referred to as noninvasive blood pressure (NIBP) units and are either electric or battery powered. An NIBP unit will give the SBP, DBP, MAP, and a pulse rate with each reading. Time intervals may be programmed from continuous to every 60 minutes. These units are convenient when serial blood pressures are indicated in the critically injured but they are not essential.

If a stethoscope is not readily available, the blood pressure may be palpated. To do this, the cuff is applied and the radial pulse is felt. The cuff is inflated to a point 15 to 20 mm Hg higher than the pressure where the pulse is no longer felt and the cuff is then slowly deflated. The pressure where the radial pulse is once again felt is the systolic pressure. The diastolic pressure is not measured using this technique, and the blood pressure is referred to as SBP over palpation. Although this is

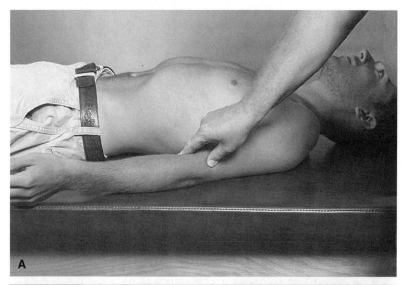

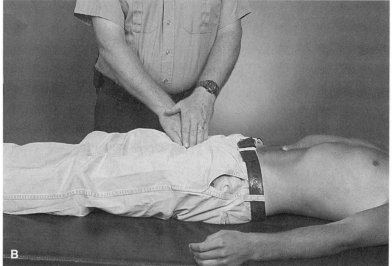

Figure 2-5. Severe bleeding in the arm or leg can be controlled using pressure points.
A: Brachial pressure point on inside of arm.
B: Femoral pressure point in groin.

a simple and convenient method, a systolic and diastolic pressure should be measured at least once during the management of the athlete to establish a baseline.

By convention a normal blood pressure is considered to be 120/80, although experience shows that this is unrealistic. Although a systolic pressure of less than 100 mm Hg is considered **hypotension** in the general population, athletes are expected to have low pressures. The significance of any blood pressure reading must be correlated with an athlete's chief complaint and a thorough physical examination. For the purpose of preseason screening, a normal systolic pressure is between 100 and 140 mm Hg, whereas a normal diastolic pressure is between 60 and 85 mm Hg.[2] The diagnosis of **hypertension** is made based on high diastolic pressure and requires additional evaluation and possible treatment.

Respiratory Rate

Counting an accurate respiratory rate is not as easy as it may seem and frequently is miscounted. An athlete will unknowingly alter his or her respiratory pattern if it is known that

his or her breathing is being monitored. Because an accurate rate requires a minimum of 30 seconds to count, it is reasonable to combine counting a pulse rate with counting the respiratory rate. To do this, when taking a pulse, tell the athlete you will be counting his or her pulse for 1 minute. Count the pulse for the first 30 seconds and the respiratory rate for the second 30 seconds.

A normal resting respiratory rate is between 10 and 20 breaths per minute. Because an athlete is involved in physical activity, a rate much greater than 20 is expected. This rate should quickly return to normal. A rapid respiratory rate (**tachypnea**) also may be caused by anxiety, pain, excitement, or acidosis. Tachypnea in the general population is a rate higher than 20, although in athletes a more reasonable definition might be a rate higher than 30. **Bradypnea** is a rate less than 10 and is always a cause for alarm in someone who is injured. Possible causes are head injury or opioid overdose. Slow respiratory rates require additional evaluation and possibly ventilatory assistance. Respiratory patterns should always exhibit a regular pattern. Irregular respirations are cause for alarm, especially if found in athletes with head

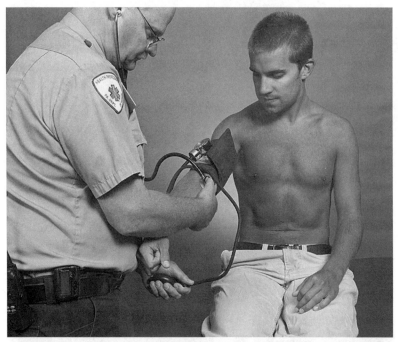

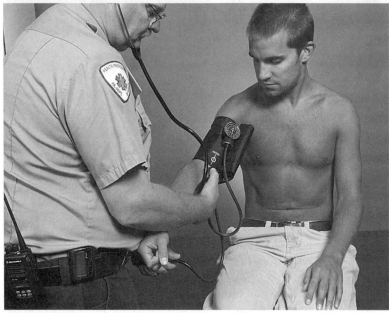

Figure 2-6. An improperly sized blood pressure cuff will yield an inaccurate blood pressure.

injuries. **Cheyne-Stokes respirations** are characterized by an increasing rate and depth followed by a period of apnea. This pattern is a sign of significant brain injury (Fig. 2-7).

It is just as important to assess the work of breathing along with the respiratory rate. Respirations at rest without breathing supplemental oxygen are referred to as easy on room air or unlabored. Symptoms of increased work of breathing include intercostal retractions, nasal flaring, pursed lip breathing, sternocleidomastoid muscle contractions, and upright posturing. A well-conditioned athlete should only manifest these symptoms if an underlying

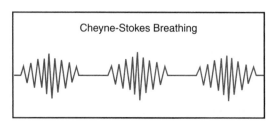

Figure 2-7. Breathing pattern exhibited during Cheyne-Stokes respirations: increasing rate and depth of respirations followed by periods of apnea.

pathology is present such as an acute asthma attack. Poorly conditioned athletes may exhibit these signs but they should resolve spontaneously with rest.

Temperature

Temperature measurement is not usually obtained in the prehospital arena but it is still important, especially if heat illness is suspected. Rectal temperatures have long been considered the gold standard for accurately measuring core body temperature but are typically not used for obvious reasons. Oral temperatures may be an accurate reflection of core temperature, and the advent of digital thermometers has made this a simple and quick task. Tympanic temperatures are easy to obtain and are strongly favored by parents of small children, but the accuracy is questionable.[3] Axillary or skin temperatures may be substituted for oral temperatures if an athlete has a decreased level of consciousness, which precludes taking an oral temperature. A recent study evaluating temperature measures taken at various sites (mouth, ear, axilla, and forehead) showed that these temperatures may be several degrees cooler than those taken rectally, calling into question their usefulness in assessing core body temperature.[4] Normal temperature for a healthy person at rest is 98.6°F (37°C). The method of taking the temperature should always be noted—for example: "The athlete's temperature is 96.5° F axillary."

Pulse Oximetry

Pulse oximetry is a relatively new vital sign and is perhaps the single most important monitor available. It is considered a mandatory monitor for any patient receiving sedation in the hospital. Pulse oximeters can be pocket sized or found as a component of much larger EKG monitors and are standard equipment on ambulances in the United States (Fig. 2-8). Oximetry operates under the principle that oxygenated

hemoglobin and deoxygenated hemoglobin absorb infrared and red light differently. Oxyhemoglobin absorbs infrared light at 990 nm, whereas deoxyhemoglobin absorbs red light at 660 nm. The gradient is measured by the pulse oximeter and provides a percentage of oxyhemoglobin. The expected value for a healthy nonsmoker is in the range of 99% to 100%. Values less than 90% require supplemental oxygen. Very large athletes who are in a supine position may have pulse oximeter readings of 90% to 95%, but a few deep breaths will easily increase the reading to the optimal range.

The pulse oximeter is a noninvasive monitor consisting of a clothespin-like probe that is placed on a fingertip, toe, or ear. Light passes through the skin and the oxyhemoglobin percentage is displayed on the screen along with a pulse rate. The pulse rate displayed must correlate with a manual pulse rate or the reading is considered inaccurate. Several factors may interfere with pulse oximeter readings including cold fingers, low blood pressure, fast or irregular pulse rates, and bright ambient light. Moving the probe to a different location may resolve interference. The probe can be placed anywhere on the body that will allow the passage of light. Time should not be lost obtaining an accurate pulse oximeter reading on an athlete in critical condition, and it is crucial to remember that pulse oximetry is not a measurement of ventilation. Pulse oximetry only measures the amount of oxyhemoglobin (saturation) and not oxygen/carbon dioxide gas exchange in the lungs (ventilation).

Although very unusual in athletics, it should be noted that patients exposed to carbon monoxide will have falsely high pulse oximeter readings because of its higher binding affinity to hemoglobin as compared to oxygen.

Pain

Although not yet widely acknowledged, many consider assessment of pain as the newest vital sign, mostly because health care providers will routinely underestimate the severity of a

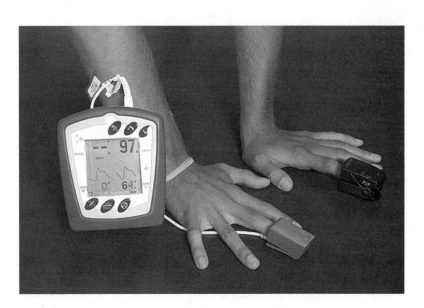

Figure 2-8. A pulse oximeter will show the pulse rate and oxygen saturation. The radial pulse must match the pulse rate on the oximeter to be considered accurate.

patient's pain. To effectively treat pain it must be quantified. The easiest method of pain assessment is to ask the athlete to rate his or her pain on a scale of zero to 10 with zero meaning no pain and 10 meaning the worst pain ever felt. Serial assessments allow the health professional to measure the effectiveness of the pain treatment regimen (Fig. 2-9). This scale is universal and gives a frame of reference to other health professionals who may take over care of the athlete at a later time. The importance of pain control can never be underestimated. "No pain, no gain" is an archaic philosophy that has no place in the treatment of acute injuries.

The effective management of any emergency situation depends on the athletic trainer remaining calm and in control of the situation. Ensure that the scene is safe, and call for help if the injury is serious or there are insufficient resources to manage the situation. Focus on the primary survey and immediately correct any deficiencies. Monitor vital signs closely and watch for trends that indicate the athlete is deteriorating. Perform the secondary survey and identify all injuries. Prepare for an efficient and expeditious transfer to EMS personnel on their arrival. Above all, follow the well-developed EAP for your institution (Box 2-6).

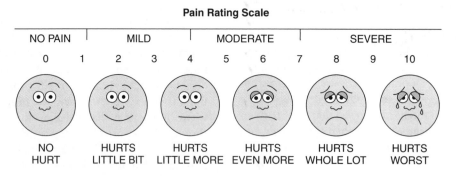

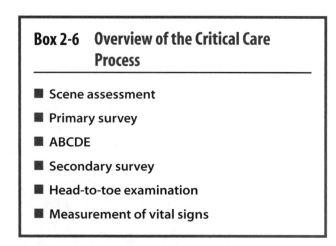

Figure 2-9. Rating of pain must use a consistent scale to gauge pain relief. A number scale is appropriate for adults, whereas the happy face scale is good for children.

Box 2-6   Overview of the Critical Care Process

- Scene assessment
- Primary survey
- ABCDE
- Secondary survey
- Head-to-toe examination
- Measurement of vital signs

EMERGENCY ACTION

The athletic trainer quickly recognizes that the cheerleader is seriously injured and the scene is not safe because of the large number of well-meaning but potentially interfering spectators. She stabilizes the cheerleader's head and neck in a neutral position and determines that the athlete is breathing and has a carotid pulse. The cheerleader coach states that the injured athlete fell about 6 feet from a pyramid stunt they were performing. Next, the athletic trainer instructs a senior cheerleader to return to the home sideline to get the team physician and the athletic training students and to tell them to activate the EAP. She then tells the cheerleader coach to start moving everybody away from the scene and back into the stands. The team physician and athletic training students quickly arrive and the doctor starts the physical examination. A senior athletic training student states EMS has been called and the spine board and immobilization equipment are on the way. Although the cheerleader has an obvious ankle fracture and elbow dislocation, the priority of care is focused on a presumed head and neck injury. The cheerleader is immobilized on a spine board with a cervical collar in place. The ankle and elbow are splinted and vital signs are taken. EMS arrives, administers oxygen, and transports the cheerleader to the local trauma center.

CHAPTER HIGHLIGHTS

- Evaluation of the injured or ill athlete consists of conducting a physical examination and obtaining a complete set of vital signs.

- A physical examination has four components: inspection, palpation, percussion, and auscultation.

- The primary survey is a rapid head-to-toe assessment designed to identify and immediately correct life- and limb-threatening injuries.

- The primary survey includes five parts: stabilize cervical spine and check the *airway*, check for *breathing*, check for *circulation*, check for neurological *disability* (or apply *defibrillator*), and check level of *exposure*.

- The secondary survey consists of a complete head-to-toe examination to rule out other injuries that may not be apparent on the primary examination.

- There are six easily measured vital signs: pulse, blood pressure, respiratory rate, temperature, pulse oximetry, and pain assessment.

Chapter Questions

1. What are the four components of a physical examination?

   A. Inspection

   B. Palpation

   C. Percussion

   D. Auscultation

   E. All of the above

2. What is the golden hour?

   A. Minimum time to get the injured athlete to a trauma center

   B. Time for an ambulance to arrive on scene

   C. Interval between vital sign measurements

   D. None of the above

3. A primary survey consists of the ABCDEs. Which of the following is not a part of the primary survey?

   A. Airway

   B. Circulation

   C. Breathing

   D. Body fat measurement

4. Snoring is a common sign of _____?

   A. Fatigue

   B. Airway compromise

   C. Intoxication

   D. All of the above

5. Which of the following is not considered one of the six vital signs?

   A. Pulse rate

   B. Blood pressure

   C. Respiratory rate

   D. Central venous pressure

6. Inadequate tissue perfusion is the definition of _____.

   A. Pulmonary embolism

   B. Shock

   C. Heart attack

   D. Stroke

7. A blood pressure cuff should cover at least what percentage of the arm?

   A. 50%

   B. 70%

   C. 80%

   D. 90%

8. Describe a common pain scale used in health care.

   A. 0–10 with 10 the worst

   B. 0–10 with 0 the worst

   C. Mild, moderate, and severe

   D. None of the above

9. Which temperature measurement is the least accurate?

   A. Oral

   B. Axillary

   C. Tympanic

   D. Rectal

10. A respiratory rate less than 10 requires _____.

    A. Further evaluation and possible assistance

    B. Nothing because this is normal

    C. Immediate cause for alarm and activation of EMS

    D. Application of a pulse oximeter

■ *Case Study 1*

During preseason practice in August, a soccer player comes into the athletic training room complaining of fatigue and dizziness. He sits on a treatment table and promptly passes out. The athletic trainer calls for help and starts his examination. He finds the athlete is breathing and has a strong carotid but weak radial pulse. The athlete sluggishly responds to questions and is confused. The skin is warm, moist, and flushed. BP is 80/50, pulse is 120, respiratory rate is 20, pulse oximetry is 99% on room air, and axillary temperature is 99.5°F. The athlete denies pain.

Case Study 1 Questions

1. Is this athlete in shock and, if so, how did you determine that?
2. Can this athlete be treated effectively in the athletic training room?
3. How often should vital signs be monitored?

■ *Case Study 2*

While rebounding during practice two basketball players violently collide and crash to the floor. As the athletic trainer approaches, he sees that one player is holding her knee and screaming in pain while the other player is lying motionless. Recognizing that the screaming player is conscious and has a patent airway, he proceeds to the motionless player. She is unresponsive and has snoring respirations so he immediately performs a jaw thrust maneuver and the snoring is relieved. The athletic trainer instructs the coach to activate the emergency action plan and call 911.

Case Study 2 Questions

1. Which athlete should be treated first?
2. Can the athletic trainer manage this situation alone?
3. What are the priorities in treating these athletes?

References

1. McManus J, Yershov A, Ludwig D, et al. Radial pulse character relationships to systolic blood pressure and trauma outcomes. Prehosp Emerg Care. 2005;9(4): 423–428.
2. The Sixth Report of the Joint National Committee on Prevention, Detection, Evaluation, and Treatment of High Blood Pressure. Arch Intern Med. 1997;157(21): 2413–2446.
3. Dickinson E, Bevilacqua J, Hill J, et al. The utility of tympanic versus oral temperature measurements of firefighters in emergency incident rehabilitation operations. Prehosp Emerg Care. 2003;7(3):363–367.
4. Casa D, Becker S, Ganio M, et al. Validity of devices that assess body temperature during outdoor exercise in the heat. J Athl Train. 2007;42(3):333–342.

Suggested Readings

1. Greenwald I, O'Shea J. Measuring and interpreting vital signs. J Emerg Med Serv. 2004;29(9):82–97.
2. Pre-Hospital Trauma Life Support Committee of the National Association of Emergency Medical Technicians in Cooperation with the Committee of Trauma of the American College of Surgeons. Pre-Hospital Trauma Life Support, 3rd Edition. St. Louis: Mosby–Year Book; 1994.

Appendix 2-1

Shock

Shock results when a person's cardiovascular system cannot supply an adequate amount of oxygenated blood to the vital organs. The tissues of the heart, lungs, brain, and kidneys are easily damaged from a lack of oxygen and the subsequent buildup of waste products. Eventually, one or more of these organs will fail and death can result. It is critical that the early signs and symptoms of shock be recognized and the victim be transported before late shock develops.

Shock can be classified into different types:

1. Hypovolemic. Lack of tissue perfusion resulting from significant reduction in blood volume (severe bleeding or general dehydration are frequent causes).

2. Cardiogenic. Lack of tissue perfusion from loss of myocardial contractility (heart attack, dysrhythmias, and myocarditis are causes).

3. Distributive. Lack of tissue perfusion as a result of venous pooling or poor blood flow distribution (neurogenic shock is one example).

4. Obstructive. Lack of tissue perfusion as a result of an external force that inhibits cardiac function (compression of the heart as a result of a tension pneumothorax or obstructed blood flow resulting from hypertension are examples).

Signs and symptoms of shock include the following:

1. Reduction in cerebral blood flow, manifested by the following:
   Restlessness, anxiety, or agitation
   Disorientation or confusion
   Combative behavior
   Inappropriate response to questions or commands

2. Increased heart rate; during practice or a game, this may show up as a heart rate that does not return to normal over several minutes after participation has stopped

3. Pale, cool, clammy skin as a result of blood being diverted away from the skin and toward vital organs; during a practice or game when an athlete's body temperature is elevated, the skin may not be cool or clammy initially

4. Nausea or vomiting

5. Thirst (hypovolemic shock)

6. Respiration changes

7. Decreased blood pressure (sign of late shock)

Emergency care for shock includes the following:

1. Immediately activate EAP; transport victim as soon as possible.

2. Maintain victim's airway.

3. Control any bleeding.

4. Maintain victim's body temperature.

5. If there is no suspected lower extremity fracture, head injury, or spinal trauma, elevate the victim's legs approximately 12 inches.

6. Provide oxygen if possible.

7. Continue to monitor victim's vital signs.

Chapter 3

Airway Management

Francis Feld, MS, MEd, CRNA, ATC, NREMT-P

KEY TERMS

Airway obstruction

Airway patency

Apnea

Aspiration *Breathing in*
pneumonitis *vomit*

Bag valve mask
(BVM)

Combitube

Endotracheal
intubation

Epiglottis

Epistaxis – *bloody nose*

Glottis

Jaw thrust maneuver

King laryngeal tube-
disposable (King LT-D)

Laryngeal mask airway
(LMA)

Larynx

Nares

Nasal cannula

Nasopharynx

Nasopharyngeal (NP)
airway

Oropharyngeal (OP)
airway

Oropharynx

Oxygen therapy

Pocket mask

Reservoir bag face mask

Simple face mask

Trachea

 EMERGENCY SITUATION

An assistant football coach runs into the athletic training room yelling that the head coach has collapsed in his office. The athletic trainer runs to the office and finds the coach sitting in his chair with his head slumped forward. The coach does not respond to shouting and prodding. The athletic trainer quickly realizes the coach is not breathing well and his skin has a bluish tint. The athletic trainer tells the assistant coach to call 911 and activate the emergency action plan. What would you do next?

Of all the components of emergency care, only cardio-pulmonary resuscitation (CPR) and defibrillation have a higher priority than airway management. Although cardiac arrest and airway compromise are rare in athletics, the results are devastating, especially if the athletic trainer is unprepared. *(See Chapter 4 for more information on sudden cardiac death.)* This chapter will discuss briefly the anatomy of the airway, how to relieve airway compromise including the use of airway adjuncts, and the administration of oxygen and will introduce techniques of advanced airway management. Although some states may have legislation precluding athletic trainers from using some of these interventions, all athletic trainers and athletic training students should be familiar with the concepts.

> ✪ *STAT Point 3-1. Only CPR and defibrillation are more important than airway management.*

Airway Anatomy

The airway can be divided into two parts: the upper and lower airway (Fig. 3-1A). The upper airway is composed of the **oropharynx** and **nasopharynx.** The nasopharynx consists of two passages through the nose and into the posterior oropharynx. Air passing through the nose is warmed and particles are filtered by the nasal hairs. The largest diameter of the nasal passages is in the inferior compartment, which is important to remember when placing a nasopharyngeal airway. The oropharynx starts at the mouth and ends at the **trachea.** The mouth includes the tongue inferiorly and the hard palate superiorly. The tongue has many functions, but for our purposes it is only a problem. The tongue is the most common reason for **airway obstruction** because in the supine unconscious athlete it can slide backward and occlude the passage of air into the trachea (Fig. 3-1B). This situation is commonly described as the tongue being "swallowed," although swallowing the tongue is not actually possible.

The lower airway consists of the **epiglottis** and the **larynx.** The epiglottis is a flap that covers the opening to the trachea (the **glottis**) when food or fluid passes into the esophagus. The larynx is composed of nine cartilages and muscles and is located anterior to the fourth, fifth, and sixth cervical vertebrae in adults. The larynx is also known as the Adam's apple. It is a dynamic structure and protects the glottis while also allowing phonation (Fig. 3-1C). Airway anatomy is much more complex than what has been presented here, but a detailed description is beyond the scope of this text. Students are encouraged to study the airway in more detail.

Airway Compromise

Airway patency is a term used to describe the status of the airway. An open and clear airway is called patent, whereas an obstructed airway is compromised. Signs of an obstructed

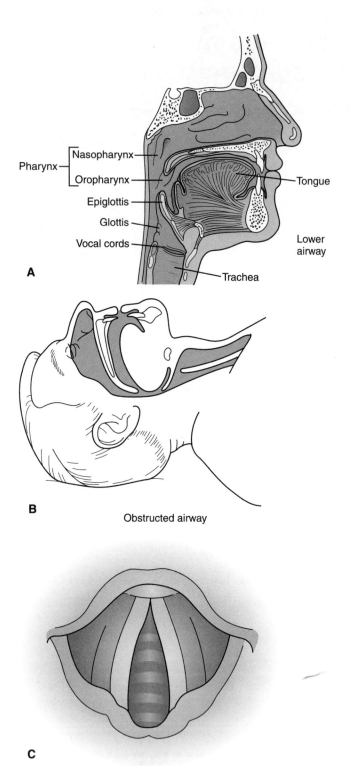

Figure 3-1. **A:** Understanding the normal airway anatomy is necessary to manage airway obstruction. **B:** The tongue is the most common reason for airway obstruction. **C:** The vocal cords mark the opening to the trachea and are a crucial landmark for endotracheal intubation.

airway include snoring respirations, sternal and intercostal retractions, accessory muscle use, and gurgling. Snoring respirations are common and indicate that the tongue is partially occluding the airway. A smooth and symmetrical expansion of the thorax indicates a normal respiratory effort. The condition in which the upper sternum sinks inward while the remainder of the sternum expands outward is called sternal retractions and very little air is exchanged with each breath. Intercostal retractions and accessory muscle use mostly describe difficulty breathing frequently seen with acute asthma attacks and may or may not be related to airway obstruction. Intercostal retractions are seen by examining the chest wall and looking at the muscles between the ribs. If the muscles sink inward while the chest is expanding outward for inhalation, retractions are present. Accessory muscle use describes the contraction of the sternocleidomastoid muscles of the neck to aid in expansion of the chest for inhalation. Gurgling always indicates fluid in the airway, typically either saliva or vomitus.

⭐ *STAT Point 3-2. Snoring is a sign of partial airway obstruction.*

Clearing an obstructed airway usually requires repositioning the head, jaw, and neck. The head tilt–chin lift technique (Fig. 3-2) will almost always result in a patent airway; however, this technique cannot be used in the unconscious athlete who is assumed to have a cervical spine injury. Therefore, the jaw thrust, or triple airway, **maneuver** is more appropriate for an athlete who is unconscious (Fig. 3-3). The jaw thrust is painful and may stimulate the athlete into consciousness. Fluid associated with gurgling must be suctioned to clear the airway. Foreign-body obstructions are relieved by either back blows or abdominal thrusts, as taught in CPR courses.

Airway Adjuncts

The **oropharyngeal (OP)** and **nasopharyngeal (NP) airways** are used to relieve an obstructed airway after the initial jaw thrust maneuver has shown its effectiveness. The athletic trainer will find the jaw thrust maneuver physically

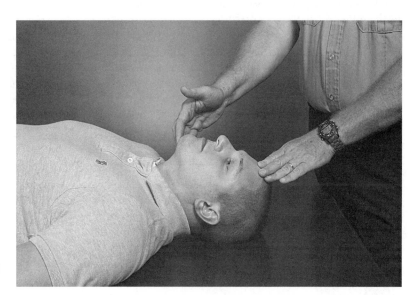

Figure 3-2. The head tilt–chin lift method is used to open the airway occluded by the tongue.

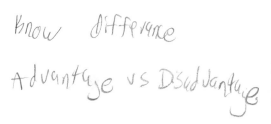

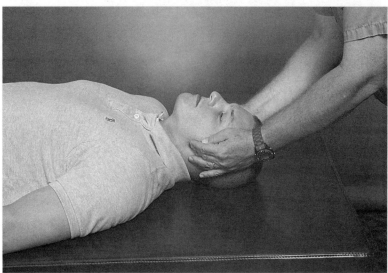

Figure 3-3. The jaw thrust maneuver is used to open the airway when a cervical spine injury is suspected.

demanding if done over an extended period, and switching to either of these airways as soon as possible is warranted. The adult OP airway comes in small, medium, and large sizes (Fig. 3-4) and is made of hard plastic. Metric sizes are sometimes found in 8, 9, and 10 mm. Proper sizing is made by holding the airway along the cheek. It should stretch from the tip of the ear to the corner of the mouth (Fig. 3-5A, B). Inserting the OP airway requires stabilizing the tongue with a tongue depressor and sliding the airway into the posterior oropharynx following the natural curve of the airway. An alternate method not requiring a tongue depressor may be used. The OP airway is inserted with the curve toward the hard palate until the tip is beyond the middle of the tongue. The airway is then rotated into its natural position with the tip downward and into the posterior pharynx. This technique is contraindicated in the pediatric population. An intact gag reflex as indicated by biting is a contraindication to placement of an OP airway. The flange of the OP airway should be at the lips if properly sized. Complications of insertion include damage to the teeth and hard palate and worsening of the airway obstruction if not positioned properly (Fig. 3-6).

✪ *STAT Point 3-3. Oral and nasal airways relieve airway obstruction.*

✪ *STAT Point 3-4. Never use an oral airway if the gag reflex is intact.*

The NP airway is made of soft rubber and comes in sizes small, medium, and large (see Fig. 3-4). Nonlatex airways are also manufactured and are firmer than the rubber airways. An alternative sizing scale is 28, 30, 32, and 34 French. Pediatric sizes are also available. A properly sized NP airway should reach from the tip of the nose to the tip of the ear (see

Fig. 3-5B). The diameter of the airway should approximate the size of the **nares.** The flange on the airway prevents losing the entire airway in the nose and is adjusted for length based on sizing. The airway is lubricated with a water-soluble gel and inserted with the bevel toward the septum and inferiorly in the left nostril. If resistance is met, the airway should be withdrawn and reinserted at a new angle. If still unable to pass the airway, withdraw and use the right nostril. When using the right side, the airway is inserted upside down so the bevel is aligned with the septum. Once approximately half the airway is into the nostril, rotate into its natural position. The NP airway can be used when the gag reflex is intact (Fig. 3-7). Contraindications to the NP airway are facial trauma and **epistaxis.** A small amount of blood may be seen with insertion, but significant bleeding is a complication and usually related to forceful insertion.

Oxygen Therapy

Airway management is not complete without the administration of supplemental oxygen. Athletic trainers need to check the scope of practice defined by their state licensure acts, but short-term oxygen administration is not contraindicated in an emergency situation. Involvement of the team physician in the decision to provide **oxygen therapy** may resolve any conflicts.

✪ *STAT Point 3-5. Oxygen administration by an athletic trainer may be restricted by state law.*

Oxygen is supplied in either steel or aluminum tanks of varying sizes, which are painted green. Aluminum tanks are superior to steel because they are lighter and will not rust. Although oxygen tanks come in various sizes, all are pressurized to 2000 psi when full. The most common-sized tanks

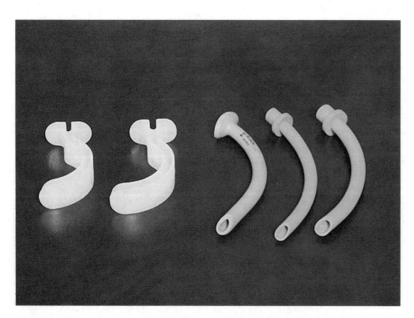

Figure 3-4. Various-sized oral and nasal pharyngeal airways.

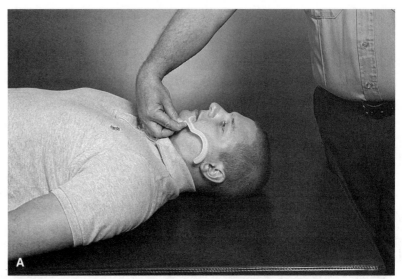

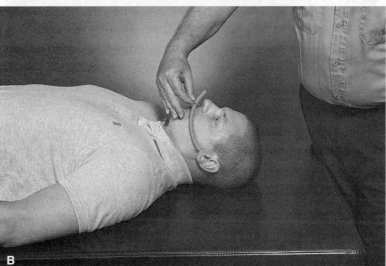

Figure 3-5. **A:** Inappropriate-sized airways are ineffective and can injure the athlete. The OP airway should extend from the corner of the mouth to the tip of the ear. **B:** The nasal pharyngeal airway should extend from the nares to the tip of the ear. The diameter of the airway should match the size of the nares.

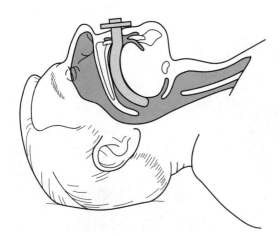

Figure 3-6. The properly sized airway will relieve an airway obstruction when the gag reflex is absent.

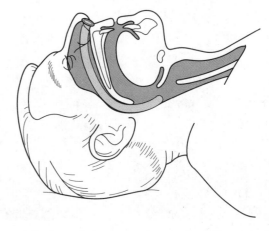

Figure 3-7. A nasal airway may be used to relieve an airway obstruction if the athlete still has a gag reflex.

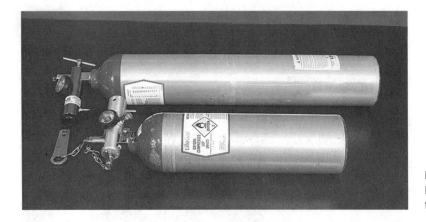

Figure 3-8. Although the compact size of the D oxygen tank is attractive, it will empty much faster than the larger E tank.

used in the prehospital arena are D and E tanks (Fig. 3-8). A D tank is 20 inches in length and holds 360 L of oxygen, whereas an E tank is 30 inches in length and holds 625 L of oxygen. A regulator is attached to the top of the tank and has three parts: a pressure gauge, a pressure-reducing valve, and a flow meter. The gauge shows the pressure in the tank (2000 psi is a full tank), the valve reduces the pressure to a usable flow, and the meter sets the oxygen flow rate. Therefore, a D tank set at 10 L/min will last 36 minutes when the tank is full, whereas an E tank will last 62.5 minutes. Oxygen tanks must be stored carefully and should always be in a holder and never left standing upright. If the regulator is knocked off, the sudden release of highly pressurized oxygen will cause the tank to fly through the air like a deadly missile. Although oxygen is not flammable, it does support combustion and should never

be used near an open flame. Smoking in the area of oxygen administration is contraindicated and dangerous.

Patients with chronic obstructive pulmonary disease (COPD) deserve special mention. COPD includes emphysema, bronchitis, asthma, and black lung disease. Oxygen administration over a long period (hours) may lead to hypoventilation or even **apnea.** For this reason there is a common misconception among health care providers that patients with COPD should never receive oxygen by any means other than a **nasal cannula** (Fig. 3-9A) at low flow rates. High-flow oxygen to any patient with difficulty breathing in an emergency situation is recommended no matter what past medical history exists. It should be noted that the incidence of COPD in a young athletic population is almost always asthma.

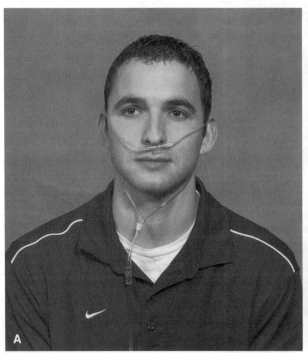
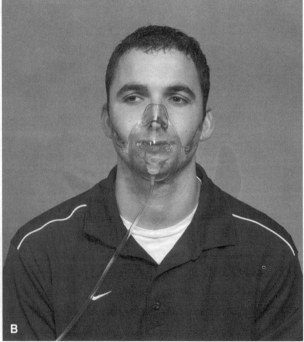

Figure 3-9. **A:** The nasal cannula will administer low flows of oxygen and is comfortable for the athlete. **B:** The simple face mask delivers a higher concentration of oxygen than the nasal cannula.

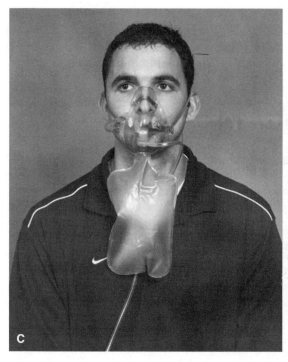
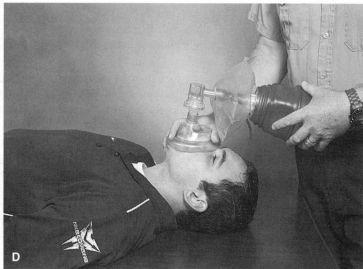

Figure 3-9, *continued* **C:** The reservoir bag oxygen mask delivers the highest concentration of oxygen and should be used for the unconscious athlete with adequate respiratory effort. **D:** The bag valve mask is used to assist respirations in the unconscious athlete with inadequate respirations.

⭐ *STAT Point 3-6. COPD is not a contraindication to short-term administration of high-flow oxygen.*

Oxygen is administered by a variety of devices. Each of these devices delivers a set amount of oxygen to the patient, referred to as the fraction of inspired oxygen (FiO_2). A nasal cannula has two prongs that are inserted in the nose and held in place by tubing wrapped around the ears. A nasal cannula can administer from 1 to 6 L/m of oxygen, which gives a FiO_2 of 25% to 40% (Box 3-1). Flow rates of 5–6 L/m are uncomfortable and, unless humidified, will dry the nasal passages and lead to nose bleeds. Oxygen by nasal cannula is only utilized with conscious and stable patients (see Fig. 3-9A).

A **simple face mask** (see Fig. 3-9B) will deliver a FiO_2 of 40% to 60% at 6 to 10 L/m, whereas a **reservoir bag face mask** will deliver 60% to 90% at 10 to 15 L/m. The reservoir bag face mask (also referred to as a partial nonbreather mask) is preferred for patients who are unconscious or unstable (see Fig. 3-9C). Although it is common for emergency medical technicians (EMT) to use 15 L/m with either type of face mask, the clinical difference in FiO_2 between 10 and 15 L/m is insignificant and will only drain the tank one third faster. This is an important consideration if using a D tank.

The **bag valve mask (BVM)** (see Fig. 3-9D) is used to either assist the breathing or ventilate a patient with apnea. An adult BVM has a capacity of approximately 1600 cc and uses a mask to maintain a seal around the face. When connected to an oxygen source and using a reservoir bag, the BVM will deliver a FiO_2 of nearly 100%. The flow rate should be sufficient to fill the bag with each ventilation or 10 to 15 L/m. The BVM may also be connected to an endotracheal tube if the patient is intubated. All artificial breathing tubes (**endotracheal**, **laryngeal mask airway [LMA]**, **combitube**, and **King laryngeal tube-disposable [King LT-D]**) have the same 15 mm connector for the BVM.

Ventilating a patient with a BVM mask is a difficult skill to master, and practice on a regular basis with a mannequin is strongly encouraged. Using the E-C technique described later in the text is important to obtain a good seal around the mouth and nose to deliver effective tidal volumes to the patient.[2] Using your left hand, place your thumb and index finger on the mask, forming a C. Then place your small, ring, and middle fingers along the mandible with your small

Box 3-1 FiO_2 and Flow Rates for Various Devices

Device	FiO_2(%)	Flow Rate (L/m)
Nasal cannula	25–40	1–6
Simple face mask	40–60	6–10
Reservoir bag face mask	60–90	10–15
BVM	100	10–15

finger at the corner of the jaw. These three fingers should form an E. Lift up on the jaw with the E and pull the mouth and nose up into the mask (Fig. 3-10). Squeeze the bag with your right hand and gauge the effectiveness of your ventilations by how high the chest rises. Good chest expansion is crucial for effective BVM mask ventilation. If air leaks around the mask, either reposition your hands or use your right hand to seal the patient's right cheek with the mask. If using both hands to obtain a good mask seal, you will need a second person to squeeze the bag. Novices are encouraged to use a two-person technique when performing BVM mask ventilation. Ventilate the patient at 10 breaths per minute. It is almost always necessary to use either an NP or OP airway when bagging a patient.

A CPR **pocket mask** may also be used in ventilating a patient (Fig. 3-11). This simple device has the same type of mask used with a BVM along with a one-way valve. Ventilations are provided by the athletic trainer through mouth-to-mask ventilation. The mask is sealed in the same manner as the BVM mask. Unless equipped with a supplemental oxygen port, the pocket mask delivers less than room air FiO_2 (21%). The pocket mask is convenient to carry and is better than mouth-to-mouth rescue breathing but is not a good substitute for a BVM and oxygen.

Advanced Airway Devices

Although effective ventilation with a BVM is possible for a short time, eventually the airway must be secured by an advanced airway device. This may occur before or after arrival at the hospital, and the gold standard has always been **endotracheal intubation.** This technique involves using a laryngoscope to directly visualize the vocal cords at the glottic opening and passing a cuffed endotracheal tube into the trachea (Fig. 3-12). Once the tube is properly placed and the cuff is inflated, the trachea is sealed and gastric aspiration is unlikely. This skill is reserved for

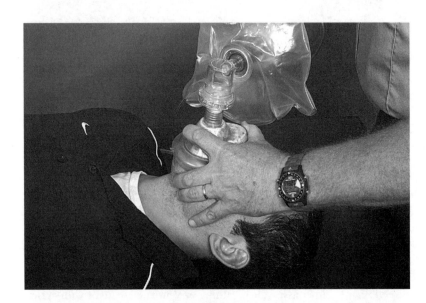

Figure 3-10. Shaping your fingers into an E and C formation allows for effective mask ventilation with a BVM.

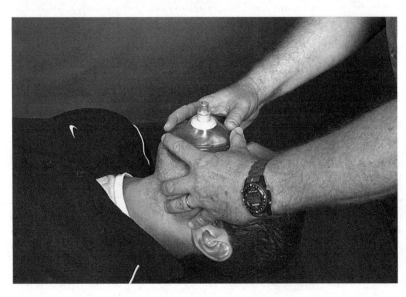

Figure 3-11. The pocket mask is a safer and more effective alternative to mouth-to-mouth respirations.

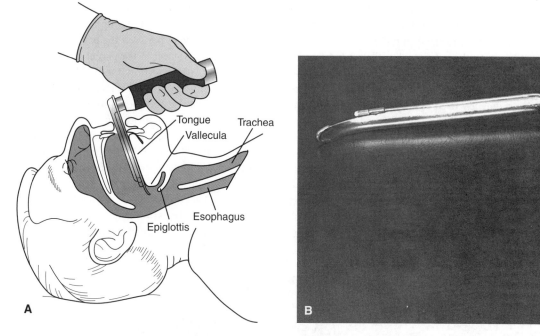

Tongue

Vallecula

Trachea

Esophagus

Epiglottis

A

B

Figure 3-12. **A:** Endotracheal intubation is an advanced skill that directly places a breathing tube into the trachea. **B:** A straight laryngoscope blade will displace the epiglottis and allow direct visualization of the vocal cords.

physicians, nurse anesthetists, paramedics, and occasionally respiratory therapists and EMT-Intermediates and requires significant training and frequency to maintain proficiency. It has recently been suggested that paramedics do not perform the skill often enough to maintain a reasonable level of proficiency.[1] Intubation is not within the athletic trainer's scope of practice, but they should be familiar with the technique. Large sports medicine staffs should consider having at least one person available who has the training and legal status to perform advanced airway techniques.

Other devices used to secure an airway require less training and frequency of use to maintain proficiency. State laws may or may not allow athletic trainers to use these devices.

Laryngeal Mask Airway

The LMA was developed in Great Britain in the late 1980s and is often used in operating rooms for minor surgical cases requiring general anesthesia (Fig. 3-13). The LMA comes in

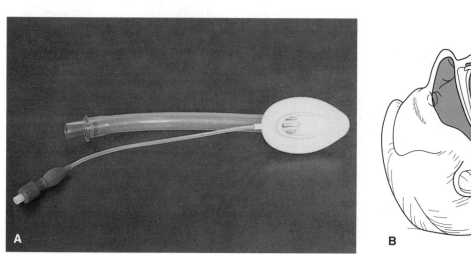

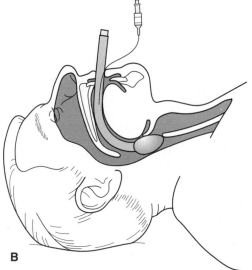

A

B

Figure 3-13. **A:** The LMA is a super-glottic airway that does not protect against gastric aspiration. **B:** The LMA in place over the glottic opening.

eight sizes based on weight, including pediatric. It is blindly inserted into the posterior oropharynx, and the cuff is inflated with 10 to 30 cc of air, creating a seal around the glottic opening. A BVM is attached and the patient is ventilated. The LMA does not prevent aspiration of gastric contents and the seal may be lost when moving the patient. Disposable LMAs are low cost and are frequently used as a backup to a failed intubation within the hospital. LMA use by paramedics is uncommon in the United States.

Combitube

The combitube is a double lumen tube that is blindly inserted into the esophagus (Fig. 3-14A). There are two balloons, each with an inflation port. The distal balloon is inflated with 15 cc of air and seals the esophagus. The proximal balloon is inflated with 60 cc of air and seals the oropharynx. Lumen 1 is closed at the tip but has holes between the balloons that allow air to enter the trachea. Lumen 2 is open at the tip but not between the balloons. After insertion, the BVM is attached to lumen 1 and the patient is ventilated (Fig. 3-14B). If properly positioned, the chest will rise and breath sounds will be heard by auscultation with a stethoscope. Rarely, the combitube may enter the trachea, in which case lumen 2 is used to ventilate the patient (Fig. 3-14C). The combitube provides some protection against gastric aspiration and is disposable. Although the combitube may be used as a primary airway device, it is most often used as a backup to a failed intubation. The combitube comes in two sizes based on height and is significantly more expensive than the disposable LMA.

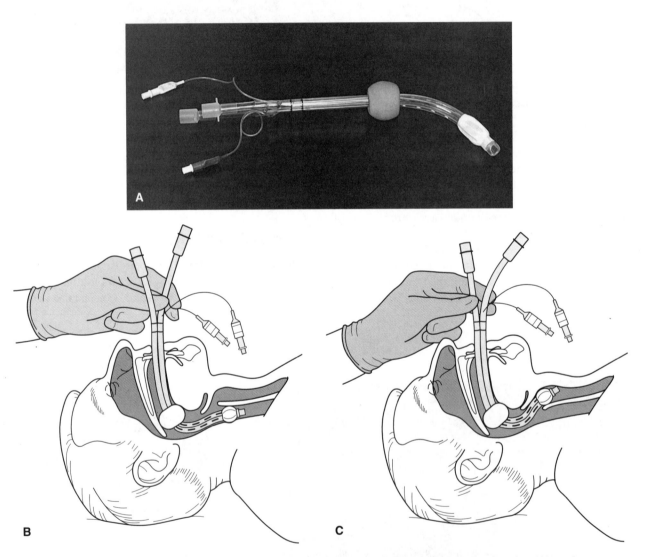

Figure 3-14. **A:** The combitube is an alternative airway device. **B:** The combitube is designed to be placed into the esophagus. **C:** On rare occasions the combitube may enter the trachea, in which case it functions as an endotracheal tube.

King LT-D

The King laryngeal tube-disposable is a new device introduced into the United States from Germany in 2005. It resembles the combitube but has only one lumen and its two balloons are filled from one inflation port (Fig. 3-15). The King LT-D is inserted blindly into the esophagus. The distal balloon is inflated, which seals the esophagus; the proximal balloon seals the oropharynx. There are three sizes based on height, and the amount of air used to inflate the balloons varies by size (45–90 cc). The King LT-D cannot be used for patients who are shorter than 4 feet tall. Pediatric sizes are under development. The area between the balloons is open and air will enter the trachea when the BVM is attached. The King LT-D provides some protection against gastric aspiration and is only slightly more expensive than the disposable LMA. The King LT-D is a new device that shows great promise.[3] Because of its simplicity, the King LT-D is featured in Box 3-2. An overview of airway management equipment is featured in Table 3-1.

Suction

The risk of vomiting exists during the management of any airway crisis, especially when advanced airway devices or a BVM are used. Aspiration of vomitus into the lungs may cause **aspiration pneumonitis,** which is a serious and sometimes fatal complication. Athletes are assumed to have a full stomach because they are consuming fluids during practice and competition; therefore, the risk of vomiting is high when the airway is compromised. Various types of portable suction equipment are available, ranging from manual to electronic. Electronic suction units are superior to manual units but are more expensive and require a battery charging system. These electronic units use a large bore yankauer suction catheter to remove vomitus. Suctioning should be limited to less than 20 seconds because all oxygen is removed from the airway during the procedure. Care must also be taken so that the athlete does not bite down on the yankauer catheter. The effectiveness of manual units is suspect. If suction equipment is not available, the athlete may be turned on his or her side while maintaining the cervical spine in a neutral position and the vomitus cleared manually with a towel. Prior to their arrival, EMS personnel should be advised that the athlete has vomited so that they may have their portable suction unit readily available. Figure 3-16 on page 46 shows a type of portable electronic suction unit, and Figure 3-17 on page 46 shows a type of manual suction unit.

Early recognition and intervention are crucial when dealing with a compromised airway. A variety of advanced techniques and equipment is available to aid in airway management. Athletic trainers must know and adhere to the scope of practice for their state and never exceed this scope. Additional training and certification may be necessary to use many of the techniques and equipment covered in this chapter. It is recommended that students and staff regularly practice on a mannequin all of the techniques available to them.

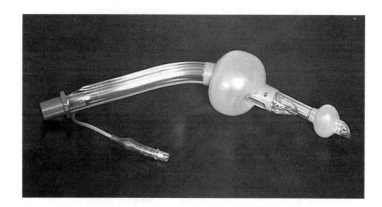

Figure 3-15. The King airway is a super-glottic airway that offers some protection against gastric aspiration and is easy to insert.

BOX 3-2   King LT-D Manufacturer Quick Reference Insert

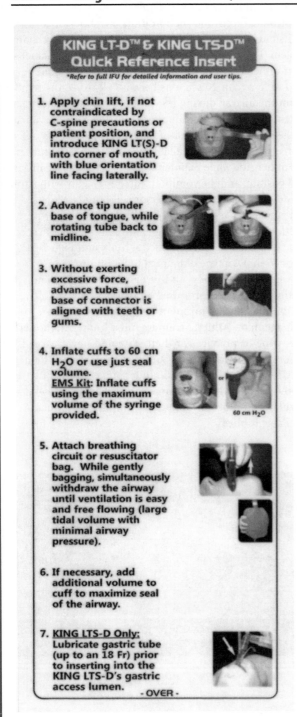

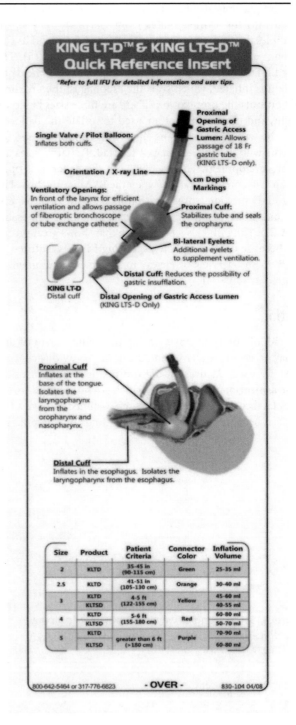

King Lt-D™. Copyright by King Systems, A Consort Medical Company. Reprinted with permission.

Table 3-1   Overview of Airway Management Equipment

Type	Name	Use	Use permissible by athletic trainer?
Airway adjuncts			
	CPR pocket mask	CPR, rescue breathing; protect rescuer from fluid exchange with victim	Yes
	Oropharyngeal airway	Control obstructed airway; use with bag valve mask (BVM)	Possible; check state practice act
	Nasopharyngeal airway	Control obstructed airway; use with BVM	Possible; check state practice act
	BVM	Ventilate victim; more effective than pocket masks; can be used alone or in conjunction with supplemental oxygen and/or intubation	Yes
Supplemental oxygen delivery			
	Nasal cannula	Used in conjunction with oxygen tank	Possible; check state practice act
	Simple face mask	Used in conjunction with oxygen tank	Possible; check state practice act
	Reservoir bag face mask	Used in conjunction with oxygen tank	Possible; check state practice act
Intubation			
	Endotracheal tube	Gold standard for intubation tubes; most effective control of airway and ventilation of victims with least risk of gastric aspiration; can be used in conjunction with BVM	No
	Laryngeal mask airway (LMA)	Effective control of airway and ventilation of victims with low risk of gastric aspiration; can be used in conjunction with BVM	No
	Combitube	Effective control of airway and ventilation of victims with low risk of gastric aspiration; can be used in conjunction with BVM	No
	King laryngeal tube-disposable (King LT-D)	Effective control of airway and ventilation of victims with low risk of gastric aspiration; can be used in conjunction with BVM	No

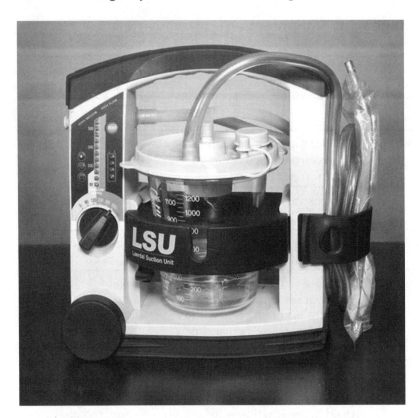

Figure 3-16. An electronic portable suction unit will clear the airway of large particulate matter but requires maintenance and regular battery charging.

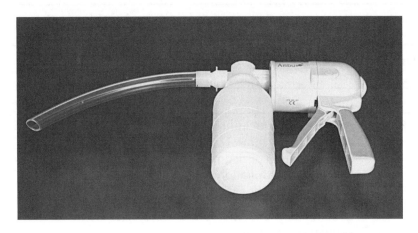

Figure 3-17. A portable manual suction unit is less effective than an electronic unit but requires no maintenance.

 EMERGENCY ACTION

Recognizing that the head coach has an obstructed airway, the athletic trainer carefully aligns the coach's head into a neutral position and does a jaw thrust maneuver. The coach immediately starts to breathe normally and his color improves. The assistant coach returns and says EMS is on the way. An athletic training student brings the oxygen tank, and oxygen is administered via a reservoir bag face mask. Vital signs are taken and history is obtained. The assistant coach states the head coach suddenly complained of the worst headache of his life and then slumped over. No trauma was involved. EMS arrives and transports the coach to the hospital for treatment of a possible stroke.

CHAPTER HIGHLIGHTS

- The airway can be divided into two parts: the upper and lower airway. The upper airway is composed of the oropharynx and nasopharynx. The lower airway consists of the epiglottis and the larynx.

- Signs of an obstructed airway include snoring respirations, sternal and intercostal retractions, accessory muscle use, and gurgling.

- The head tilt–chin lift technique will almost always result in a patent airway; this technique cannot be used in the unconscious athlete who is assumed to have a cervical spine injury. Therefore, the jaw thrust or triple airway maneuver is more appropriate for the unconscious athlete.

- The oropharyngeal (OP) and nasopharyngeal (NP) airways are used to relieve an obstructed airway after the initial jaw thrust maneuver has shown its effectiveness.

- Although athletic trainers need to check the scope of practice defined by their state licensure acts, there are no contraindications to short-term oxygen administration in an emergency situation.

- Oxygen can be administered by a variety of devices, including nasal cannulas, simple face masks, reservoir bag face masks, and bag valve masks.

Chapter Questions

1. Which anatomical structure is most commonly associated with airway compromise?
   A. Tongue
   B. Teeth
   C. Nose
   D. Epiglottis

2. Gurgling sounds indicate _____ in the airway.
   A. Air
   B. Fluid
   C. Foreign body
   D. Blood

3. _____ is a common symptom of airway obstruction.
   A. Stuttering
   B. Apnea
   C. Bradypnea
   D. Snoring respirations

4. Opening the airway in the presence of a cervical spine injury is accomplished by using the _____.
   A. Bag valve mask
   B. Pocket mask
   C. Jaw thrust maneuver
   D. Oxygen mask

5. The NP airway should span the distance between _____ and _____.
   A. Ear and jaw
   B. Ear and tip of nose
   C. Jaw and nose
   C. Corner of mouth and nose

6. What is the range of FiO_2 for a simple face mask?
   A. 40% to 60%
   B. 100%
   C. 20% to 40%
   D. More than 100%

7. How should oxygen tanks be stored?
   A. Upright
   B. Near the smoking area
   C. On a shelf
   D. In a holder away from flame

8. What letters describe the hand placement technique for using a BVM mask?
   A. X-Y
   B. Z-W
   C. E-C
   D. A-B-C

9. A pocket mask without a supplemental oxygen port delivers a FiO_2 of _____.

   A. About 16%

   B. 21%

   C. 25%

   D. 30%

10. _____ is considered the gold standard for advanced airway techniques.

    A. Combitube

    B. Endotracheal intubation

    C. LMA

    D. King LT-D

■ *Case Study 1*

During football practice a defensive back tackles a receiver but does not get up after the play. The athletic trainer runs to his side and sees the player is not moving and has snoring respirations. While calling for help from the staff, the athletic trainer kneels at the player's head and stabilizes the cervical spine in a neutral position. The jaw thrust maneuver relieves the snoring, but the player remains unconscious. A staff member runs to call 911 and activate the emergency action plan.

Case Study 1 Questions

1. What are your priorities in treating this seriously injured athlete?
2. Is oxygen indicated for this athlete? Why?
3. Is an airway adjunct indicated for this athlete? Which would you choose?

■ *Case Study 2*

A wrestler with a known history of asthma enters the athletic training room complaining of difficulty breathing. He is unable to speak in full sentences but indicates he has been using his inhaler without relief. The athletic trainer notes accessory muscle use and intercostal retractions with each breath. The emergency action plan is activated and EMS is called. The wrestler suddenly leans backward on a treatment table and passes out. The athletic trainer notes that the wrestler's respiratory effort is minimal.

Case Study 2 Questions

1. Should a BVM be used to assist the athlete's respirations?
2. Which airway adjunct would you choose? Is one better than the other?
3. Should oxygen be administered?

References

1. Wang H, Kupas D, Hostler D, et al. Procedural experience with out-of-hospital endotracheal intubation. Crit Care Med. 2005;33(8):1718–1721.

2. American Heart Association. ACLS Provider Manual. Dallas, TX: 2001; 25.

3. Fowler R. King LT-D to the rescue. J Emerg Med Serv. 2005;30(7):90–92.

Suggested Readings

1. Slovis C, High K. Ten commandments of airway management. J Emerg Med Serv. 2005;30(7):42–54.

2. For information regarding the combitube, go to www.combitube.org

3. For information regarding the King LT-D, go to www.kingsystems.com

4. For information regarding the LMA, search for "LMA" online.

Chapter 4

Sudden Cardiac Death

Vincent N. Mosesso, Jr., MD, FACEP

KEY TERMS

Agonal respirations

Asystole

Automated external
   defibrillator

Cardioversion

Commotio cordis

Critical
   Incident Stress
   Management

Defibrillation

Dyspnea

Echocardiography

Electrocardiographic

Exercise-related SCA

Hyperkalemia

Hypovolemia

Postictal state

Pulseless electrical activity

Sudden cardiac arrest

Sudden cardiac death

Syncope

Ventricular fibrillation

 EMERGENCY SITUATION

It is a cool but sunny afternoon at the Newton North High School football stadium where the Newts are taking on the Laketon Blue Devils. After a hard-fought first half, the Newts begin their first play from scrimmage of the second half. You, the athletic trainer for the Laketon team, see the referee suddenly collapse in the backfield. You watch for a second as you hear the whistle blow to end the play but do not see the referee move or attempt to get up. You rush onto the field, and when you call his name or shake him, he does not answer. You observe a brief, deep gasp but cannot feel a carotid pulse with your cold hands.

Overview

Sudden death in athletes has an ancient legacy. Perhaps the first reported case was Pheidippides. He was the Greek soldier who ran 24 miles from Marathon to Athens to announce victory over the Persians. On arrival, legend has it, he dropped dead.

Unfortunately, sudden death in athletes is not just of historic interest and remains a very real problem, as evidenced by the sudden death of these more modern athletes: Hank Gathers (22 years old), Loyola Marymount University basketball player, at the free throw line; John McSherry (51), Major League Baseball umpire, behind home plate; Reggie Lewis (27), during an NBA playoff game; Louis Acompora (14), while playing lacrosse; Mindy Alpeter (16), while performing on stage; and Thomas Herrion (23), Minnesota Vikings football player, immediately after a preseason game.

Sudden cardiac arrest (SCA) is the sudden and unexpected cessation of the heart's pumping activity. The resultant lack of blood flow to the brain leads to unconsciousness in about 20 to 30 seconds. If flow is not resumed, permanent brain damage will begin to occur in 4 to 6 minutes, and the condition is generally fatal if not treated in 10 minutes.[1-4] When the heart is not pumping blood, there is no delivery of oxygen or glucose to any of the body's tissue—including the heart itself because the heart tissue is perfused by blood flowing from the aorta into the coronary arteries. When sudden cardiac arrest results in death, it is termed **sudden cardiac death.**

The survival rate from SCA varies widely dependent on the specific setting and the geographic location. Different studies may also use different denominators, such as all cardiac arrests in the community, all treated by emergency medical services (EMS), and those that were witnessed only; there are also variable methods for determining which patients are considered dead on arrival (DOA). The generally accepted overall survival rate is about 5% to 7%.[5,6] SCA presents with one of three cardiac rhythms:

- **Ventricular fibrillation** (VF)
- **Pulseless electrical activity**
- **Asystole**

Ventricular fibrillation is the most common initial rhythm, occurring in about 60% of cases when assessed by an on-site **automated external defibrillator** (AED) and likely even higher among athletes.[7] This rhythm represents electrical chaos and usually not a mechanical problem with the heart (Fig. 4-1). It is the rhythm most amenable to treatment, which is a high-energy shock delivered to the heart called **defibrillation.** In community-based reports, survival from patients initially in VF varies greatly from about 10% to as high as 49%.[8,9] Studies have found survival rates as high as 74% when defibrillation occurs within 3 minutes from the time of collapse and report that AEDs added to an on-site response plan can double survival rates.[7,10] The survival rate decreases between 5% and 10% for every minute that passes from the time of collapse until defibrillation is achieved, but immediate cardiopulmonary resuscitation (CPR) can ameliorate this decrease (Fig. 4-2).[11,12] Thus, early defibrillation and on-site defibrillators are vital.

Pulseless electrical activity (PEA) is the term used for any other **electrocardiographic** (ECG) rhythm, including normal sinus rhythm, when there is no associated cardiac contraction. This may be amenable to treatment when a reversible condition is the cause, such as **hypovolemia** or **hyperkalemia,** but the mortality from this condition is higher than for VF. Asystole, or "flatline," means the absence of any cardiac electrical activity and therefore the absence of any mechanical cardiac function. Patients found in this rhythm have a grim prognosis, with most studies reporting survival of only 0% to 2%.[13,14]

SCA should be differentiated from a "heart attack." The medical term for a heart attack is myocardial infarction. This condition results in the death of some heart muscle resulting from total (or near total) occlusion of a coronary artery. This

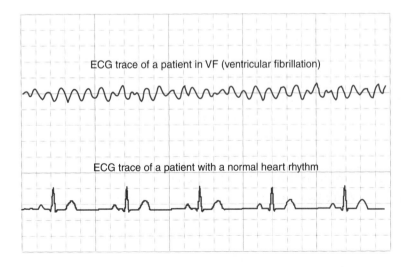

Figure 4-1. ECG recording of ventricular fibrillation.

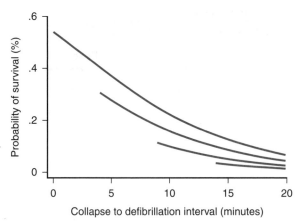

Figure 4-2. Effect of delay to CPR and defibrillation on survival. Relation of collapse to CPR and defibrillation to survival: simplified model. Graphic representation of simplified (includes collapse to CPR and collapse to defibrillation only) predictive model of survival after witnessed, out-of-hospital cardiac arrest from ventricular fibrillation. Each curve represents change in probability of survival as delay (minutes) to defibrillation increases for a given collapse-to-CPR interval (minutes). From Valenzuela TD, Roe DJ, Cretin S, et al. Estimating effectiveness of cardiac arrest interventions: A logistic regression survival model. Circulation. 1997;96(10):3308–3313.

is almost always a result of the acute formation of a blood clot at a site of preexisting narrowing (atherosclerosis) in a coronary artery. A heart attack predisposes to SCA but should be distinguished as a distinct process. The risk of SCA is greatest in the first 2 hours after a myocardial infarction and gradually diminishes over time.

Incidence and Etiology of Sudden Death in the General Population

Because SCA is not a reportable disease and because there is no standard criteria for listing the cause of death on death certificates, the actual incidence of SCA is not precisely known. Studies of specific communities suggest that the incidence in North America is likely 0.5 to 1/1000 persons, with the lower rate reflective of more recent studies.[15,16] Estimates ranging from 460,000/year to 200,000/year have been published.[17,18] Despite this wide range, it is clear that SCA is the leading cause of death in the United States, claiming more deaths than motor vehicle crashes, fires, lung cancer and breast cancer *combined*!

In the general population, SCA most often occurs in people age 50 to 75 years, which is consistent with the development of ischemic heart disease and congestive heart failure. About two thirds of people who experience SCA have coronary artery disease; SCA is often the first manifestation of underlying heart disease. Despite the

common misconception, more women die of SCA than men. In fact, SCA can strike anyone of any age, any gender, and any race—it is truly nondiscriminatory.

Sudden Cardiac Arrest in Athletes

Exercise-related SCA has been defined as sudden cardiac arrest occurring within 1 hour of participation in sport or exercise.[19] Consistent with the low prevalence of cardiovascular disease in people younger than 35 years of age, the frequency of sudden death in athletes is considered to be very low but not precisely known. One report estimates 300 deaths annually in the United States among 10 to 15 million athletes participating in competitive sports.[20] Another report estimated there to be 25 to 125 deaths each year among 25 million competitive athletes.[21]

Still, SCA is the leading cause of death in athletes.[22,23] One study noted that sudden cardiac collapse was the cause of twice as many fatalities as trauma among high school and college athletes.[24] The death of a competitive athlete is usually an event of high visibility, is emotionally disturbing, and may create significant liability concerns.

The vast majority (85%) of sudden deaths in athletes are a result of underlying cardiovascular conditions.[25] However, in contrast to sudden death in the general population, which is usually a result of ischemic heart disease, congenital abnormalities are most often to blame in athletes younger than age 35. Most deaths occur in athletes with structural heart disease, as noted in Table 4-1.[25] Hypertrophic cardiomyopathy is most common, followed by congenital coronary artery anomalies, aortic dissection or aneurysm from Marfan syndrome, and valvular deformities.

In about 2% of deaths, no structural abnormality can be found, and these are considered primary arrhythmic deaths (often referred to as sudden arrhythmic death syndrome [SADS] or autopsy-negative sudden unexplained death [SUD]). These cases result from conditions that disrupt the electrical system on the cellular level, including long QT, short QT, and Brugada syndromes and familial catecholaminergic polymorphic ventricular tachycardia.

One series found 90% of athletes who died of SCA in the United States were males and that 68% of cases were related to football and basketball.[26] Most of our knowledge in this area is from case series; thus, incidence and demographic findings may be skewed.

External factors may also directly cause or predispose to SCA in athletes. Most prominent is the condition called **commotio cordis,** which is the provocation of ventricular fibrillation or ventricular tachycardia by a blow to the anterior chest over or near the heart. The impact must occur at a specific point in the cardiac electrical cycle, called the vulnerable period of repolarization (during the second half of the T wave). This is usually caused by a solid object such as a baseball and may occur with only mild or moderate force. This seems to occur most commonly in the early teens.[27]

Table 4-1   Causes of Sudden Death in 387 Young Athletes*

Cause	No. of Athletes	Percent
Hypertrophic cardiomyopathy	102	26.4
Commotio cordis	77	19.9
Coronary artery anomalies	53	13.7
Left ventricular hypertrophy of indeterminate causation[†]	29	7.5
Myocarditis	20	5.2
Ruptured aortic aneurysm (Marfan syndrome)	12	3.1
Arrhythmogenic right ventricular cardiomyopathy	11	2.8
Tunneled (bridged) coronary artery[‡]	11	2.8
Aortic valve stenosis	10	2.6
Atherosclerotic coronary artery disease	10	2.6
Dilated cardiomyopathy	9	2.3
Myxomatous mitral valve degeneration	9	2.3
Asthma (or other pulmonary condition)	8	2.1
Heat stroke	6	1.6
Drug abuse	4	1.0
Other cardiovascular cause	4	1.0
Long QT syndrome[§]	3	0.8
Cardiac sarcoidosis	3	0.8
Trauma causing structural cardiac injury	3	0.8
Ruptured cerebral artery	3	0.8

*Data are from the registry of the Minneapolis Heart Institute Foundation (3).
[†]Findings at autopsy were suggestive of HCM but were insufficient to be diagnostic.
[‡]Tunneled coronary artery was deemed the cause of death in the absence of any other cardiac abnormality.
[§]The long QT syndrome was documented on clinical evaluation.
Source: Reproduced from Maron BJ[20] with permission of the Massachusetts Medical Society.

⭐ *STAT Point 4-1. Commotio cordis: The impact must occur at a specific point in the cardiac electrical cycle, called the vulnerable period of repolarization (during the second half of the T wave).*

An important predisposing factor to SCA, particularly in the setting of sports and exercise, is the use of performance-enhancing and recreational substances, including anabolic steroids, Ma Huang, bitter orange, cocaine, and other stimulants. It should also be recognized that sports venues and fitness facilities have been identified as one of the most common locations where SCA occurs in general.[28,29]

Preventive Measures: Screening and Recognition of Cardiac Warning Signs

Preparticipation Screening

Every person who intends to participate in vigorous physical activity, especially competitive sports, should receive thorough screening for cardiovascular and other disorders that might predispose to illness or even death.[30,31] This "preparticipation physical" or screening examination should be performed by a medical practitioner with training and experience in this specific field. The screening should consist of a careful assessment of the athlete's medical history to identify symptoms that might indicate the presence of underlying conditions. Symptoms include **syncope,** palpitations, episodic or exertional **dyspnea,** exertional chest pain, and early fatigue, among others. A physical examination focusing on the cardiovascular examination and phenotypic evidence of congenital syndromes is also warranted. Findings causing concern should trigger testing such as ECG and **echocardiography.** Family history and cardiovascular disease in siblings should also be investigated.

⭐ *STAT Point 4-2. Preseason physical health history symptoms for possible cardiac problems. Symptoms include syncope, palpitations, episodic or exertional dyspnea, exertional chest pain, and early fatigue.*

Despite widespread policy requiring some level of screening, this process has been of low yield in general.[20] This is likely because of the low incidence of abnormalities, the occult nature of some heart conditions, and suboptimal performance of the screening. However, a number of studies of rigorous screening efforts including routine echocardiography also had a very low detection rate.[32–35]

Recognition of Warning Signs

Athletic trainers should maintain constant vigilance for signs of underlying cardiovascular disease and should be able to recognize the signs and symptoms when they do present. Particular symptoms of concern that should prompt further evaluation are listed in Box 4-1. Symptoms occurring during or immediately after exertion are most worrisome, as are symptoms that occur repeatedly. Athletes of all ages are often reluctant to admit to the presence or seriousness of physical illness. Therefore, it is up to the athletic trainer and medical staff to identify such episodes and arrange for appropriate evaluation. Such evaluation for competitive athletes should be conducted by a physician trained or experienced in sports medicine or a cardiologist with expertise in this field.

Although a full discussion of prevention is beyond the scope of this chapter and currently many episodes of SCA are not preventable, some common sense measures are in order. These include counseling on avoidance of performance-enhancing drugs and supplements (especially androgenic steroids), alcohol, and caffeine and other stimulants and excessive use of vitamin supplements; ensuring proper nutrition, hydration, and rest; and paying attention to environmental stress. As mentioned earlier, athletic trainers and coaches must maintain vigilance for potential signs and symptoms of an underlying medical condition and assure proper evaluation is performed when identified. Athletes must be encouraged to report any symptoms despite the associated fear of withdrawal from participation.

Box 4-1   Symptoms of Concern in Athletes

- ■ Lightheadedness
- ■ Dizziness
- ■ Syncope or near-syncope
- ■ Chest pain or pressure
- ■ Palpitations (fluttering in chest)
- ■ Nausea/vomiting (unrelated to other illness)
- ■ Fatigue/weakness (disproportionate to baseline or to others)
- ■ Shortness of breath

Note: These symptoms are particularly worrisome if they occur during or immediately after exertion.

Preparation for Cardiac Emergencies

SCA Awareness

The first step in preventing death from SCA is adequate awareness of and the ability to recognize the condition, the dire emergency that it represents, and the need for immediate bystander action. Everyone in any way involved with the athletic program, including the athletes themselves, should receive education on SCA and the program's emergency action plan (EAP). It is strongly recommended that all receive formal training in basic CPR and use of an AED.

Such awareness and training should extend to the entire school or applicable community as well. This is an opportunity for athletic trainers to make a contribution to the community beyond the athletic program. Many athletic trainers team with the school nurse or other medical staff and other interested faculty and staff to promote SCA awareness, CPR training, and AED deployment throughout the campus and community.

Training and Education for Responders

Response Planning

Every athletic program should develop a written EAP.[36] *(For more information on EAP, see Chapter 1.)* It is worth repeating that having an effective plan is most critical for time-sensitive conditions, and none is more time sensitive than SCA. Whether the SCA victim lives or dies is often determined by whether the EAP was properly designed and implemented. The EAP should identify responders who will be available for all potential situations, including practices. All of these responders, which might include coaches and other staff especially for practices, should have formal training in CPR, AED use, and basic first aid and a thorough knowledge of the EAP, how to contact local EMS, and location of the nearest AED. The plan should be tested and verified in a variety of situations. Do not wait for a real SCA to find out whether your plan works.

Equipment and Supplies

Again, a comprehensive discussion of this topic is covered in Chapter 1. Here we will focus on equipment and supplies specific to management of SCA. These include the following:

- ■ Defibrillators
- ■ Ventilation aids
- ■ Telephone or other communications equipment to call 911 and other resources

Defibrillators

Defibrillators are of two main types: manual and automated (also called automatic). Manual defibrillators must be used by medical personnel with specific training in cardiac rhythm recognition and management and in operation of the defibrillator. This type of defibrillator requires the user to interpret the ECG rhythm and determine if an electric countershock should be delivered; if so, the user must be able to set the energy level, activate the charging process, and then push a button to deliver the shock.

The other type is typically referred to as automated external defibrillator or AED (Fig. 4-3). These devices can be used by virtually anyone, even without prior training, although training is highly advised. These portable, battery-powered devices provide verbal and visual prompts to the user once the device is turned on. The most important user action is to place the two ECG sensing defibrillation pads onto the proper locations on the patient's chest (Fig. 4-4). Some models require the user to push an "analyze" button

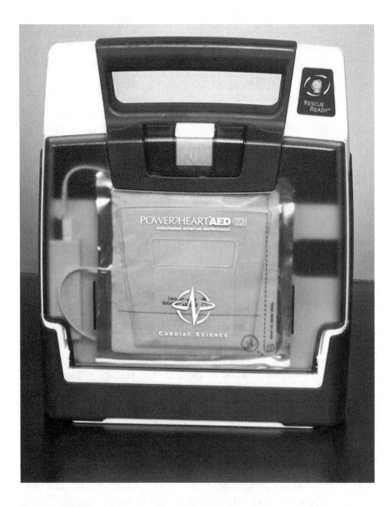

Figure 4-3. Automated external defibrillator.

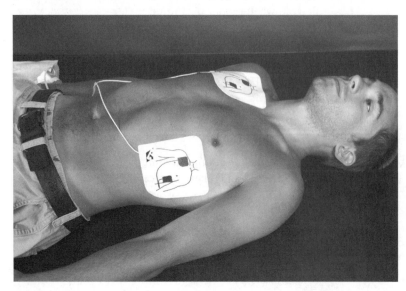

Figure 4-4. Standard location of defibrillation pads on an adult.

and/or a "shock" button to deliver the electric shock (semiautomatic) and some perform analysis, charging, and shock delivery without further user action (fully automatic).

All AEDs use a sophisticated computer algorithm to analyze the ECG waveform and determine whether a shock is appropriate (Fig. 4-5). All models shock VF and rapid ventricular (wide complex) tachycardia (VT). At least one model has the capability to also perform synchronized **cardioversion** of supraventricular (narrow complex) tachycardia. The specificity of these algorithms approaches 100% (i.e., it is extremely rare that a shock is advised or delivered inappropriately), whereas the sensitivity is generally more than 90% (i.e., the device will recommend shock at least 90% of the time when a shockable rhythm is present).[37] The high specificity at a modest cost in sensitivity assures a greater safety margin should the device be applied to a person who is not really in cardiac arrest.

Models also vary in the prompts provided. Some newer models are specifically designed for laypersons with minimal (or no) training and have ergonomic advancements to facilitate layperson use. Others are designed for trained first responders who receive regular training with the device. Some have specific features that might apply to special circumstances, such as a high degree of water resistance or the capability to function in "manual" mode (like the manual defibrillators described earlier.) We suggest reviewing all available models and features to determine which best meets your specific needs. Additional information about AEDs and links to descriptions and photos of specific models can be found at www.suddencardiacarrest.org.

⭘ *STAT Point 4-3. Additional information about AEDs and links to descriptions and photos of specific models can be found at www. suddencardiacarrest.org*

Whereas in some settings the AED may be kept with the team medical equipment, in others it may be appropriate to install the AED at a fixed specific location. Wall mount and freestanding cabinets are available that have optional features including audible and visible alarms and auto-dialers that can call 911 and/or an on-site dispatch center when the cabinet is opened. It is recommended that an AED cabinet not be locked except in rare situations when it is certain there will be no need for the device.

Some ancillary supplies kept with the AED may be helpful, such as a towel, scissors (to cut clothing), disposable razor (for excessive chest hair removal), and pocket mask with one-way valve.

Ventilation Aids

In the strictest sense, ventilation adjuncts are not absolutely necessary because mouth-to-mouth resuscitation can be performed. However, when advance planning is possible, it is prudent to have adjuncts readily available that provide the rescuer with some protection from blood and body fluid exposure and that may facilitate better ventilation.

The simplest adjuncts are a variety of face shields and masks that cover the victim's mouth and nose and provide a port for the rescuer's mouth (Fig. 4-6). Many of these have a one-way valve either incorporated or as an attachment to prevent air and fluid exchange from the victim to the rescuer. These devices can be used by laypersons with minimal training and in most cases should be kept in the case with the AED.

More advanced airway adjuncts should only be used after proper training. These include nasopharyngeal and oropharyngeal airways (which help to maintain an open airway in an unresponsive person) and ventilation bags that attach to the face mask (commonly called bag mask, or bag valve mask, devices). Some masks have a port for the connection of supplemental oxygen. This is discussed in more detail in Chapter 3.

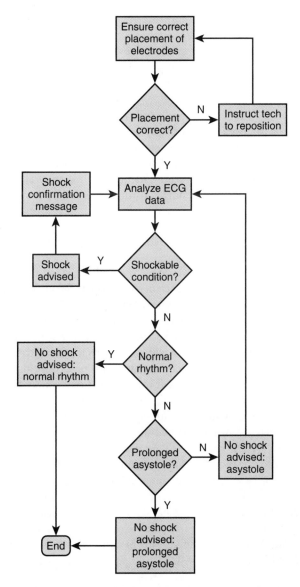

Figure 4-5. Function of the automated external defibrillator. From Medronics Inc., with permission.

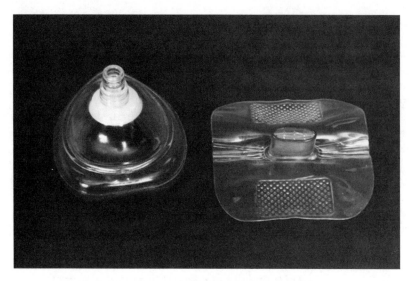

Figure 4-6. Example of a pocket mask (left) and a face shield (right).

Management of Sudden Cardiac Arrest

Successful resuscitation of the victim of SCA requires the proper interventions to be provided in a very short time. The actions that must occur have been called the "Chain of Survival."

- Early recognition of SCA and call to 911
- Early CPR
- Early defibrillation
- Early Advanced Life Support[38]

The first three steps can—and in most situations *must*—be provided by bystanders, who may or may not be medical professionals. These steps as they apply to athletic settings are described further later in this chapter. An interorganizational consensus panel has developed an algorithm for the management of SCA in athletic programs, as described in Figure 4-7.[39]

Recognition of SCA and Activation of Local EMS

Time to intervention is the most important determinant of survival from sudden cardiac arrest. Therefore, immediate recognition of this condition followed by prompt action is the key to survival. The astute athletic trainer will maintain constant surveillance for a player (or spectator) that suddenly collapses. SCA should be of high concern if such collapse occurs without contact and whenever the fall occurs in an "unprotected" manner, which usually indicates the subject is already unconscious.

As soon as a collapsed person is spotted, the athletic trainer should immediately and quickly move to the person's side and determine if the person is conscious. This can be done by calling the person by name or asking if he or she is okay. If there is no response to this verbal stimulus, then the athletic trainer should gently shake or physically stimulate the person's body to see if this elicits a response. If there is concern for spinal trauma, be careful not to cause movement

of the head and neck. If there is no response, local EMS should be summoned immediately, CPR should be started, and the AED should be brought to the victim.

A presentation of cardiac arrest that may confuse rescuers and lead to delay in providing CPR and AED use is seizure-like activity. This may occur immediately after the onset of the heart stoppage as a result of low blood flow to the brain. The seizure usually lasts only a minute or two and may be followed by **agonal respirations,** which are intermittent gasping breaths. These should not be confused with a normal breathing effort and do not indicate that the person has a heartbeat or is breathing adequately. It is imperative to recognize that the patient is in cardiac arrest and not simply in a **postictal state.**

CPR

If the victim does not respond to either verbal or physical stimuli, then the athletic trainer must open the airway and determine if spontaneous breathing is present. If there is no concern for trauma, then the rescuer should tilt the head back by pushing on the forehead and pulling up on the bony part of the lower jaw (head tilt–chin lift maneuver). If cervical trauma is a concern, then the modified jaw thrust procedure should be performed. These procedures pull the tongue away from the posterior pharyngeal wall, thereby removing obstruction to airflow. Checking for breathing is best done by leaning over and placing your face close to the victim's face while looking to see the chest rise and fall, listening for air movement, and feeling for air movement against your cheek (look, listen, and feel). The latter will be difficult in an outdoor environment.

If the athletic trainer does not find regular breathing, then rescue breathing should be started. This can be done mouth to mouth initially, but a barrier device or bag valve mask device should be used if trained. Two breaths for 1 second each should be provided, with each breath just large enough to make the victim's chest rise.

After these two breaths, the rescuer should begin chest compressions. Good-quality chest compressions and few

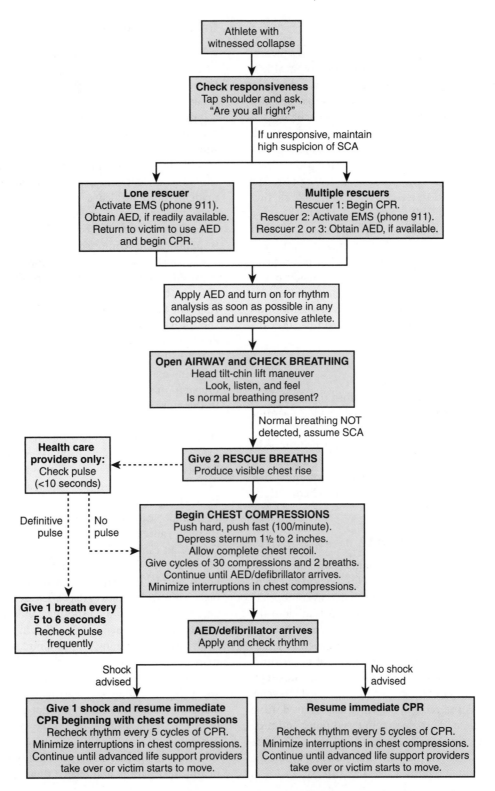

Figure 4-7. Inter-Association Task Force Algorithm for Management of Sudden Cardiac Arrest.

interruptions in compressing are critical for success. Rescuers trained as health professionals should check for a carotid pulse and, if not found within 10 seconds, begin chest compressions. Determining whether a pulse is present can be difficult, and if there is any doubt and no other signs of life are present, it is better to perform chest compressions. The athletic trainer should be familiar with the current guidelines for basic life support for health care professionals developed by the American Heart Association (www.americanheart.org/cpr) or another recognized authority.[38]

AED Use

As noted previously, it would be ideal if an AED was present at all athletic competitive events and practices. If an AED is present or known to be available on the premises, it should be brought to the victim and used as soon as possible. The athletic trainer should be well trained in the use of the AED. If the AED advises NOT to shock, the athletic trainer must realize the need to begin or resume chest compressions immediately. The AED can only recognize whether the patient has a shockable rhythm, not whether the person has a pulse. The AED should be allowed to reassess for a shockable rhythm after every 2 minutes of CPR or as per current guidelines.

Some AEDs have specific defibrillation pads or other modification to decrease the delivered energy for use in children, generally defined as age 1 to 8 years. Use of the pediatric dose for defibrillation is preferred when possible in this age group. However, if this capability is not immediately available, then the AED should be used as it would for an adult. Defibrillation should not be withheld because the pediatric modification is not available.[38–41]

Transfer of Care

The athletic trainer must continue performing CPR along with using the AED until more advanced providers assume care of the patient. The athletic trainer should report to the EMS personnel or care providers what happened immediately prior to the collapse and, in the case of a player or coach, if the patient had reported any ill symptoms earlier that day and any known underlying medical conditions and medications.

Documentation and Reporting

As part of the emergency action plan, all organized programs should have a reporting system for medical emergencies. The athletic trainer and other responders as appropriate should document any known circumstances leading to the event, exactly what the examination findings were, what care was rendered, and who assumed care of the victim. Times for key events should be documented as best as possible, which can be facilitated by the times recorded by the AED if the AED is synchronized to a known time source. Key events include time collapse recognized, time help arrived, time AED was used, time of any specific interventions, and time when advanced help arrived. The record of the AED (ECG recording and time stamping of AED actions) should be saved with the written report.

Debriefing and Follow-Up

After every incident, once the documentation of every involved party has been completed and the AED data have been retrieved, a thorough review of the incident should occur. This should involve the team physician, the EMS medical director or another physician experienced in emergency care, the team athletic trainers, and other responders and support personnel. All aspects of the EAP should be reviewed specific to the incident. The response and actions taken should be evaluated to determine if improvements could be made in future incidents. This should include assessment of system factors, such as communication capabilities and accessibility of the AED. Feedback should be provided to the responders. This comprises commendation for actions well done, constructive recommendations for areas of improvement, and information on the disposition of the patient.

The benefit of responders participating in a **Critical Incident Stress Management** (CISM) or similar program should be considered, especially for incidents involving a death or other significant stressors.

Finally, it is important that everyone involved in the planning and response to SCA realizes that despite the best preparation and treatment, many victims will still die. Even in the most ideal situations, it is likely that only about one third of those in shockable rhythms and even fewer in nonshockable rhythms will survive this life-threatening event. Everyone involved should be made aware of this during initial orientation and training to avoid unmet and unrealistic expectations. *(For more information on debriefing and follow-up, see Chapter 13.)*

Sudden cardiac arrest is uncommon but is still the most frequent cause of death among young athletes, claiming the lives of an estimated 300 athletes each year in the United States. Many of those stricken had no preceding symptoms and a normal preparticipation screening. SCA most often occurs during or immediately after exertion in persons with an often undetected predisposing condition. Sudden cardiac arrest is a life-threatening condition in which the heart suddenly stops functioning properly, no longer pumping blood to the brain, other organs, and the heart itself. If not reversed immediately, death is certain. Immediate bystander action consisting of calling 911, starting CPR, and using an AED can prevent death in many, but not all, cases. Proper planning and preparation is necessary to assure these actions occur in a timely fashion to avoid unnecessary deaths. Athletic trainers bear the responsibility to lead these efforts in athletic programs and related venues.

EMERGENCY ACTION

You suspect the referee is in SCA. Fortunately, your school had just purchased an AED, and, in accordance with your emergency action plan, it is on the sideline with the other emergency equipment. As you begin CPR, you ask one of the officials to get the AED from your team bench. He returns with it about a minute later and you immediately turn it on; apply the pads to the referee's chest; and, when the AED advises to shock, you push the shock button. You resume CPR and do not see any movement or breathing effort. After 2 minutes of CPR you stop and again have the AED analyze the heart rhythm. Again it advises shock is needed and you again push the shock button. As you are resuming CPR you notice the referee makes a weak cough, then a few gasps. You assist with a few more breaths and your patient begins breathing normally. You feel a regular carotid pulse as the EMS crew arrives on the scene.

The referee was transported to the local hospital. Evaluation determined the patient had likely suffered a heart attack the previous day but had ignored the symptoms. His SCA was likely a result of ventricular fibrillation triggered by the recent myocardial infarction. Fortunately, because of the athletic trainer's prompt response, initiation of CPR, and rapid use of the defibrillator, the patient suffered no significant neurological or cardiac damage. The patient went through a cardiac rehabilitation program and resumed officiating football games the next season.

CHAPTER HIGHLIGHTS

- Sudden cardiac arrest (SCA) is the sudden and unexpected cessation of the heart's pumping activity. The resultant lack of blood flow to the brain quickly leads to unconsciousness; if flow is not resumed, permanent brain damage will begin to occur soon thereafter, with death occurring within a few minutes.

- SCA presents with one of three cardiac rhythms: ventricular fibrillation, pulseless electrical activity, or asystole.

- SCA is the leading cause of death in athletes.

- External factors may also directly cause or predispose to SCA in athletes. Most prominent is the condition called *commotio cordis,* which is the provocation of ventricular fibrillation or ventricular tachycardia by a blow to the anterior chest over or near the heart.

- An important predisposing factor to SCA, particularly in the setting of sports and exercise, is the use of performance-enhancing and recreational substances, including anabolic steroids, Ma Huang, bitter orange, cocaine, and other stimulants.

- Having an effective emergency action plan is most critical for time-sensitive conditions, and none is more time sensitive than SCA. Whether the SCA victim lives or dies is often determined by whether the emergency action plan was properly implemented.

- Successful resuscitation of the athlete with SCA requires the proper interventions to be provided in a very short time. The actions that must occur are known as the "Chain of Survival" and include early recognition of

SCA and call to 911, early CPR, early defibrillation, and early Advanced Life Support.

- Victims of SCA sometimes exhibit agonal respirations. These should not be confused with a normal breathing effort and do not indicate that the person has a heartbeat or is breathing adequately.
- After every incident a thorough review should occur. This should involve the team physician, the EMS medical director or another physician experienced in emergency care, the team athletic trainers, and other responders and support personnel. All aspects of the emergency action plan should be reviewed specific to the incident, constructive feedback should be supplied, and the emergency action plan should be amended if necessary.

Chapter Questions

1. Which of the following conditions causes the most deaths annually in the United States?

   A. Breast cancer

   B. Motor vehicle crashes

   C. Sudden cardiac arrest

   D. Lung cancer

2. When you see a person collapse, you should first:

   A. Go to the person and assess him or her

   B. Begin mouth-to-mouth breathing

   C. Call 911

   D. Run get the nearest AED

3. The most common cause of death among athletes is:

   A. Head injury

   B. Heat stroke

   C. Sudden cardiac arrest

   D. Drug overdose

4. All of the following are recognized causes of SCA except:

   A. Long QT syndrome

   B. Commotio cordis

   C. Hypertrophic cardiomyopathy

   D. Sudden fibrillation syndrome

5. The following is a characteristic of all AEDs:

   A. Requires external power source

   B. Performs ECG rhythm analysis

   C. Requires user to push button to deliver shock

   D. Requires user to initiate ECG analysis

6. The following is NOT a characteristic of an AED:

   A. Must be operated by professional medical personnel

   B. Provides shock for SVT in addition to VF

   C. Automatically charges and shocks after VF detection

   D. Can be used on adults and children

7. The ECG rhythm associated with the highest likelihood of survival in persons who collapse in sudden cardiac arrest is:

   A. Asystole

   B. Normal sinus rhythm

   C. Pulseless electrical activity

   D. Ventricular fibrillation

8. When treating a person in cardiac arrest, you should:

   A. Call 911 if the person does not regain consciousness in 3 to 5 minutes

   B. Interrupt chest compressions as little as possible

   C. Repeat ECG analysis immediately if the AED advises no shock

   D. Avoid touching the patient if you observe occasional gasping

9. Proper response to sudden cardiac arrest at an athletic event requires all the following except:

   A. Written emergency action plan

   B. On-site EMS crew

   C. On-site defibrillation capability

   D. Training of targeted responders

10. After a sudden cardiac arrest event has transpired, the athletic trainer should:

    A. Determine if any responders require CISM

    B. Avoid restocking the AED until authorized by local police

    C. Accompany the patient to the hospital in the ambulance

    D. Cancel all athletic events until athletes receive additional screening

■ *Case Study 1*

You are the athletic trainer for the local college basketball team. At a routine practice, you notice one of the freshman players falling behind the others while running and almost stopping at times. He is usually in front of the pack. You go over to him, and he tells you that he is just fatigued today. He says he is getting a cold and didn't sleep well. You notice he is breathing hard and appears just a little shaky. You know he completed appropriate preseason screening and has no record of any prior medical problems.

Case Study 1 Discussion

1. What should you do now? Should you pull him from practice? What if this occurred during a game?
2. What further questions should you ask the player? What physical examination should you do?
3. What follow-up or further evaluation is indicated?

■ *Case Study 2*

You are the lead athletic trainer for a large area high school. As you are entering the gym for the annual father–son basketball game, your assistant informs you that the AED is beeping. She wants to know what she should do and whether she still should bring the device to the event.

Case Study 2 Discussion

1. What are the possible reasons why the AED is beeping? How can you determine the exact cause?
2. You check the AED and determine that the cause of the beeping is a low battery. You know the AED showed ready status without alarms yesterday. Do you need to replace the battery immediately (before the event)? Is it acceptable to take the AED as is to the event?
3. What procedures should you have in place for checking and maintaining the school's AEDs?

References

1. Baum RS, Alvarez H, Cobb LA. Survival after resuscitation from out-of-hospital ventricular fibrillation. Circulation. 1974;50:1231.

2. Olson DW, LaRochelle J, Fark D, et al. EMT-defibrillation: The Wisconsin experience. Ann Emerg Med. 1989;18(8): 806–811.

3. Eisenberg MS, Horwood BT, Cummins RO, et al. Cardiac arrest and resuscitation: A tale of 29 cities. Ann Emerg Med. 1990;19(2):179–186.

4. Thompson RJ, McCullough PA, Kahn JK, et al. Prediction of death and neurologic outcome in the emergency department in out-of-hospital cardiac arrest survivors. Am J Cardiol. 1998;81(1):17–21.

5. Callaway CW. Improving neurologic outcomes after out-of-hospital cardiac arrest. Review Prehosp Emerg Care. 1997;1:45–57.

6. Stiell G, Wells GA, Field BJ, et al. Improved out-of-hospital cardiac arrest survival through the inexpensive optimization of an existing defibrillation program: OPALS study phase II. Ontario Prehospital Advanced Life Support. JAMA. 1999;281:1175–1181.

7. Hallstrom AP, Ornato JP, Weisfeldt M, et al. Public-access defibrillation and survival after out-of-hospital cardiac arrest. N Engl J Med. 2004;351(7):637–646.

8. Myerburg RJ, Velez M, Rosenberg DG, et al. Automatic external defibrillators for prevention of out-of-hospital

sudden death: Effectiveness of the automatic external defibrillator. J Cardiovasc Electrophysiol. 2003;14(Suppl): 108–116.

9. White RD, Asplin BR, Bugliosi TF, et al. High discharge survival rate after out-of-hospital ventricular fibrillation with rapid defibrillation by police and paramedics. Ann Emerg Med. 1996;28(5):480–485.

10. Valenzuela TD, Roe DJ, Nichol G, et al. Outcomes of rapid defibrillation by security officers after cardiac arrest in casinos. N Engl J Med. 2000;343(17): 1206–1209.

11. Valenzuela TD, Roe DJ, Cretin S, et al. Estimating effectiveness of cardiac arrest interventions: A logistic regression survival model. Circulation. 1997;96(10):3308–3313.

12. Larsen MP, Eisenberg MS, Cummins RO, et al. Predicting survival from out-of-hospital cardiac arrest: A graphic model. Ann Emerg Med. 1993;22(11): 1652–1658.

13. Engdahl J, Bang A, Lindqvist J, et al. Can we define patients with no and those with some chance of survival when found in asystole out of hospital? Am J Cardiol. 2000;86(6):610–614.

14. Gray WA, Capone RJ, Most AS. Unsuccessful emergency medical resuscitation—Are continued efforts in the emergency department justified? N Engl J Med. 1991;325(20):1393–1398.

15. Vickers C, Dogra V, Daya M, et al. Current burden of sudden cardiac death: Multiple source surveillance versus retrospective death certificate-based review in a large U.S. community. J Am Coll Cardiol. 2004;44:1268–1275.

16. Rea TD, Eisenberg MS, Sinibaldi G, et al. Incidence of EMS-treated out-of-hospital cardiac arrest in the United States. Resuscitation. 2004;63(1):17–24.

17. Zheng ZJ, Croft JB, Giles WH, et al. Sudden cardiac death in the United States, 1989 to 1998. Circulation. 2001;104:2158–2163.

18. Cobb LA, Fahrenbruch CE, Olsufka M, et al. Changing incidence of out-of-hospital ventricular fibrillation, 1980–2000. JAMA. 2002;288:3008–3013.

19. Basilico F. Current concepts: Cardiovascular disease in athletes. Am J Sports Med. 1999;27:108–121.

20. Maron BJ, Zipes DP. Introduction: Eligibility recommendations for competitive athletes with cardiovascular disease—General considerations. J Am Coll Cardiol. 2005;45:735–1097.

21. Futterman LG, Myerburg R. Sudden death in athletes: An update. Sports Med. 1998;26:335–350.

22. Maron BJ. Sudden death in young athletes. N Engl J Med. 2003;349(11):1064–1075.

23. Van Camp SP, Bloor CM, Mueller FO, et al. Nontraumatic sports death in high school and college athletes. Med Sci Sports Exerc. 1995;27(5):641–647.

24. Cantu RC. Congenital cardiovascular disease: The major cause of athletic death in high school and college. Med Sci Sports Exerc. 1992;24:279–280.

25. Maron BJ, Zipes DP. Introduction: Eligibility recommendations for competitive athletes with cardiovascular abnormalities-general considerations. J Am Coll Cardiol.2005;45:735–1097.

26. Maron BJ. Sudden death in young athletes. N Engl J Med. 2003;349(11):1064–1075.

27. Maron BJ, Gohman TE, Kyle SB, et al. Death in a young athlete due to commotio cordis. JAMA. 2002;287(9): 1142–1146.

28. Becker L, Eisenberg M, Fahrenbruch C, et al. Public locations of cardiac arrest: Implications for public access defibrillation. Circulation. 1998;97:2106–2109.

29. Frank RL, Rausch MA, Menegazzi JJ, et al. The locations of nonresidential out-of-hospital cardiac arrests in the City of Pittsburgh over a three-year period: Implications for automated external defibrillator placement. Prehosp Emerg Care. 2001;5:247–251.

30. Maron BJ, Thompson PD, Puffer JC, et al. Cardiovascular preparticipation screening of competitive athletes. A statement for health professionals from the Sudden Death Committee (clinical cardiology) and Congenital Cardiac Defects Committee (cardiovascular disease in the young), American Heart Association. Circulation. 1996;94(4):850–856.

31. American Academy of Family Physicians, American Academy of Pediatrics, American College of Sports Medicine, American Medical Society for Sports Medicine, American Orthopaedic Society for Sports Medicine, American Osteopathic Academy of Sports Medicine. Preparticipation physical evaluation, 3rd ed. New York: McGraw-Hill; 2005.

32. Fuller CM, McNulty CM, Spring DA, et al. Prospective screening of 5,615 high school athletes for risk of sudden cardiac death. Med Sci Sports Exerc. 1997;29: 1131–1138.

33. Mehrotra, Curry CL. Preparticipation echocardiographic screening for cardiovascular disease in a large, predominantly black population of collegiate athletes. Am J Cardiol. 1989;64:1029–1033.

34. Maron BJ, Bodison SA, Wesley YE, et al. Results of screening a large group of intercollegiate competitive athletes for cardiovascular disease. J Am Coll Cardiol. 1987;10:1214–1221.

35. Weidenbener EJ, Krauss MD, Waller BF, et al. Incorporation of screening echocardiography in the preparticipation exam. Clin J Sport Med. 1995;5:86–89.

36. Andersen J, Courson RW, Kleiner DM, et al. National Athletic Trainers' Association Position Statement: Emergency planning in athletics. J Athl Train. 2002; 37(1):99–104.

37. Kerber RE, Becker LB, Bourland JD, et al. Automatic external defibrillators for public access defibrillation: Recommendations for specifying and reporting arrhythmia analysis algorithm performance, incorporating new waveforms, and enhancing safety. A statement for health professionals from the American Heart Association Task Force on Automatic External Defibrillation, Subcommittee on AED Safety and Efficacy. Circulation. 1997;95(6):1677–1682.

38. 2005 American Heart Association Guidelines for Cardiopulmonary Resuscitation and Emergency Cardiovascular Care. Circulation. 2005;112 (24 Suppl):IV–203.

39. Drezner JA, Courson RW, Roberts WO, et al. Inter-Association Task Force Recommendations on Emergency Preparedness and Management of Sudden Cardiac Arrest in High School and College Athletic Programs: A Consensus Statement. J Athl Train. 2007;42(1):143–158.

40. Atkins DL, Kenney MA. Automated external defibrillators: Safety and efficacy in children and adolescents. Pediatr Clin N Am. 2004;51:1443–1462.

41. Samson RA, Berg RA, Bingham R, et al. Use of automated external defibrillators for children: An update: An advisory statement from the pediatric advanced life support task force, International Liaison Committee on Resuscitation. Circulation. 2003;107:3250–3255.

Suggested Readings and Websites

1. AHA Guidelines for CPR and ECC 2005: www.americanheart.org/presenter.jhtml?identifier=3035517

2. Inter-Association Task Force Recommendations on Emergency Preparedness and Management of Sudden Cardiac Arrest in High School and College Athletic Programs: A Consensus Statement: www.nata.org/jat/readers/archives/42.1/i1062-6050-41-4-143.pdf. NATA position statements: www.nata.org/statements.

3. Ornato JP, Peberdy MA, eds. Cardiopulmonary resuscitation. Totowa, NJ: Humana Press; 2005.

Nonprofit Organizations

1. American Red Cross: www.redcross.org
2. American Heart Association: www.americanheart.org
3. Cardiac Arrhythmias Research & Education (CARE) Foundation: www.longqt.org
4. Children's Cardiomyopathy Foundation: www.childrenscardiomyopathy.org
5. Heart Rhythm Foundation: www.heartrhythmfoundation.org
6. Hypertrophic Cardiomyopathy Association: www.4hcm.org
7. Mended Hearts: www.mendedhearts.org
8. Louis J. Acompora Memorial Foundation: www.la12.org
9. Matthew Krug Foundation: www.matthewkrugfoundation.org
10. Project Adam: www.chw.org/projectadam
11. Parent Heart Watch: www.parentheartwatch.org
12. Sudden Arrhythmia Death Syndrome (SADS) Foundation: www.sads.org
13. Sudden Cardiac Arrest Association: www.suddencardiacarrest.org

Appendix 4-1

The Visit to the Emergency Room: Tips for the Student Athletic Trainer

At some point, one of the athletes (or coaches or staff) from your team will require a visit to the local hospital Emergency Department (formerly called the "emergency room" but now more properly referred to as the "ED"). This section intends to provide you with a small glimpse of what to expect during your visit to the ED and some tips for facilitating your experience during the visit.

Brief Outline of What to Expect on Arrival

1. Check in by a clinical technician who will ask for the patient problem and age.

2. Brief assessment by the triage nurse, who will determine whether the patient needs immediate attention or can wait in the waiting room.

3. On placement in the treatment room, another nurse will do a more complete assessment and begin basic care based on protocols, such as clean and dress wounds, draw labs, and start an IV line.

4. Physician (perhaps a resident or medical student first if you are at a teaching hospital) will then do an evaluation (history and physical examination) and order tests such as X-rays and labs. Treatments such as pain control and stabilization will be initiated.

5. After test results are received, the physician will provide a report to the patient and discuss recommended treatments, including consultations. Treatments in the ED may include reduction of fractures and dislocations (often with procedural sedation) and other procedures.

6. After discussion with consultants and often the team physician, a decision will be made regarding whether the patient will require admission to the hospital or will be discharged. If the patient is discharged, thorough instructions about what the patient should do, including follow-up appointments and prescriptions, should be provided.

Tips to Enhance Your Interaction with the ED Staff

- First, realize that, although your athlete's injury or illness is the most important concern to you at the moment, there are likely many other patients in the ED who are just as or even more seriously ill. The staff may not be able to provide you with their full attention immediately.

- A prearrival call from the team physician or athletic trainer will help the ED physician understand the context of the illness or injury and provide important background information and preferred specialty consultants.

However, do not expect that the athlete will be ushered in and cared for ahead of others who have been waiting for care.

- If the athlete is transported by EMS, it is usually best to let the EMS and ED staff interact as per their usual routines and let them guide you. Listen to the EMS report; after they leave, you can provide the ED staff with any additional information or corrections you feel are pertinent.

- If the athlete is brought to the ED with any nondisposable supplies (splints, spine board, etc.) belonging to the team or school, it is probably best for you to take them with you once they are removed. If not removed while in the ED, ask the nurse how you might eventually retrieve them. Different EDs assign different personnel to this task.

- Remember the Health Insurance Portability and Accountability Act (HIPAA)—ED staff will not be able to provide you any information about the athlete's condition unless he or she gives explicit permission. Having athletes sign a form in advance may be helpful; keep in mind that you will need those forms with you.

- You will find yourself walking a fine line regarding discussions with medical and nursing personnel. You should speak intelligently but avoid coming off like you think you know more about the condition or injury (even if in some respects, such as mechanisms or long-term care, you might). You and the ED staff should speak professionally to each other, but realize you are a student and are on "their turf." Respect their right to direct care as they see fit.

- That being said, don't be afraid to bring up issues you don't think were adequately addressed. This might include a missed injury or symptom, some past history, or inadequate pain control. However, do not do this in a confrontational or condescending manner; rather, politely but firmly make your point.

- Make sure staff knows you can get in contact with the team physician if needed. This can often be very helpful and prevent delays.

- Don't be afraid to offer to help with splint application and similar procedures, but let the physician guide you as to what to do.

- If the athlete is discharged, make sure the ED staff provides clear and thorough instructions to the athlete and that the athlete clearly understands them. This should include limitations of activity, specific care measures, and who to see for and when to obtain follow-up care.

Make sure the athlete is provided with an adequate regimen for pain control and other symptoms.

- With permission of the athlete, you might want to provide a brief report to the ATC or team physician prior to leaving the ED to make sure they are comfortable with the plan and have no further questions for the ED physi-

cian. This is unnecessary if the ED physician spoke directly to the team physician.

- When leaving, consider a thank you or expression of appreciation to the staff who cared for your athlete. ED staff often work long hours at a hectic pace without much expressed gratitude.

Chapter 5

Head Injuries

Kevin M. Guskiewicz, PhD, ATC
Johna Register-Mihalik, MA, ATC

KEY TERMS

Anterograde
  amnesia
Balance error
  scoring system
Battle's sign
Cerebral concussion
Cerebral contusions
Cerebral hematomas
Cerebral infarction
Cognitive functions

Consciousness
Contrecoup injury
Coup injury
Diffuse brain injuries
Focal brain injuries
Lucid
Mental status
Morbidity rate
Mortality rate
Neuropsychological testing

Otorrhea
Postconcussion syndrome
Racoon eyes
Retrograde amnesia
Romberg test
Rhinorrhea
Second impact syndrome
Traumatic brain injury

 EMERGENCY SITUATION

A high school soccer goalkeeper attempts to make a save and is kicked in the head by an opposing player. The goalkeeper falls to the ground and does not get up. When the athletic trainer arrives on the field, the athlete is bleeding from a laceration on his forehead but is conscious. However, as the athletic trainer begins the evaluation, the athlete begins to become less **lucid.** The athlete is confused and soon loses **consciousness.** What actions should the athletic trainer take?

Cerebral concussion is an injury associated with virtually every sport and with a host of work and recreational activities. Whether on the sideline, athletic training room, or clinical/hospital environment, a thorough and consistent approach to evaluating athletes suspected of a concussion will aid in improving clinical diagnoses and return-to-play decisions. However, when a head injury is suspected, the nature and severity of the injury must first be determined in order to develop an appropriate management plan. An injury that at first appears to be a concussion could actually involve more serious pathology. The athletic trainer should be skilled in the early detection and diagnosis of these injuries and in follow-up evaluation procedures.

Pathomechanics of Brain Injuries

Cerebral concussion can be defined as any transient neurological dysfunction resulting from an applied force to the head.[1] A forceful blow to the resting movable head usually produces maximum brain injury beneath the point of cranial impact. This is known as a coup injury. A moving head hitting against an unyielding object usually produces maximum brain injury opposite the site of cranial impact (contrecoup injury) as the brain rebounds within the cranium. When the head is accelerated prior to impact, the brain lags toward the trailing surface, thus squeezing away the cerebrospinal fluid (CSF) and allowing for the shearing forces to be maximal at this site (Fig. 5-1). This brain lag actually thickens the layer of CSF under the point of impact, which explains the lack of coup injury in the moving head injury. However, when the head is stationary prior to impact, there is neither brain lag nor disproportionate distribution of CSF, accounting for the absence of contrecoup injury and the presence of coup injury. Many sport-related concussions involve a combined coup–contrecoup mechanism but are not considered to be necessarily more serious than an isolated coup or contrecoup injury.[2] If a skull fracture is present, the first two scenarios do not pertain because the bone itself may absorb much of the trauma energy or may directly injure the brain tissue. If the energy absorption is transient, a linear fracture may result; if the absorption is permanent, a depressed fracture may result (Table 5-1). Focal lesions are most common at the anterior tips and the inferior surfaces of the frontal and temporal lobes because the associated cranial bones have irregular surfaces.[3–7]

Three types of stresses can be generated by an applied force when considering injury to the brain: compressive, tensile, and shearing. *Compression* involves a crushing force whereby the tissue cannot absorb any additional force or load. *Tension* involves pulling or stretching of tissue, and *shearing* involves a force that moves across the parallel organization of the tissue (Fig. 5-2). Uniform compressive stresses are fairly well tolerated by neural tissue, but shearing stresses are very poorly tolerated.[5,6,8]

Types of Pathology

Several other terms are used to describe the injury, the most global being traumatic brain injury (TBI), which can be classified into two types: focal and diffuse. Focal brain injuries are posttraumatic intracranial mass lesions that may include subdural hematomas, epidural hematomas, cerebral contusions, and intracerebral hemorrhages and hematomas (Box 5-1). These are considered uncommon in sport but are serious injuries. The athletic trainer must be able to detect signs of clinical deterioration or worsening symptoms during serial assessments to classify the injury and manage it appropriately. Signs and symptoms of these focal vascular emergencies can include loss of consciousness, cranial-nerve deficits, mental-status deterioration, and worsening symptoms (Box 5-2). Concern for a significant focal injury should also be raised if the signs or symptoms arise after an initial lucid period in which the athlete seemed normal.

⭐ *STAT Point 5-1. Concern for a significant focal injury should also be raised if the signs or symptoms arise after an initial lucid period in which the athlete seemed normal.*

Diffuse brain injuries can result in widespread or global disruption of neurological function and are not usually associated with macroscopically visible brain lesions except in the most severe cases. Most diffuse injuries involve an acceleration–deceleration motion, either within a linear plane or in a rotational direction, or both. In these cases, lesions are caused by the brain essentially being shaken within the skull.[9,10] The brain is suspended within the skull in CSF and has several dural attachments to bony ridges that make up the inner contours of the skull. With a linear acceleration–deceleration mechanism (side to side or front to back), the brain experiences a sudden momentum change that can result in tissue damage. The key elements of injury mechanism are the velocity of the head before impact, the time over which the force is applied, and the magnitude of the force.[9,10] Rotational acceleration–deceleration injuries are believed to be the primary injury mechanism for the most severe diffuse brain injuries (Box 5-3).

Structural diffuse brain injury (diffuse axonal injury, or DAI) is the most severe type of diffuse injury because axonal disruption occurs, typically resulting in disturbance of cognitive functions, such as concentration and memory. In its most severe form, DAI can disrupt the brain stem centers responsible for breathing, heart rate, and wakefulness.[9,10]

Cerebral concussion, the most common sport-related TBI, can best be classified as a mild diffuse injury and is often referred to as mild traumatic brain injury (MTBI). The injury involves an acceleration–deceleration mechanism in which a blow to the head or the head striking an object results in one or more of the following conditions: headache, nausea, vomiting, dizziness, balance problems, feeling "slowed down," fatigue, trouble sleeping, drowsiness,

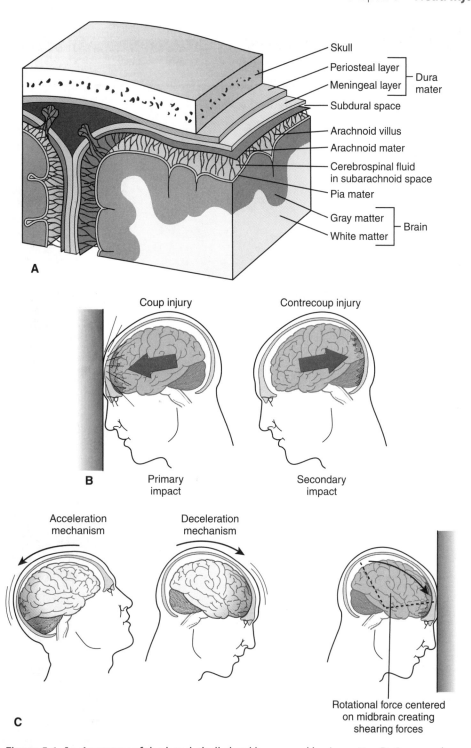

Figure 5-1. **A:** Anatomy of the head; skull, dural layers, and brain matter. **B:** Coup and contrecoup injury mechanism. **C:** Acceleration, deceleration, and rotational mechanisms of injury.

sensitivity to light or noise, loss of consciousness, blurred vision, difficulty remembering, or difficulty concentrating.[11,12] It is often reported that there is no universal agreement on the standard definition or nature of concussion; however, agreement does exist on several features that incorporate clinical, pathologic, and biomechanical injury constructs associated with head injury:

⭐ *STAT Point 5-2. There is no universal agreement on the standard definition or nature of concussion; however, agreement does exist on several features that incorporate clinical, pathological, and biomechanical injury constructs associated with head injury.*

Table 5-1   Types of Skull Fractures

Type	Description	
Depressed	Portion of the skull is indented toward the brain	Depressed fracture
Linear	Minimal indentation of skull toward the brain	Linear fracture
Nondepressed	Minimal indentation of skull toward the brain	
Comminuted	Multiple fracture fragments	Comminuted fracture
Basal/basilar	Involves base of skull	Basilar fracture

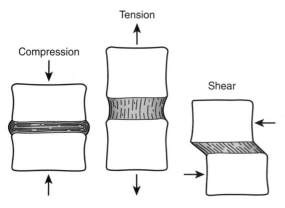

Figure 5-2. Illustration of tension, compression, and shearing forces on brain.

Box 5-1   Focal Brain Injuries

- Subdural hematomas
- Epidural hematomas
- Cerebral contusions
- Intracerebral hemorrhages
- Intracerebral hematomas

---

1. Concussion is caused by a direct blow to the head or elsewhere on the body, resulting in a sudden mechanical loading of the head that generates turbulent rotatory and other movements of the cerebral hemispheres.

2. These collisions or impacts between the cortex and bony walls of the skull typically cause an immediate and short-lived impairment of neurological function involving a variety of symptoms. In some cases the symptomatology is longer lasting and results in a condition known as **postconcussion syndrome**.

3. Concussion may cause neuropathological changes or temporary deformation of tissue; however, the acute clinical symptoms largely reflect a functional disturbance rather than a structural injury.

4. Concussion may cause a gradient of clinical syndromes that may or may not involve loss of consciousness (LOC). Resolution of the clinical and cognitive symptoms often follows a sequential course but is dependent on a number of factors including magnitude of the impact to the head and the individual's concussion history.

5. Concussion is most often associated with normal results on conventional neuroimaging studies, such as magnetic resonance imaging (MRI) or computed tomography (CT) scan.[3,4,9,13–16]

Box 5-2   Signs and Symptoms of Focal Vascular Emergencies

- Loss of consciousness
- Cranial-nerve deficits
- Mental-status deterioration
- Worsening symptoms

Box 5-3   Diffuse Brain Injuries

- Diffuse axonal injury (DAI)
- Mild traumatic brain injury (cerebral concussion)
- Mild
- Moderate
- Severe

✪ *STAT Point 5-3. Concussion is most often associated with normal results on conventional neuroimaging studies.*

Occasionally, players sustain a blow to the head, resulting in a stunned confusional state that resolves within minutes. The colloquial terms "got dinged" or "got his bell rung" are often used to describe this initial state. However, the use of this type of terminology is not recommended because this stunned confusional state is still considered a concussion resulting in symptoms, although only very short in duration, and should not be regarded in a casual manner.[16] It is essential that this injury be reevaluated frequently to determine if a more serious injury has occurred because often the evolving signs and symptoms of a concussion are not evident until several minutes to hours later.

✪ *STAT Point 5-4. The evolving signs and symptoms of a concussion are often not evident until several minutes to hours later. It is therefore imperative that the athlete be reassessed over time.*

Although it is important for the athletic trainer to recognize and eventually classify the concussive injury, it is equally important for the athlete to understand the signs and symptoms of a concussion and the potential negative consequences, such as **second-impact syndrome** or higher predisposition to future concussions, of not reporting a concussive injury. Once the athlete has a better understanding of the injury, he or she can provide a more accurate report of the concussion history.[16]

Classification of Cerebral Concussion

Several grading scales have been proposed for classifying and managing cerebral concussions.[11,17–25] None of the scales have been universally accepted or followed with any consistency by the sports medicine community. Although some of the scales are more conservative than others, they all are believed to be safe when used appropriately for managing concussion. Although most scales are based primarily on level of consciousness and amnesia, it is very important to consider other signs and symptoms associated with concussion because the majority of concussions will *not* involve loss of consciousness or observable amnesia. For example, it has been reported that only 8.9% involve loss of consciousness and only 27.7% involve amnesia.[26] Regardless of the grade of injury, clinicians should focus on the duration of any and all symptoms associated with the injury. Table 5-2 contains a list of signs and symptoms associated with cerebral concussion that can be checked off or graded for severity on an hourly or daily basis following an injury. The graded symptom checklist (GSC) is best used in conjunction with the Cantu Evidence-Based grading system for concussion[17] (Table 5-3), which very appropriately emphasizes signs and symptoms other than LOC and amnesia in the grading of the injury. It is also important to grade the concussion *after* the athlete's symptoms have resolved because the duration of symptoms are believed to be a good indicator of overall outcome.[12,16,17]

⭐ *STAT Point 5-5. The majority of concussions will not involve loss of consciousness or observable amnesia.*

Mild Concussion

The mild concussion, which is the most frequently occurring (approximately 85%), is the most difficult head injury to recognize and diagnose.[12,26,27] The force of impact causes a transient aberration in the electrophysiology of the brain substance, creating an alteration in **mental status.** Although mild concussion involves no loss of consciousness, the athlete may experience impaired cognitive function, especially in remembering recent events (posttraumatic amnesia) and in assimilating and interpreting new information.[17,27–29] Dizziness and tinnitus (ringing in the ears) may also occur, but there is rarely a gross loss of coordination that can be detected with a **Romberg test.** The clinician should never underestimate the presence of a headache, which presents to some degree in nearly all concussions.[26] The intensity and duration of the headache can be an indication of whether the injury is improving or worsening over time.

Moderate Concussion

The moderate concussion is often associated with transient mental confusion, tinnitus, moderate dizziness, unsteadiness. and prolonged posttraumatic amnesia (>30 minutes). A momentary loss of consciousness often results, lasting from several seconds up to 1 minute. Blurred vision, dizziness, balance disturbances, and nausea may also be present. Moderate concussions demand careful clinical observation and skillful judgment, especially regarding return to play at a later date.

Severe Concussion

It is not difficult to recognize a severe concussion because these injuries present with signs and symptoms lasting significantly longer than those of mild and moderate concussions. Additionally, the athlete will often experience more signs and symptoms than described for a mild or moderate concussion, and blurred vision, nausea, and tinnitus are more likely to be present. Most experts agree that a concussion resulting in prolonged loss of consciousness should be classified as a severe concussion. Some authors[16,20] classify *brief* loss of consciousness (including momentary blackout) as a severe concussion instead of the more widely accepted moderate classification. The severe concussion may also involve posttraumatic amnesia lasting longer than 24 hours and some **retrograde amnesia** (memory loss of events occurring prior to the injury). In addition, neuromuscular coordination is markedly compromised, with severe mental confusion, tinnitus, and dizziness. *Again, despite the emphasis often placed on LOC and amnesia, it is important to consider the duration of all signs and symptoms when classifying the injury.* Serial observations (repeated assessments) for signs and symptoms should be conducted in an attempt to identify progressive underlying brain damage.

Management of the three types of concussive injuries is not all that different—rest and serial evaluations are the standards of care. In the event of prolonged LOC (severe concussion), the athlete should be evaluated by a physician, with consideration given to neuroimaging of the brain. *No athlete should be returned to participation while still experiencing symptoms.* More specific assessment guidelines are presented in the management section of this chapter.

⭐ *STAT Point 5-6. No athlete should be returned to participation while still experiencing symptoms.*

Cerebral Contusion

The brain substance may suffer a cerebral contusion (bruising) when an object hits the skull or visa versa. The impact causes injured vessels to bleed internally, and there is a concomitant loss of consciousness. A cerebral contusion may be associated with partial paralysis or hemiplegia (paralysis of one side of the body), one-sided pupil dilation, or altered

Table 5-2   Graded Symptom Checklist for Concussion

Symptom	Time of Injury	2–3 Hours Postinjury	24 Hours Postinjury	48 Hours Postinjury	72 Hours Postinjury
Blurred vision					
Dizziness					
Drowsiness					
Excess sleep					
Easily distracted					
Fatigue					
Feel " in fog"					
Feel "slowed down"					
Headache					
Inappropriate emotions					
Irritability					
Loss of consciousness					
Loss of orientation					
Memory problems					
Nausea					
Nervousness					
Personality change					
Poor balance/coordination					
Poor concentration					
Ringing in ears					
Sadness					
Seeing stars					
Sensitivity to light					
Sensitivity to noise					
Sleep disturbance					
Vacant stare/glassy eyed					
Vomiting					

NOTE: A postconcussion signs and symptoms (PCSS) checklist is used not only for the initial evaluation but for each subsequent follow-up assessment, which is periodically repeated until all PCSS have returned to baseline or cleared at rest and during physical exertion.

Table 5-3   Cantu Evidence-Based Grading System for Concussion[6]

Grade 1 (Mild)	No LOC PTA <30 minutes, PCSS <24 hours
Grade 2 (Moderate)	LOC <1 minute **or** PTA ≥30 minutes <24 hours **or** PCSS ≥24 hours <7 days
Grade 3 (Severe)	LOC ≥1 minute **or** PTA ≥24 hours **or** PCSS ≥7 days

LOC, loss of consciousness; PTA, posttraumatic amnesia (anterograde/retrograde); PCSS, postconcussion signs/symptoms other than amnesia.

vital signs and may last for a prolonged period. Progressive swelling (edema) may further compromise brain tissue not injured in the original trauma. Even with severe contusions, however, eventual recovery without intercranial surgery is typical. The prognosis is often determined by the supportive care delivered from the moment of injury, including adequate ventilation and cardiopulmonary resuscitation if necessary.

Cerebral Hematoma

The skull fits the brain like a custom-made helmet, leaving little room for space-occupying lesions like blood clots. Blood clots, or **cerebral hematomas,** are of two types, epidural and subdural, depending on whether they are outside or inside the dura mater. Each of these can cause an increase in intracranial pressure and shifting of the cerebral hemispheres away from the hematoma. The development of the hematoma may lead to deteriorating neurological signs and symptoms typically related to the intracranial pressure.

Epidural Hematoma

An epidural hematoma in the athlete most commonly results from a severe blow to the head that typically produces a skull fracture in the temporoparietal region. These are usually isolated injuries involving acceleration–deceleration of the head, with the skull sustaining the major impact forces and absorbing the resultant kinetic energy. The epidural hematoma involves an accumulation of blood between the dura mater and the inner surface of the skull as a result of an arterial bleed—most often from the middle meningeal artery. The hemorrhage results in the classic CT scan appearance of a biconvex or lenticular shape of the hematoma (Fig. 5-3).[6] These are typically fast-developing hematomas leading to a deteriorating neurological status within 10 minutes to

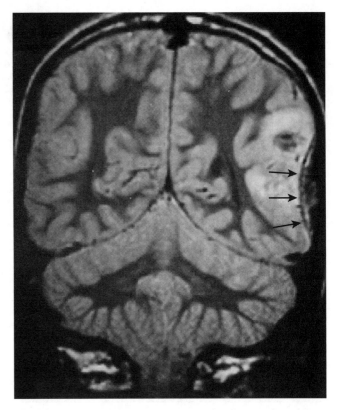

Figure 5-3. Epidural hematoma compressing the underlying brain tissue.

2 hours. The athlete may or may not lose consciousness during this time but will most likely have at least an altered state of consciousness. The athlete may subsequently appear asymptomatic and have a normal neurological examination; this is known as a lucid interval.[6]. The problem arises when the injury leads to a slow accumulation of blood in the epidural space, causing the athlete to appear asymptomatic (lucid) until the hematoma reaches a critically large size and begins to compress the underlying brain.[28] Immediate surgery may be required to decompress the hematoma and to control the hemorrhage. The clinical manifestations of epidural hematoma depend on the type and amount of energy transferred, the time course of the hematoma formation, and the presence of concurrent brain injuries. Often the size of the hematoma determines the clinical effects.[29,30]

Subdural Hematoma

The mechanism of the subdural hematoma is more complex. The force of a blow to the skull thrusts the brain against the point of impact. As a result, the subdural vessels stretch and tear, leading to the development of a hematoma in the subdural space. Bleeding into the subdural space is typically venous in origin; the resultant hematoma will therefore accumulate over a longer period of time compared to an epidural hematoma. This pathology has been divided into acute subdural hematoma, which presents in 48 to 72 hours after injury, and chronic subdural hematoma, which occurs in a later time frame with more variable clinical manifestations.[6] As bleeding produces low pressure with slow clot formation, symptoms may not become evident until hours or days (acute) or even weeks later (chronic), when the clot may absorb fluid and expand. The clinical presentation of an athlete with acute subdural hematoma can vary and includes those who are awake and alert with no focal neurological deficits, but typically individuals with any sizeable acute subdural hematoma have a significant neurological deficit. This may consist of alteration of consciousness, often to a state of coma or major focal neurological deficit.[6] Treatment for any athlete who has suffered loss of consciousness or altered mental status should include prolonged (several days) observation and monitoring because slow bleeding will cause subsequent deterioration of mental status. In such a case, surgical intervention may be necessary to evacuate (drain) the hematoma and decompress the brain.

Intracerebral Contusion and Hemorrhage

A cerebral contusion is a heterogenous zone of brain damage that consists of hemorrhage, **cerebral infarction**, necrosis, and edema. Cerebral contusion is a frequent sequela of head injury and is often considered the most common traumatic lesion of the brain visualized using imaging studies.[6,31] Typically, these are a result of an inward deformation of the skull at the impact site. Contusions can vary from small, localized areas of injury to large, extensive areas of involvement. Intracerebral hematomas are similar in pathophysiology and imaging appearance to a cerebral contusion. The intracerebral hematoma, which is a localized collection of blood within the brain tissue itself, is usually caused by a torn artery from a depressed skull fracture, penetrating wound, or large acceleration–deceleration force. These injuries are not usually associated with a lucid interval and are often rapidly progressive; however, there can be a delayed traumatic intracerebral hematoma. Intracerebral hematomas are the most common cause of sport-related lethal brain injuries, along with subdural hematoma.[6]

Second Impact Syndrome

A special condition involves that of **second impact syndrome (SIS)**. There has been much discussion and debate over the past two decades about SIS in sport.[5,8,11,23,25,32–34] SIS occurs when an athlete who has sustained an initial head trauma, most often a concussion, sustains a second injury before symptoms associated with the first have totally resolved. Often, the first injury was unreported or unrecognized. SIS usually occurs within 1 week of the initial injury and involves rapid brain swelling and herniation as a result of the brain losing autoregulation of its blood supply. Brain stem failure develops in 2 to 5 minutes, causing rapidly dilating pupils, loss of eye movement, respiratory failure, and eventually coma. On-field management of SIS should include rapid removal of any helmet or pads so the athlete can be rapidly intubated (*see Chapter 3 for more information on airway management and Chapter 6 for more information about equipment removal*). Unfortunately, the **mortality rate** of SIS is 50%, and the **morbidity rate** is 100%. Although the number of reported cases is relatively low, the potential for SIS to occur in athletes with mild head injuries should be a major consideration when making return-to-play decisions.[19]

Although the involved structures of these nonconcussive head injuries may vary depending on the impact acceleration–deceleration and the mechanism, the presentation of signs and symptoms and recommended care are standard (Table 5-4).

Immediate Management of Sport-Related Concussion

Recognition of a concussion is straightforward if the athlete has a loss of consciousness. Unfortunately, 90% to 95% of all cerebral concussions involve no loss of consciousness, only a transient loss of alertness or the presence of mental confusion. The athlete will likely appear dazed, dizzy, and disoriented. These injuries are more difficult to recognize and even more challenging to classify, given the numerous grading scales available and inability to quantify most of the signs and symptoms.

> ✪ *STAT Point 5-7. Of all cerebral concussions, 90% to 95% involve no loss of consciousness but rather only a transient loss of alertness or the presence of mental confusion.*

There are three primary objectives for the clinician dealing with an athlete with a head injury (Box 5-4):

1. Recognizing the injury and its severity
2. Determining if the athlete requires additional attention and/or assessment
3. Deciding when it is safe for the athlete to return to sports activity.

The first of these objectives can be met by performing a thorough initial evaluation. A well-prepared protocol is the key to the successful initial evaluation of an athlete who has suffered a head injury or any other type of trauma. During the secondary survey, a seven-step protocol (history, observation, palpation, special tests, active/passive range of motion, strength tests, and functional tests) should be strictly followed to ensure that nothing has been overlooked.

Initial On-Site Assessment

Your approach to the initial assessment may differ depending whether you are dealing with an *athlete-down* or *ambulatory* condition. *Athlete-down* conditions are signified by the athletic trainer and/or team physician responding to the athlete

Table 5-4   Traumatic Intracranial Lesions

Type	Mechanism	Injured Structures	Signs and Symptoms	Care/Other
Cerebral contusion	Object impacts skull	Injured vessels bleed internally	LOC, partial paralysis, hemiplegia, unilateral pupil dilation, altered vital signs	Adequate ventilation, CPR if necessary, proper transport, expert evaluation. May not require surgery
	Skull impacts object	Progressive swelling may injure brain tissue not originally harmed		
Cerebral hematoma				
Epidural	Severe blow to head; skull fracture	Middle meningeal artery	Neurological status deteriorates in 10 min–2 hr	Transport and expert evaluation Immediate surgery may be required
Subdural	Force of blow thrusts brain against point of impact	Subdural vessels tear and result in venous bleeding	Neurological status deteriorates in hours, days, or weeks	Prolonged observation/ monitoring. Surgical intervention may be required.
Intracerebral	Depressed skull fracture, penetrating wound, acceleration– deceleration injury	Torn artery bleeds within brain substance	Rapid deterioration of neurologic status	Immediate transport to ER; death may occur before athlete can be transported
Second impact syndrome (SIS)	Sustains second injury before symptoms from first injury resolve	Brain loses autoregulation of blood supply; rapidly swells and herniates	Typically occurs within 1 wk of first injury; pupils rapidly dilate, loss of eye movement, respiratory failure, eventual coma	Rapid intubation; 50% morbidity rate

---

Box 5-4   Objectives for Managing the Athlete with a Head Injury

1. Recognition of the injury and its severity

2. Determining if the athlete requires additional attention and/or assessment

3. Deciding when it is safe for the athlete to return to sports activity

---

on the field or court. *Ambulatory* conditions involve the athlete being seen by the clinician at some point following the injury. Head trauma in an athletic situation requires immediate assessment for appropriate emergency action, and, if at all possible, the athletic trainer or team physician should perform the initial evaluation of the athlete at the site of injury.

A *primary survey* involving basic life support should be performed first. This is easily performed and usually takes only 10 to 15 seconds as respiration and cardiac status are assessed to rule out a life-threatening condition (*see Chapter 2 for more information about the primary survey*).

Once life-threatening conditions have been ruled out, the *secondary survey* can begin.

The *secondary survey* specific to head injuries begins with the clinician performing a thorough history. The history is thought to be the most important step of the evaluation because it can narrow down the assessment very quickly. The clinician should attempt to gain as much information as possible about any mental confusion, loss of consciousness, and amnesia. Confusion can be determined quickly by noting facial expression (dazed, stunned, "glassy-eyed") and any inappropriate behavior such as running the wrong play or returning to the wrong huddle. Some physicians monitor level of consciousness through the use of a neural watch chart (Table 5-5).

If the athlete is unconscious or is regaining consciousness but is still disoriented and confused, the injury should be managed similar to that of a cervical spine injury because the clinician may not be able to rule out an associated cervical spine injury. (See Chapter 6 for more information about managing potential cervical spine injuries.) Therefore, the unconscious athlete should be transported from the field or court on a spine board with the head and neck immobilized. Vital signs should be monitored at regular intervals (1–2 minutes), as the clinician talks to the athlete in an attempt to help bring about full consciousness. If the athlete is in a state of lethargy or stupor or appears to be unconscious, do not attempt to arouse the individual by shaking. Shaking the athlete is contraindicated when a cervical spine injury is suspected. If loss of consciousness is brief, lasting less than 1 minute, and the remainder of the examination is normal, the athlete may be observed on the sideline and referred to a physician at a later time. Prolonged unconsciousness, lasting 1 minute or longer, requires immobilization and transfer to an emergency facility so the athlete can undergo a thorough neurological examination.

Table 5-5   Neural Watch Chart

Unit		Time
1. Vital signs	Blood pressure	_____
	Pulse	_____
	Respiration	_____
	Temperature	_____
	Pulse oximetry	_____
2. Conscious and...	Oriented	_____
	Disoriented	_____
	Restless	_____
	Combative	_____
3. Speech	Clear	_____
	Rambling	_____
	Garbled	_____
	None	_____
4. Will awaken to...	Name	_____
	Shaking	_____
	Light pain	_____
	Strong pain	_____
5. Nonverbal reaction	Appropriate	_____
	Inappropriate	_____
	"Decerebrate"	_____
	None	_____
6. Pupils	Size on right	_____
	Size on left	_____
	Reacts on right	_____
	Reacts on left	_____
7. Ability to move	Right arm	_____
	Left arm	_____
	Right leg	_____
	Left leg	_____

✪ *STAT Point 5-8. Prolonged unconsciousness, lasting 1 minute or longer, requires immobilization and transfer to an emergency facility so the athlete can undergo a thorough neurological examination.*

The clinician can perform amnesia testing by first asking the athlete simple questions directed toward recent memory and progressing to more involved questions. Asking the athlete for the first thing he or she remembered after the injury will test for length of posttraumatic amnesia, also known as **anterograde amnesia.** Asking what the play was before the injury or who the opponent was last week will test for retrograde amnesia. Retrograde amnesia is generally associated with a more serious head injury. Questions of orientation (name, date, time, and place) may be asked; however, research suggests that orientation questions are not good discriminators between injured and non-injured athletes.[35] Facing the athlete away from the field and asking the name of the team being played may be helpful. The athlete should also be asked if he or she is experiencing any tinnitus, blurred vision, or nausea. The clinician should use a concussion symptom checklist similar to that found in Table 5-2 to facilitate the follow-up assessment of signs and symptoms.

Portions of the *observation* and *palpation* plan should take place during the initial on-site evaluation. The clinician should observe for any deformities and abnormalities in facial expressions (indicating possible compromise of cranial nerve VII), speech patterns, respirations and movement of the extremities; all of this can be performed while asking the athlete questions. Additionally, gentle palpation of the skull and cervical spine should be performed to rule out an associated fracture. The athlete who is conscious or who was momentarily unconscious should be transported to the sidelines or locker room for further evaluation after the initial on-site evaluation. If the athlete is unconscious,

Table 5-6   On-Site Assessment

Primary Survey	Secondary Survey	
Rule out life-threatening condition Check respirations (breathing) Check cardiac status	History	Mental confusion Loss of consciousness Amnesia
	Observation	Monitor eyes Graded symptom checklist Deformities, abnormal facial expressions, speech patterns, respirations, extremity movement
	Palpation	Skull and cervical spine abnormalities Pulse and blood pressure (if deteriorating)

moving and positioning should be done carefully, assuming possible associated cervical injury. A helmet does not have to be removed at this time unless in some way it compromises maintenance of adequate ventilation. Often an adequate airway can be maintained just by removing the face mask or strap. Any unconscious player must be moved with care, avoiding motion of the neck by gentle, firm support, and transported on a spine board (*see Chapter 6 for more details*). Table 5-6 highlights the primary and secondary survey.

Sideline Assessment

A more detailed examination can be conducted on the sideline or in the athletic training room once the helmet has been removed. At this time, the clinician can proceed with the remainder of the observation and palpation. A quick cranial nerve assessment should first be conducted. Visual acuity (cranial nerve II: optic) can be checked by asking the athlete to read or identify selected objects (at near range and far range). Eye movement (cranial nerves III and IV: oculomotor and trochlear) should be checked for coordination and a purposeful appearance by asking the athlete to track a moving object (Table 5-7). The pupils also should be observed to determine if they are equal in size and equally reactive to light; the pupils should constrict when light is shined into the eyes. Observation of the pupils also assesses the oculomotor nerve. Abnormal movement of the eyes, changes in pupil size, or reaction to light often indicate increased intracranial pressure. The clinician should also look for any signs indicating a potential basilar skull fracture, including "**battle's sign**" (posterior auricular hematoma), **otorrhea** (CSF draining from the ear canal), **rhinorrhea** (CSF draining from the nose), and "**raccoon eyes**" (periorbital ecchymosis secondary to blood leaking from the anterior fossa of the skull). If the athlete's condition appears to be worsening, the pulse and blood pressure should be taken. The development of an

unusually slow heart rate or an increased pulse pressure (increased systolic and decreased diastolic) after the athlete has calmed down may be signs of increasing intracranial involvement. The overwhelming majority of cerebral concussions will not reveal positive results for these tests; however, they are important considerations for detecting a more serious injury such as an epidural or subdural hematoma. The clinician must be capable of identifying deteriorating conditions that would warrant immediate physician referral or transfer to the emergency department. A physician referral checklist is presented in Box 5-5.

Special Tests for the Assessment of Coordination

The inclusion of objective balance testing in the assessment of concussion is recommended. The **Balance Error Scoring System (BESS)** is recommended over the standard Romberg test, which for years has been used as a subjective tool for the assessment of balance. The BESS was developed to provide clinicians with a more objective test that is a rapid and cost-effective method of objectively assessing postural stability in athletes on the sports sideline or athletic training room after a concussion. Research has found the BESS to be a reliable and valid assessment tool for the management of sport-related concussion.[36–38] Three different stances (double, single, and tandem) are completed twice, once while on a firm surface and once while on a 10-cm–thick piece of medium density foam (Airex, Inc) for a total of six trials (Fig. 5-4). The total test time is approximately 6 minutes—the athlete is asked to assume the required stance by placing their hands on the iliac crests and on eye closure the 20-second test begins. During the single-leg stances, subjects are asked to maintain the contralateral limb in 20 to 30 degrees of hip flexion and 40 to 50 degrees of knee flexion. Additionally, the athlete is asked to stand quietly and as motionless as possible

Table 5-7 Cranial Nerves: Function and Assessment

Nerve	Name	Function	Assessment
I	Olfactory	Sense of smell	Identify odor
II	Optic		Check for blurred or double vision
III	Oculomotor	Control size of pupil, some eye motions	Check pupil reactivity; check upward and downward eye motion
IV	Trochlear	Some eye motions	Check lateral eye motion
V	Trigeminal	Jaw muscles	Check ability to keep mouth closed
VI	Abducens	Some eye motions	Check lateral and medial eye motion
VII	Facial	Some facial muscles	Check ability to squeeze eyes closed tightly or "big smile"
VIII	Vestibulocochlear	Hearing; balance	Check for loss of hearing on one side; balance testing
IX	Glossopharyngeal	Gag reflex	Check ability to swallow
X	Vagus	Controls voice muscles	Check ability to say "ahhh"
XI	Accessory	Innervate trapezius muscles	Check resisted shoulder shrug
XII	Hypoglossal	Motor function of tongue	Check ability to stick out tongue

in the stance position keeping his or her hands on the iliac crests and eyes closed. The single-limb stance tests are performed on the nondominant foot. This same foot is placed toward the rear on the tandem stances. Subjects are told that, on losing their balance, they are to make any necessary adjustments and return to the testing position as quickly as possible. Performance is scored by adding one error point for each error committed (Box 5-6). Trials are considered to be incomplete if the athlete is unable to sustain the stance position for longer than 5 seconds during the entire 20-second testing period. These trials are assigned a standard maximum error score of "10." Balance test results during injury recovery are best used when compared to baseline measurements, and clinicians working with athletes or patients on a regular basis should attempt to obtain baseline measurements when possible.

More sophisticated balance assessment using computerized forceplate systems and sensory organization testing (SOT) has identified balance deficits in athletes up to 3 days following a mild concussion.[36,39,40] These tests are recommended for making return-to-play decisions, especially when preseason baseline measurements are available for comparison.

The finger-to-nose test is also considered to be a good test for combining cognitive processing and balance. The clinician asks the athlete to stand with his or her eyes closed and arms out to the side. The athlete is then asked to touch the index finger of one hand to the nose and then to touch the index finger of the other hand to the nose. The athlete is then asked to open his or her eyes and touch the index finger of the evaluator (placed at varying ranges in the peripheral view) to test acuity and depth of perception. Inability to perform any of these tasks may be an indication of physical disorientation secondary to intracranial involvement.

Special Tests for Assessment of Cognition

The cognitive evaluation should begin by giving the athlete three unrelated words (e.g., pig, blue, hat) to remember; they will be asked to recall the words at the conclusion of the assessment. A brief mental status examination should be conducted using the Standardized Assessment of Concussion (SAC). The SAC is a brief screening instrument designed for the neurocognitive assessment of concussion by a medical professional who has no prior expertise in **neuropsychological testing**.[41,42] Studies have demonstrated the psychometric properties and clinical sensitivity of the SAC in assessing concussion and tracking postinjury recovery.[43–46] The SAC requires approximately 5 minutes to administer and assesses four domains of cognition, including orientation, immediate memory, concentration, and

Box 5-5   Physician Referral Checklist

DAY-OF-INJURY REFERRAL

1. Loss of consciousness on the field

2. Amnesia lasting longer than 15 minutes

3. Deterioration of neurological function*

4. Decreasing level of consciousness*

5. Decrease or irregularity in respirations*

6. Decrease or irregularity in pulse*

7. Increase in blood pressure

8. Unequal, dilated, or unreactive pupils*

9. Cranial-nerve deficits

10. Any signs or symptoms of associated injuries, spine or skull fracture, or bleeding*

11. Mental-status changes: lethargy, difficulty maintaining arousal, confusion, agitation*

12. Seizure activity*

13. Vomiting

14. Motor deficits subsequent to initial on-field assessment

15. Sensory deficits subsequent to initial on-field assessment

16. Balance deficits subsequent to initial on-field assessment

17. Cranial-nerve deficits subsequent to initial on-field assessment

18. Postconcussion symptoms that worsen

19. Additional postconcussion symptoms as compared with those on the field

20. Athlete is still symptomatic at the end of the game (especially at high school level)

DELAYED REFERRAL (AFTER THE DAY OF INJURY)

1. Any of the findings in the day-of-injury referral category

2. Postconcussion symptoms worsen or do not improve over time

3. Increase in the number of postconcussion symptoms reported

4. Postconcussion symptoms begin to interfere with the athlete's daily activities (e.g., sleep disturbances, cognitive difficulties)

*Requires the athlete be transported immediately to the nearest emergency department.

delayed recall. A composite total score of 30 possible points is summed to provide an overall index of cognitive impairment and injury severity. The SAC also contains a brief neurological screening and documentation of injury-related signs and symptoms (e.g., LOC, posttraumatic amnesia, retrograde amnesia).[16] Equivalent alternate forms of the SAC are available and should be used to minimize practice effects from serial testing after an injury. Significant differences have been shown between concussed athletes and nonconcussed controls and between preseason baselines and postinjury scores.[44,46] In lieu of using the SAC, the clinician can consider using a series of questions for concentration (Box 5-7) and recent memory (Box 5-8). The SAC is most helpful when baseline scores have been obtained prior to injury.

Computerized Neuropsychological Tests

A number of computerized neuropsychological testing programs have been designed for the assessment of athletes after concussion. The Automated Neuropsychological Assessment Metrics (ANAM), CogState, Concussion Resolution Index,

and Immediate Postconcussion Assessment and Cognitive Testing (ImPACT) are all currently available and have shown promise as reliable and valid concussion assessment tools (Table 5-8).[47–60] The primary advantages to computerized testing include the ability to assess reaction time, the ability to baseline test a large number of athletes in a short time, and the multiple forms used within the testing paradigm to reduce the practice effects.

However, computerized neuropsychological testing faces some of the same challenges that the traditional testing faces. Despite gaining increased popularity since the late 1990s, issues still exist surrounding the best follow-up assessment protocol, interpretation of results—especially regarding practice effects—, and the cost—especially for the high school setting. Once a decision has been made to institute a testing program, baseline measures should be captured during the athlete's preseason so that in the event of a concussive injury comparisons can be made between preinjury and postinjury measures. These comparisons are most useful in making return-to-play decisions if the athlete is assessed after the athlete has become asymptomatic.[16,61] Prior to instituting a neuropsychological testing program,

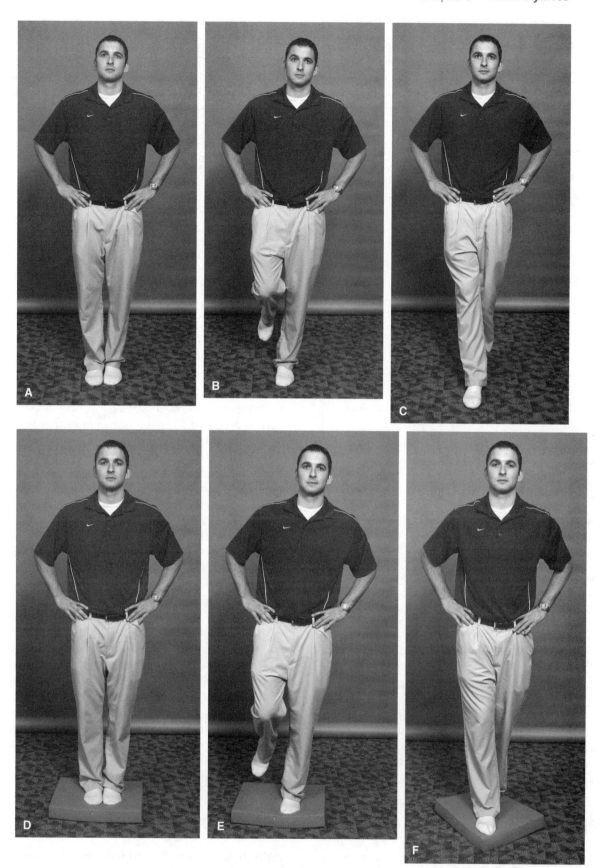

Figure 5-4. Six testing conditions for the Balance Error Scoring System (BESS). **A:** Double-leg stance on firm surface. **B:** Single-leg stance on firm surface. **C:** Tandem on firm surface. **D:** Double-leg stance on foam surface. **E:** Single-leg stance on foam surface. **F:** Tandem on foam surface.

Box 5-6 **Balance Error Scoring System (BESS)**

ERRORS

Hands lifted off iliac crests

Opening eyes

Step, stumble, or fall

Moving hip into more than 30 degrees of flexion or abduction

Lifting forefoot or heel

Remaining out of testing position for more than 5 seconds

The BESS score is calculated by adding one error point for each error or any combination of errors occurring during a movement.

Box 5-8 **Tests of Recent Memory**

Questions	Correct Response?
1. Where are we playing (name of field or site)?	
2. Which quarter (period, inning, etc.) is it?	
3. Who scored last?	
4. Who did we play last week?	
5. Who won last week?	
6. Recite the three words given at the start of the examination.	

Box 5-7 **Tests of Concentration**

Questions	Correct Response?
1. Recite the days of the week backward beginning with today.	
2. Recite the months of the year backward beginning with this month.	
3. Serial 3s—count backward from 100 by 3s until you get to single digits.	
4. Serial 7s—count backward from 100 by 7s until you get to single digits.	

clinicians should be trained in the administration of the tests and identify a licensed neuropsychologist in their community who will assist in clinical interpretation of postinjury test results.

Other Tests

If the athlete successfully completes the special tests and return to participation on the same day is anticipated, sensory (dermatome) testing and range of motion (ROM) testing should be performed followed by strength testing. These tests are performed to ensure that the athlete has normal sensory and motor function, which could have been compromised as a result of an associated brachial plexus injury. These tests can be performed in a systematic order, as described for upper and lower quarter screenings.

If the athlete has been asymptomatic for at least 20 minutes and has been cleared on all tests to this point, functional tests may be performed to assess the athlete's readiness to return to participation.[16] Functional testing should include exertional tests on the sideline such as situps, pushups, short sprints, and sport-specific tasks. The objective of these tests is to seek evidence of early postconcussive symptoms. Often these exercises will increase intracranial pressure in the athlete with a head injury and cause symptoms to reappear.

It is essential that the clinician document and record the initial findings and subsequent monitoring of any athlete with a head injury. Depending on the severity of the injury, return-to-participation decisions can be considered on the same day of the injury or could perhaps take days or even weeks. Regardless, a sound clinical evaluation combining the results from the Graded Symptom Checklist (GSC), BESS, and neuropsychological testing should be conducted prior to making the decision. A recommended assessment and return-to-participation protocol is presented in Figure 5-5. It is worth reinforcing that return-to-play decisions should include the team physician.

Medications

At this time, there are no evidence-based pharmacologic treatment options for an athlete with a concussion.[62] Most pharmacologic studies have been performed in patients with severe head injuries. It has been suggested that athletes with concussion avoid medications containing

Table 5-8   Computerized Neuropsychological Tests

Neuropsychological Test	Developer (Contact Information)	Cognitive Tests
Automated Neuropsychological Assessment Matrix (ANAM)	National Rehabilitation Hospital Assistive Technology and Neuroscience Center, Washington, DC (84) (jsb2@mhg.edu)	Simple Reaction Metrics, Sternberg Memory, Math Processing, Continuous Performance, Matching to Sample, Spatial Processing, Code Substitution
CogSport	CogState Ltd, Victoria, Australia (cogsport.com)	Simple Reaction Time, Complex Reaction Time, One-Back, Continuous Learning
Concussion Resolution Index	HeadMinder Inc, New York, NY (www.headminder.com)	Reaction Time, Cued Reaction Time, Visual Recognition 1, Visual Recognition 2, Animal Decoding, Symbol Scanning

aspirin or non-steroidal antiinflammatory drugs, which decrease platelet function and potentially increase intracranial bleeding, mask the severity and duration of symptoms, and possibly lead to a more severe injury. It is also recommended that acetaminophen (Tylenol, McNeil Consumer & Specialty Pharmaceuticals, Fort Washington, PA) be used sparingly in the treatment of headache-like symptoms in the athlete with a concussion because of its pain-relieving effect, which could mask the severity and duration of these symptoms. Other medications to avoid during the acute postconcussion period include those that adversely affect central nervous function—in particular, alcohol and narcotics.

Wake-Ups and Rest

Once it has been determined that a concussion has been sustained, a decision must be made as to whether the athlete can return home or should remain for overnight observation or admission to the hospital. For more severe injuries, the athlete should be evaluated by the team physician or emergency room physician if the team physician is not available. If the athlete is allowed to return home or to the dormitory room, the athletic trainer should counsel a friend, teammate, or parent to closely monitor the athlete. Traditionally, part of these instructions included a recommendation to wake up the athlete every 3 to 4 hours during the night to evaluate changes in symptoms and rule out the possibility of an intracranial bleed, such as a subdural hematoma. This recommendation has raised some debate about unnecessary wake-ups that disrupt the athlete's sleep pattern and may increase symptoms the next day from the combined effects of the injury and sleep deprivation. It is further suggested that the athlete with a

concussion have a teammate or friend stay during the night and that the athlete not be left alone. No documented evidence suggests what severity of injury requires this treatment. However, a good rule to use is if the athlete experienced LOC, had prolonged periods of amnesia, or is still experiencing significant symptoms, he or she should be awakened during the night.[16] Both oral and written instructions should be given to both the athlete and caregiver regarding waking.[16,63] The use of written and oral instructions increases the compliance to 55% for purposeful waking in the middle of the night. In the treatment of concussion, complete bed rest was ineffective in decreasing postconcussion signs and symptoms.[64] The athlete should avoid activities that may increase symptoms (e.g., staying up late studying, exertional activities) and should resume normal activities of daily living, such as attending class or driving, once symptoms begin to resolve or decrease in severity. As previously discussed, a graded test of exertion should be used to determine the athlete's ability to safely return to full activity.[16]

Return to Competition after Sport-Related Concussion

Over the past two decades a number of grading scales for severity of concussion and return to play have been proposed.[11,17,19–25] The lack of consensus among experts lies in the fact that few of the scales or guidelines are derived from conclusive scientific data; instead, they have been developed from anecdotal literature reports and clinical experience. The Cantu Evidence-Based Grading Scale presented earlier (Table 5-3) is currently recommended because it emphasizes all signs and symptoms, without placing undue emphasis on

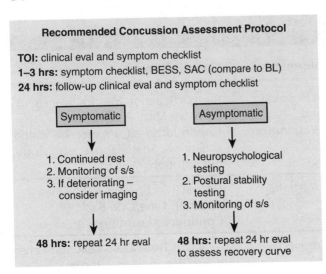

Recommended Concussion Assessment Protocol

TOI: clinical eval and symptom checklist
1–3 hrs: symptom checklist, BESS, SAC (compare to BL)
24 hrs: follow-up clinical eval and symptom checklist

Symptomatic	Asymptomatic
1. Continued rest 2. Monitoring of s/s 3. If deteriorating – consider imaging	1. Neuropsychological testing 2. Postural stability testing 3. Monitoring of s/s
48 hrs: repeat 24 hr eval	**48 hrs:** repeat 24 hr eval to assess recovery curve

TOI: Time of injury
BL: Baseline
s/s: signs and symptoms

Once Asymptomatic:

- Determine where athlete is relative to baseline scores (NP tests and PS tests)
- Require another 24 hrs. of rest, followed by a reassessment of symptoms, NP tests, and PS tests
- If 24 hrs. of asymptomatic rest and baseline or better on all tests

Conduct exertional tests to assess for increase in s/s

- If remain asymptomatic for 24 hrs. after exertional tests and baseline or better on all tests ⟶ Consider RTP

- If athlete becomes symptomatic within 24 hrs. after exertional testing or NP/PS decline ⟶ More rest required

- NOTE: This protocol is recommended for 1st time injuries; Repeat injuries may require more conservative management.

NP, Neuropsychologic; PS, Postural stability; RTP, Return to play

Figure 5-5. Recommended protocol for serial assessments and return to participation following concussion.

LOC and amnesia. This scale should be used to grade the injury only after the athlete is declared symptom-free because duration of symptoms is important in grading the injury. *No athlete should return to participation while still symptomatic.* Figure 5-5 offers a guide to making return-to-play decisions following concussion.

The question of return to competition after a head injury is handled on an individual basis, although a conservative approach seems the wisest course in all cases. The athlete whose confusion resolves promptly (within 20 minutes) and has no associated symptoms at rest or during or following functional testing may be considered a candidate to return to play. *Any loss of consciousness should eliminate a player from participation that day.* The following factors should also be considered when making decisions regarding an athlete's readiness to return following head injury:

- Athlete's previous history of concussion.
- The sport of participation (contact versus noncontact).
- Availability of experienced personnel to observe and monitor the athlete during recovery.
- Early follow-up to determine when a disqualified athlete can return to participation.

Repeated assessment should be the rule. The athletic trainer and team physician must be assured that the athlete is asymptomatic before a return to participation is permitted. This can be done through the use of neuropsychological testing and postural stability assessment.

Any athlete who has experienced loss of consciousness should not be permitted to return to play on that day. Any concussion that evolves downward should be sent for neurological evaluation and/or hospital admission. Athletes who are unconscious for a period of time or those who have headaches require evaluation and monitoring by a physician; refer again to Box 5-5.

Although the majority of people with head trauma recover without any permanent neurologic deficit or need for surgery, head trauma can be very serious and perhaps life-threatening. Several guidelines have been proposed for return to play following *multiple* head injury in the same season.[11,19,20] Most experts agree that athletes should be held from competition for extended periods (1–3 additional weeks) following a second concussion to ensure that all postconcussive symptoms have resolved and that participation in contact sports should be terminated for the season after three concussions.

Traumatic brain injury may be associated with practically every sport; therefore, it is important for clinicians to understand the evaluation, treatment, and management of various forms of sport-related brain injury. Although cerebral concussions or mild traumatic brain injuries are the most common, it is essential that other forms of brain injuries including cerebral contusions and hematomas be considered. Clinicians should be able to recognize and determine the severity of the injury for proper management to occur. Return-to-play and management decisions involving sport-related head injury can be ambiguous; however, these decisions should be made on a case-by-case basis and should be determined by the athlete's history, duration of signs and symptoms, time between injuries, and availability of experienced personnel to conduct repeated assessments and monitor recovery.

EMERGENCY ACTION

The athletic trainer should immediately activate the emergency action plan for the facility and continue to monitor the athlete until emergency medical services (EMS) arrives. The brain is possibly being compressed, which is evidenced by the deterioration in neurological function. The athletic trainer should continue to conduct a primary survey assessing respiration and cardiac status while being prepared to perform any necessary cardiopulmonary resuscitation/automatic external defibrillator techniques. The athletic trainer should control the bleeding and continue to monitor vital signs (including level of consciousness) until EMS arrives. Moving the athlete should not be attempted unless absolutely necessary because a cervical spine injury may be a possibility.

CHAPTER HIGHLIGHTS

- Cerebral concussion is an injury associated with virtually every sport and a host of work and recreational activities.

- Cerebral concussion can be defined as any transient neurological dysfunction resulting from an applied force to the head. Several other terms are used to describe the injury, the most global being traumatic brain injury (TBI), which can be classified into two types: focal and diffuse.

- Cerebral concussions are basic injuries to the brain itself and are classified by severity as mild, moderate, and severe. These injuries should be graded only after the athlete is asymptomatic.

- The majority of concussions will *not* involve loss of consciousness or observable amnesia.

- Cerebral hematomas are blood clots that form when the middle meningeal artery is damaged (epidural hematoma) or when subdural vessels tear, causing a clot to form several hours, days, or even weeks later (subdural hematoma).

- Decisions about when and if a concussed athlete can return to competition have to be made on an individual basis, depending on the athlete's concussion history, the severity of the injury, duration of signs and symptoms, time between injuries, and availability of experienced personnel to conduct repeated assessments and monitor recovery.

- It is important to combine tests of cognitive function, postural stability, and symptomatology to determine the athlete's status.

- The injury should be graded or classified only after the athlete has become asymptomatic, whether it is 5 minutes, 5 hours, 5 days, or 5 weeks following the injury.

Chapter Questions

1. Which of the following are key elements of injury mechanisms for cerebral concussion?

   A. Velocity of head before impact

   B. Time over which force is applied

   C. Magnitude of force

   D. None of the above

   E. All of the above

2. During the secondary survey, the clinician should attempt to gain as much information about all of the following except:

   A. Mental confusion

   B. Loss of consciousness

   C. History (including mechanism of injury)

   D. Amnesia

   E. All include information the clinician should obtain.

3. An epidural hematoma is:

   A. A venous bleed

   B. A subarachnoid bleed

   C. An arterial bleed

   D. An intracerebral bleed

   E. None of the above

4. Signs and symptoms of focal vascular emergencies include:

   A. Loss of consciousness and cranial nerve deficits

   B. Overall improvement in neurological function

   C. Mental status and worsening symptoms

   D. All of the above

   E. Both A and C

5. Second impact syndrome:

   A. Does not produce brain damage

   B. Produces minimal brain damage

   C. May produce brain stem failure

   D. None of the above

   E. All of the above

6. Two types of global brain injury include:

   A. Small and large

   B. Simple and complicated

   C. Focal and diffuse

   D. Uncomplicated and complex

   E. Mild and severe

7. If an athlete loses consciousness following a sport-related concussion:

   A. He or she should be allowed to return to play that day

   B. He or she should see the team physician

   C. He or she should be allowed to return whenever ready

   D. None of the above

   E. All of the above

8. Headache following a concussion:

   A. Is a minor detail

   B. Can be an indication of whether the injury is improving or worsening over time

   C. Should not be considered when making a return-to-play decision

   D. It not a common symptom

   E. None of the above

9. The three primary objectives for a clinician dealing with a head injured athlete are:

   A. Returning the athlete to play quickly, following a coach's guidelines, and grading the injury

   B. Returning the athlete to play quickly, determining if the athlete needs additional assessment, and following having the athlete participate in physical activity daily

   C. Recognizing the injury and its severity, determining whether the athlete requires additional attention or assessment, and deciding when the athlete may return to sport activity

   D. All of the above are correct

   E. None of the above are correct

10. Which of the following best represents an appropriate secondary survey:

    A. History, active/passive range of motion, strength test, and cognitive tests

    B. History, observation, range of motion, strength test, and cognitive test

    C. History, palpation, special test, strength test, functional tests, and range of motion

    D. History, observation, palpation, special test, active/passive range of motion, strength tests, and functional tests

    E. History, observation, palpation, special test, active/passive range of motion, and strength tests

■ *Case Study 1*

A 20-year-old female lacrosse player was hit in the side of the head with a lacrosse ball during a game. The athlete fell to the ground and did not get up. When the athletic trainer arrived on the field, the athlete was conscious but disoriented and complained of a headache and nausea. The athlete has no previous history of concussion or other head trauma. The athlete states she can get up, and the athletic trainer assists her off the field. On completion of the secondary survey the athlete is feeling a little better but still complains of a headache, nausea, and dizziness. The athlete is not allowed to return to play in that game and is instructed to report back to the athletic trainer the next day. The athletic trainer gives home care instructions and educates the parents. The next day, she is significantly worse. The athletic trainer refers the athlete to the team physician.

Case Study 1 Questions

1. Discuss the components the athletic trainer should have included in his or her sideline assessment (secondary survey).

2. What are the key elements the athletic trainer should have included in his or her home education/instructions to the athlete and her parents?

3. When the athlete returns the next day and is significantly worse, what is the athletic trainer most concerned about and why?

■ *Case Study 2*

A 14-year-old male football player is tackled from behind during a middle school football game. He does not get up at first, but approximately 15 seconds after the injury he gets up and walks to the sideline. He does not come over to the athletic trainer; however, the athletic trainer observed the play and walks over to evaluate the player. The player is obviously confused and is having difficulty balancing. The athletic trainer begins her assessment, and it is obvious that the athlete is concussed. After 20 minutes, the athlete is still confused and having trouble balancing. The athletic trainer informs the athlete he will not be returning to the game. The athlete gets upset and states: "It's just a ding. I don't understand why I can't play. My dad said when he played football there are games he doesn't even remember because he was hit so hard!"

Case Study 2 Questions

1. Why is it important the athlete not be returned to play while he is symptomatic?

2. Why is it important the athletic trainer pay attention throughout the game? Discuss the importance of the athletic trainer in this scenario being aware of the situation.

3. What could the athletic trainer do to help the players, parents, and coaches understand the significance of sport-related head injury? Discuss the actions the athletic trainer should take.

References

1. Giza C, Hovda D. The neurometabolic cascade of concussion. J Athl Train. 2001;36(3):228–235.

2. Barr W B, McCrea M. Sensitivity and specificity of standardized neurocognitive testing immediately following sports concussion. J Int Neuropsychol Soc. 2001;7(6):693–702.

3. Povlishock JT, Coburn TH. Morphological change associated with mild head injury. In Levin HS, Eisenberg HM, Benton Al, eds. Mild head injury. New York: Oxford University Press; 1989:37–53.

4. Povlishock JT. An overview of brain injury models. In Narayan RK, Wilberger JE, Povlishock JT, eds. Neurotrauma. New York: McGraw-Hill; 1995:1325–1336.

5. Cantu R. Reflections on head injuries in sport and the concussion controversy. Clin J Sports Med. 1997;7: 83–84.

6. Bailes JE, Hudson V. Classification of sport-related head trauma: A spectrum of mild to severe injury. J Athl Train. 2001;36(3):236–243.

7. Meaney DF, Smith DH, Shreiber DI, et al. Biomechanical analysis of experimental diffuse axonal injury. J Neurotrauma. 1995;12:689–694.

8. Cantu R. Athletic head injuries. Clin Sports Med. 1997;16(3):531–542.

9. Gennarelli T. Mechanisms of brain injury. J Emerg Med. 1993;11(suppl 1):5–11.

10. Schneider RC. Head and neck injuries in football: Mechanisms, treatment and prevention. Baltimore: Williams & Wilkins; 1973.

11. Practice parameter: The management of concussion in sports (summary statement). Report of the Quality Standards Subcommittee. Neurology. 1997;48:581–585.

12. Guskiewicz KM, McCrea M, Marshall SW, et al. Cumulative consequences of recurrent concussion in collegiate football players: The NCAA Concussion Study. JAMA. 2003;290:2549–2555.

13. Aubry M, Cantu R, Dvorak J, et al. Summary and agreement statement of the First International Conference on Concussion in Sport, Vienna 2001: Recommendations for the improvement of safety and health of athletes who may suffer concussive injuries. Br J Sports Med. 2002;36:6–10.

14. Shaw NA. The neurophysiology of concussion. Progress Neurobiol. 2002;67:281–344.

15. Foltz EL, Schmidt RP. The role of the reticular formation in the coma of head injury. J Neurosurg. 1956;13:145–154.

16. Guskiewicz KM, Bruce SL, Cantu RC, et al. National Athletic Trainers' Association Position Statement: Management of sport-related concussion. J Athl Train. 2004;39:280–297.

17. Cantu R. Posttraumatic retrograde and anterograde amnesia: Pathophysiology and implications in grading and safe return to play. J Athl Train. 2001;36(3): 244–248.

18. Ommaya A. Biomechanical aspects of head injuries in sports. In Jordan B, Tsairis P, Warren R, eds. Sports Neurology. Rockville, MD: Aspen Publishers, Inc.; 1990.

19. Cantu R. Guidelines for return to contact sports after a cerebral concussion. Physician Sportsmed. 1986;14:75–83.

20. Colorado Medical Society. Report of the Sports Medicine Committee: Guidelines for the Management of Concussion in Sports (revised). Paper Presented at the Colorado Medical Society, Denver; 1991.

21. Jordan B. Head injuries in sports. In Jordan B, Tsairis P, Warren R, eds. Sports Neurology. Rockville, MD: Aspen Publishers, Inc.; 1989.

22. Nelson W, Jane J, Gieck J. Minor head injuries in sports: A new system of classification and management. Physician Sportsmed. 1984;12:103–107.

23. Roberts W. Who plays? Who sits? Managing concussion on the sidelines. Physician Sportsmed. 1992;20(6): 66–72.

24. Torg J, ed. Athletic injuries to the head, neck and face. St. Louis: Mosby-Year Book; 1991.

25. Wilberger JJ, Maroon J. Head injuries in athletes. Clin Sports Med. 1989;8(1):1–9.

26. Guskiewicz KM, Weaver N, Padua DA, et al. Epidemiology of Concussion in Collegiate and High School Football Players. Am J Sports Med. 2000;28(5): 643–650.

27. Lovell M, Maroon JC. Does loss of consciousness predict neuropsychological decrements of concussion. Clin J Sports Med. 1999;9:193–198.

28. Jamieson KG, Yelland JDN. Extradural hematoma: Report of 167 cases. J Neurosurg Neurosurg. 1968;29: 13–23.

29. Bricolo A, Pasut LM. Extradural hematoma: Toward zero mortality, a prospective study. Neurosurg. 1984;14:8–12.

30. Servadei F. Prognostic factors in severely head injured adult patients with epidural hematomas. Acta Neurochir (Wien). 1997;139:273–278.

31. Schonauer M, Schisano G, Cimino R, et al. Space occupying contusions of cerebral lobes after closed head brain injury: Considerations about 51 cases. J Neurosurg Sci. 1979;23:279–288.

32. Mueller FO. Catastrophic head injuries in high school and collegiate sports. J Athl Train. 2001;36(3):312–315.

33. Kelly J, Nichols J, Filley C, et al. Concussion in sports: Guidelines for the prevention of catastrophic outcome. JAMA. 1991;226:2867–2869.

34. Saunders R, Harbaugh R. The second impact in catastrophic contact-sports head injuries. JAMA. 1984;252:538–539.

35. Maddocks D, Saling M. Neuropsychologial sequelae following concussion in Australian rules footballers. 1991; J Clin Exp Neuropsychol. 1991;13:439–442.

36. Guskiewicz KM, Ross SE, Marshall SW. Postural stability and neuropsychological deficits after concussion in collegiate athletes. J Athl Train. 2001;36(3):263–273.

37. Riemann BL, Guskiewicz KM, Shields EW. Relationship between clinical and forceplate measures of postural stability. J Sport Rehabil. 1998;8(2):71–82.

38. Riemann BL, Guskiewicz KM. Objective assessment of mild head injury using a clinical battery of postural stability tests. J Athl Train. 2000;35(1):19–25.

39. Guskiewicz K, Perrin D, Gansneder B. Effect of mild head injury on postural sway. J Athl Train. 1996;31(4): 300–306.

40. Guskiewicz K, Riemann V, Perrin D, et al. Alternative approaches to the assessment of mild head injuries in athletes. Med Sci Sports Exerc. 1997;29(7): S213–S221.

41. McCrea M, Kelly JP, Randolph C, et al. Standardized assessment of concussion (SAC): On-site mental status evaluation of the athlete. J Head Trauma Rehabil. 1998;13:27–35.

42. McCrea M, Randolph C, Kelly JP. The Standardized Assessment of Concussion (SAC): Manual for Administration, Scoring and Interpretation, 2nd ed. Waukesha, WI: CNS, Inc.; 2000.

43. McCrea M. Standardized mental status assessment of sports concussion. Clin J Sport Med. 2001;11:176–181.

44. McCrea M. Standardized mental status testing on the sideline after sport-related concussion. J Athl Train. 2001;36(3):274–279.

45. McCrea M, Kelly JP, Randolph C, et al. Immediate neurocognitive effects of concussion. Neurosurgery. 2002;50:1032–1042.

46. McCrea M, Kelly JP, Kluge J, et al. Standardized assessment of concussion in football players. Neurology. 1997;48:586–588.

47. Bleiberg J, Halpern E, Reeves D, et al. Future directions for neuropsychological assessment of sports concussion. J Head Trauma Rehabil. 1998;13:36–44.

48. Erlanger D, Saliba E, Barth J, et al. Monitoring resolution of postconcussion symptoms in athletes: Preliminary results of a web-based neuropsychological test protocol. J Athl Train. 2001;36(3):280–287.

49. Lovell MR, Collins MW, Iverson GL, et al. Recovery from mild concussion in high school athletes. J Neurosurg. 2003;98:296–301.

50. Bleiberg J, Garmoe W, Halpern E, et al. Consistency of within-day and across-day performance after mild brain injury. Neuropsychiatr Neuropsychol Behav Neurol. 1997;10:247–253.

51. Erlanger DM, Kutner KC, Barth JT, et al. Development and validation of a web-based protocol for management of sports-related concussion. [Abstract] Arch Clin Neuropsychol. 2000;15:675.

52. Erlanger D, Kaushik T, Cantu R, et al. Symptom-based assessment of the severity of a concussion. J Neurosurg. 2003;98:477–484.

53. Bleiberg J, Cernich AN, Cameron K, et al. Duration of cognitive impairment after sports concussion. Neurosurgery. 2004;54(5):1073–1080.

54. Collie A, Darby D, Maruff P. Computerised cognitive assessment of athletes with sports related head injury. Br J Sports Med. 2001;35:297–302.

55. Collie A, Maruff P, Makdissi M, et al. CogSport: Reliability and correlation with conventional cognitive tests used in postconcussion medical evaluations. Clin J Sport Med. 2003;13:28–32.

56. Makdissi M, Collie A, Maruff P, et al. Computerised cognitive assessment of concussed Australian Rules footballers. Br J Sports Med. 2001;35:354–360.

57. Bleiberg J, Kane RL, Reeves DL, et al. Factor analysis of computerized and traditional tests used in mild brain injury research. Clin Neuropsychol. 2000;14:287–294.

58. Collie A, Maruff P, Darby DG, et al. The effects of practice on the cognitive test performance of neurologically normal individuals assessed at brief test-retest intervals. J Int Neuropsychol Soc. 2003;9:419–428.

59. Daniel JC, Olesniewicz MH, Reeves DL, et al. Repeated measures of cognitive processing efficiency in adolescent athletes: Implications for monitoring recovery from concussion. Neuropsychiatry Neuropsychol Behav Neurol. 1999;12:167–169.

60. Reeves D, Thorne R, Winter S, et al. Cognitive Performance Assessment Battery (UTC-PAB). Report 89-1. San Diego: Naval Aerospace Medical Research Laboratory and Walter Reed Army Institute of Research; 1989.

61. McCrea M, Barr WB, Guskiewicz KM, et al. Standard regression-based methods for measuring recovery after sport-related concussion. J Int Neuropsychol Soc. 2005;11;58–69.

62. McCrory P. New treatments for concussion: The next millennium beckons. Clin J Sport Med. 2001;11:190–193.

63. de Louw A, Twijnstra A, Leffers P. Lack of uniformity and low compliance concerning wake-up advice following head trauma. Ned Tijdschr Geneeskd. 1994;138:2197–2199.

64. de Kruijk JR, Leffers P, Meerhoff S, et al. Effectiveness of bed rest after mild traumatic brain injury: A randomised trial of no versus six days of bed rest. J Neurol Neurosurg Psychiatr. 2002;73(2):167–172.

Suggested Readings

1. Aubry M, Cantu R, Dvorak J, et al. Summary and agreement statement of the First International Conference on Concussion in Sport, Vienna 2001: Recommendations for the improvement of safety and health of athletes who may suffer concussive injuries. Br J Sports Med. 2002;36:6–10.

2. Kelly JP. Loss of consciousness: Pathophysiology and implications in grading and safe return to play. J Athl Train. Sep 2001;36(3):249–252.

3. Cantu RC. Posttraumatic retrograde and anterograde amnesia: Pathophysiology and implications in grading and safe return to play. J Athl Train. Sep 2001;36(3): 244–248.

4. Guskiewicz KM, Bruce SL, Cantu RC, et al. National Athletic Trainers' Association Position Statement: Management of sport-related concussion. J Athl Train. Sep 2004;39(3):280–297.

5. National Athletic Trainers' Association: www.nata.org

Chapter 6

Emergency Care of Cervical Spine Injuries

Robert O. Blanc, MS, ATC, EMT-P

KEY TERMS

Apneic

Axial load

Blood–brain barrier

Dislocation

Fluid challenge

Ischemia

Lateral flexion

Manual stabilization

Motor function

Neuropraxia

Paraplegia

Priapism

Quadriplegia

Sagittal plane

Sensory function

Subluxation

Transect

Vasoconstriction

Vasodilation

Vasopressor

 EMERGENCY SITUATION

You are the staff athletic trainer covering a wrestling match. Your team's wrestler is picked up and thrown to the mat by his opponent, and he lands on the top of his head. The opponent falls on top of the athlete but immediately jumps up and waves for assistance. As you approach the mat you note that the downed wrestler has not moved and is lying prone with his head turned to the left. He is unconscious and does not respond to your calls or to your touch. He is breathing at a rate of 20 breaths per minute and has a pulse rate of 100 beats per minute. There is no obvious bleeding. What should you do next?

Injuries to the spinal cord can be devastating, often because they are fatal or result in significant lifelong disabilities. Each year approximately 15,000 injuries cause permanent spinal cord injury, approximately 14% of which are related to sports activities. The overwhelming majority of spinal cord injuries in sports occur in collision sports such as football and ice hockey or in high-risk sports such as gymnastics. Because of the debilitating nature of most spinal cord injuries the cost of long-term care is extremely high. This monetary cost does not take into account the emotional toll on the injured individual and his or her family and friends. Injuries to the spinal cord of athletes have been reduced in recent decades by placing greater emphasis on the prevention of such injuries by education with regard to rules changes (e.g., spearing in football, hitting from behind in ice hockey), improvements in protective equipment, and the teaching of proper and safe sport-specific techniques (e.g., tackling with the head up in football).

Anatomy

The anatomy of the cervical spine is complex, designed to allow large ranges of motion in all planes while still affording protection for the spinal cord. The *spinal column* in the cervical spine consists of the seven vertebrae and their respective intervertebral discs (Fig. 6-1). It functions in part to provide a framework for the axial skeletal system and to protect the spinal cord, which is housed within the column. The anatomy of the cervical spine pertinent to this chapter also includes a ligamentous system providing stability; a complex muscular system for movement; and nerve roots coming from the spinal cord to provide innervation of the head, neck, shoulders, and arms. All of these anatomical structures are tightly packed into a small area. Because of this, damage to one structure is likely to have an effect on nearby structures. For example, if a vertebra is fractured, the potentially sharp fragments will be very close to or even in contact with the spinal cord, presenting opportunity for a possible catastrophic injury.

Mechanisms of Injury

Normal functioning of the anatomy of the cervical spine allows for flexion, extension, rotation, and lateral flexion (Fig. 6-2). Athletes who are subjected to extremes of these motions or to axial forces of either loading or distraction are at high risk of experiencing permanent neurological deficit, paralysis, or death. Injury may also be caused by direct or penetrating trauma or may occur indirectly as a result of swelling compressing the spinal cord and disrupting its blood supply.

Hyperextension (abnormal outward extension as if the individual is looking toward the sky) and hyperflexion (increased flexion as if the individual's chin is tucked to the chest) cause the cervical spine to bend in the **sagittal plane.** In these movements the ligaments, muscles, and bony anatomy are all at risk for injury. If hyperextension is the mechanism for injury, the posterior vertebral structures are compressed and the anterior soft tissues (i.e., the anterior vertebral ligaments) will be stretched. Disruption of the disc, along with compression of the interspinous ligaments and/or fracture of the posterior vertebrae, is possible. Instability of the cervical spine may be present if there is injury to the ligaments and/or fracture of the vertebrae.

Hyperflexion may cause fractures to the anterior body of the vertebrae, stretching or rupture of the posterior longitudinal and interspinous ligaments, compression of the spinal cord, and disruption of the disc. As in hyperextension, instability is always a concern.

Rotational injuries are much less common. Injuries incurred with rotational forces most often manifest themselves in the upper cervical spine or the lumbar spine. This mechanism may cause stretching or tearing of ligaments, **subluxation** or **dislocation,** and/or fracture.

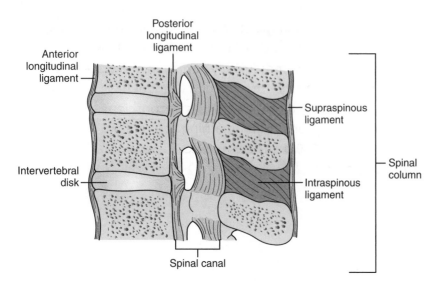

Figure 6-1. Spinal column: vertebrae, spinal canal, intervertebral disks; anterior longitudinal ligament, posterior longitudinal ligament, supraspinous ligament.

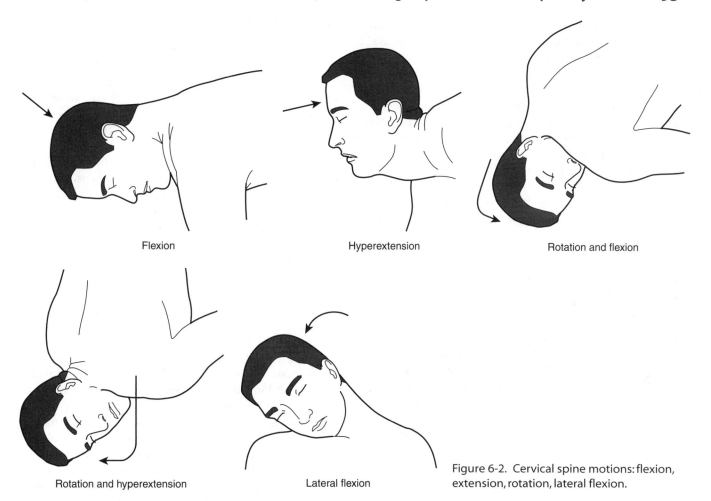

Flexion

Hyperextension

Rotation and flexion

Rotation and hyperextension

Lateral flexion

Figure 6-2. Cervical spine motions: flexion, extension, rotation, lateral flexion.

Lateral flexion occurs when a force is applied to the side of the head, forcing the ear toward the shoulder. Injuries from this mechanism would cause compression fractures of the vertebrae on one side and stretching or tearing of the ligaments and muscle tissue on the opposite side. This may also lead to instability of the spine. The amount of force necessary to cause injury with lateral flexion is generally less than that needed with extension or flexion injuries.

An **axial load** is one in which a force is applied through the length of the spine, as is the case when an athlete is struck on the top of the head with the body fixed (Fig. 6-3). The

forces are generated along the long axis of the spine, most often causing compression fractures of the vertebrae, herniation of the disc, and compression of the spinal cord.

Distraction of the cervical spine is the opposite of loading and is much less likely in the athletic setting. This mechanism is most commonly seen in hangings and causes stretching of the soft tissues including the spinal cord.

Combinations of any or all of these mechanisms of injury are likely and compound the severity of the injury. Understanding and identifying the actual mechanism may be helpful in evaluating and caring for the injured athlete.

Injuries to the Spinal Cord

The spinal column is vulnerable to many types of injuries, which in turn may lead to injury to the spinal cord. Damage to the soft tissues (i.e., ligaments, muscles, or tendons) may adversely affect the stability of the vertebral column, allowing either a dislocation or subluxation of one or more vertebrae to occur, thus causing damage to the spinal cord. Fractures to any of the bony structures may also cause instability, as described earlier; in addition, sharp bone fragments could lacerate or completely **transect** the spinal cord, resulting in permanent neurological deficit or even death.

Axial load

Figure 6-3. Axial load through the cervical spine.

Injuries to the spinal cord can occur from a variety of mechanisms and may be categorized as either primary or secondary. Primary injuries are those that occur as a direct result of a traumatic event for which the effects are immediate (e.g., a compression, stretching, or transection of the spinal cord). This will have an immediate impact on the functioning of the nervous system distal to the site of the injury. Some primary injuries, such as a **neuropraxia,** are temporary in nature (Box 6-1). Others, such as a partial or total transection, are permanent. *Concussion* of the spinal cord is a condition that, much like a cerebral concussion, results in immediate but temporary disruption of the spinal cord function. The spinal cord usually returns to normal function with no lasting adverse effects.

✪ *STAT Point 6-1. Injuries to the spinal cord can be categorized as either primary or secondary.*

A secondary injury is one in which the effect of the initial injury is not immediately apparent. Typically, secondary injuries occur after swelling and **ischemia** have developed as a result of the trauma (Box 6-2). The spinal cord can be *contused,* in which there is bruising of the tissue of the spinal cord. The damage is usually minimal and mostly from the effects of swelling or bleeding. A spinal cord contusion usually produces symptoms that last longer than those of a spinal cord concussion but typically does not result in long-term deficits.

✪ *STAT Point 6-2. Secondary injuries to the spinal cord occur after swelling and ischemia have developed as a result of trauma.*

Spinal cord compression is a secondary injury that can result from any number of injuries including fractures of the vertebrae, herniation of the intervertebral disc, or swelling from soft-tissue damage. The edema around the spinal cord places pressure on the spinal cord itself, causing ischemia as a result of limited circulation. The ischemia results in impaired function of the spinal cord. If the compressive force is large enough, it can cause physical damage to the spinal cord beyond that of the ischemia itself.

Spinal cord hemorrhage may be seen any time the spinal cord is injured. The hemorrhaging may cause increased pressure on the spinal cord, disruption of the blood flow to the spinal cord, or irritation by blood crossing the **blood–brain barrier.** The amount of hemorrhaging and the length of time

---

Box 6-1   Neuropraxia

Commonly known as "stingers" or "burners," this injury typically involves either a stretching or a compression of one or more nerves of the brachial plexus as a result of a combination of cervical and shoulder girdle motions. The force imparted to the nerve creates a temporary disruption of nerve function. Signs and symptoms include the following:

- Immediate onset of burning pain, numbness, or tingling in the supraclavicular region that typically extends down into the arm, sometimes as far as the hand.

- Some degree of motor function disruption in the shoulder and arm, manifesting along a continuum from mild weakness to complete loss of function.

- Cervical range of motion is typically pain free and full.

Two main characteristics of a stinger distinguish it from a more serious injury to the spinal cord:

1. Signs and symptoms of a stinger are unilateral and only in the upper extremity. Bilateral signs and symptoms, or signs and symptoms that are felt in the upper *and* lower extremity on the same side, are *not* consistent with a stinger and should be regarded as very serious.

2. Signs are symptoms are transient, usually lasting only a few seconds to a few minutes. Signs and symptoms that persist longer than several minutes should be regarded as more serious.

Box 6-2   Primary and Secondary Injuries to the Spinal Cord

PRIMARY INJURIES

Immediate effect on function as a result of:

- Compression
- Stretching
- Laceration
- Concussion of the spinal cord

SECONDARY INJURIES

Delayed effect on function, usually as a result of progressive or ongoing ischemia.

- Spinal cord contusion
- Spinal cord compression
- Spinal cord hemorrhage

that pressure is placed on the spinal cord will determine the significance of the damage and the potential for recovery.

Transection

Transection of the spinal cord occurs when the spinal cord is either completely or partially severed. A complete transection is one in which the spinal cord is totally cut and the ability to send and receive nerve impulses is therefore entirely lost. If the transection is incomplete, some fibers of the spinal cord remain intact, which may allow for some function. The amount of disability suffered by the victim is determined by the level of the transection on the spinal cord. Nerve roots exiting the spinal cord below the level of the transection will no longer provide for function in the areas they innervate. For example, injury below the T1 level will result in incontinence and **paraplegia** and injuries in the cervical region will result in **quadriplegia,** incontinence, and possible respiratory paralysis.

Partial transections may be described in three types: anterior cord syndrome, central cord syndrome, or Brown-Sequard's syndrome. Anterior cord syndrome is caused by a disruption of the blood supply to the spinal cord as a result of compromise of the arterial supply. This is usually secondary to bone fragments or a compressive force preventing the supply of blood to the spinal cord. The prognosis in these cases is poor. Athletes suffering anterior cord syndrome will present with a loss of pain sensation and motor function, loss of light touch sensation, and loss of temperature control distal to the level of the injury.

Central cord syndrome is most commonly seen as the result of a hyperextension injury. It is often associated with a preexisting condition of arthritis or a narrowing of the vertebral canal. The results are motor weakness of the upper extremities rather than the lower extremities and, possibly, loss of bladder control. Of the three syndromes associated with incomplete transections of the spinal cord, central cord syndrome has the best potential for recovery.

Brown-Sequard's syndrome is caused by a penetrating injury that severs one side of the spinal cord. The athlete will present with loss of sensory and motor function on the affected side and loss of pain and temperature perception on the opposite side. Unless the penetration is direct, some recovery may be expected.

Spinal shock may be present when there is trauma to the spinal cord. Spinal shock is a temporary condition triggered as the body's response to injury. It is identified when the body becomes flaccid and without sensation, causing the athlete to be unable to move and appear to be paralyzed below the level of the injury. It may be accompanied by loss of bladder and bowel control and, in males, **priapism.** It is common for hypotension to be present as a result of **vasodilation** (also known as *vasodilatation*). Spinal shock is a transient condition unless the spinal cord has been seriously damaged.

Neurogenic shock occurs when the brain loses its ability to maintain control over the rest of the body as a result of damage to the spinal cord. When the brain loses the ability to control the sympathetic nervous system, it also loses control of the vascular system. **Vasoconstriction** is limited, causing changes in the skin color and temperature below the level of the injury. The lack of sympathetic tone allows the arteries and veins to dilate, which expands the vascular space and in effect causes hypotension. This will not allow the atria to fill adequately, which in turn reduces cardiac output because the ventricle does not fill completely. In a healthy individual this would cause a sympathetic response by the autonomic nervous system to trigger the release of epinephrine and norepinepherine. These hormones would cause the heart rate to increase to overcome the decrease in cardiac output. The body normally responds to hypovolemia by increasing peripheral vascular resistance through vasoconstriction. This response is not possible in an individual with a spine injury. Therefore, the athlete in neurogenic shock will present with bradycardia; hypotension; shocklike symptoms above the injury and warm, dry, and flushed skin below the injury level; and priapism in males. *(For more information on neurogenic shock, see the section later in this chapter and Chapter 2.)*

✪ *STAT Point 6-3. Signs and symptoms of neurogenic shock include bradycardia; hypotension; shocklike symptoms above the level of the injury; warm, dry, and flushed skin below the injury level; and priapism in males.*

Assessment

Assessment of an athlete with a potential spinal cord injury should begin with trying to determine the mechanism of injury (Box 6-3). If the mechanism of injury is not known, then one should always assume the cervical spine is injured until proven otherwise, especially in athletes with a decreased level of consciousness or that are unconscious. Because the athlete may not be able to appropriately answer or respond to questions, knowing the mechanism of injury is the most critical piece of information needed to make treatment decisions when a cervical spine injury is possible. Any athlete with a head injury should also be treated as if he or she has a cervical spine injury until a thorough evaluation can be completed and injury to the cervical spine is no longer suspected.

During the approach toward a downed athlete, the athletic trainer can observe many things that help form a picture of the potential problem. Note the positioning of the athlete and if the athlete is moving any extremities. The reaction of teammates may also help determine the severity of the injury. If the athlete is unconsciousness, on your arrival immediately consider a cervical spine injury and apply **manual stabilization** to the head and neck in the position found (Fig. 6-4). If the athlete is supine, maintain the cervical spine position by placing your hands on either side of the head

Box 6-3   On-Field Assessment of an Athlete with a Potential Cervical Spine Injury

1. Determine mechanism of injury if possible.

2. While moving to athlete, determine level of consciousness of athlete if possible (is the athlete moving?).

3. Manually stabilize head and neck of injured athlete.

4. Determine level of consciousness; if unconscious, activate EMS.

5. Check ABCs. This may require rolling a prone athlete.

6. Activate EMS, manage airway, and begin rescue breathing or CPR if necessary.

7. Perform secondary assessment.

8. Continue to monitor vital signs for changes.

suspect a spinal injury, immediately apply manual stabilization in the position found. Activation of the local emergency medical service (EMS) should be initiated immediately if there is any suspicion of spinal injury.

Once you have effectively stabilized the head and neck, proceed with an assessment of the ABCs. *(See Chapter 2 for more details.)* If the athlete is found in the prone position, he or she may need to be log rolled to properly assess the ABCs. *(See later section on log rolling procedure.)* Any abnormal findings with regard to the ABCs must be treated immediately. Airway maneuvers are more difficult when cervical spine precautions are indicated; practice of these skills is therefore essential. If the athlete is found to be **apneic,** an oral airway should be inserted and ventilations with a bag valve mask should be initiated. *(See Chapter 3 for more details.)* Advanced airway procedures including intubation with cervical spine precautions may be indicated. If the athlete is wearing a helmet, the face mask or even the helmet itself will need to be removed for advanced airway procedures. *(See later section on equipment removal.)* In the athlete who does not have a pulse, chest compressions should be performed while manual stabilization of the cervical spine is maintained. Standard cardiopulmonary resuscitation (CPR) and automatic external defibrillator (AED) protocols should be followed in all cases of cardiac arrest. *(See Chapter 4 for more details.)*

If the athlete is breathing and has a steady pulse, then proceed with your evaluation. Maintaining a neutral, in-line position of the cervical spine is most important because this allows the spinal cord to have the maximum amount of space in case there is bleeding or swelling. If the cervical spine is not in a neutral position, the athletic trainer should gently attempt to move the head to get the spine to neutral. If any resistance is felt, or the conscious athlete indicates significant apprehension and/or an increase in pain, immediately stop the movement and immobilize in that position. It is critical to discontinue movement at the first sign of resistance, athlete apprehension, or increased pain; failure to do so may cause

with the heel of the hands resting just laterally to the occiput while spreading the fingers out over the side of the face. Care should be taken not to apply traction or compression to the spine. If the athlete is prone, he or she will need to be stabilized and rolled, as described in a later section. If the athlete is wearing a helmet, the hand placement will be on the helmet in a similar fashion to that described earlier. If the athlete is conscious, quickly assess the level of consciousness and the major complaint. It bears repeating that, regardless of the findings, if the mechanism of injury is such that you

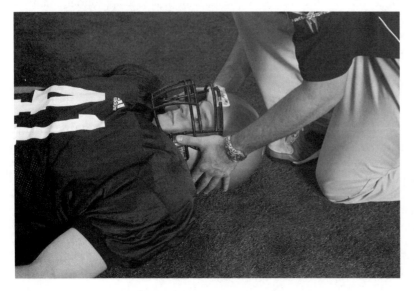

Figure 6-4. Manual stabilization of the cervical spine. Hands should be on both sides of the head with fingers spread to provide the most control over head and neck movements. Traction is not recommended.

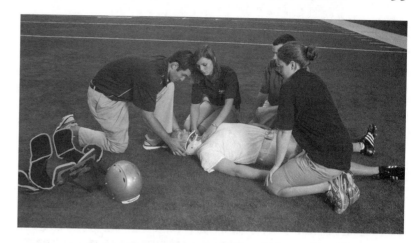

Figure 6-5. Application of a rigid cervical collar. Manual stabilization is maintained while the second rescuer applies the collar.

further damage to the cervical spinal column and/or spinal cord. At this time examine the cervical spine for rigidity, painful palpation, sensation changes, and deformity.

⭐ *STAT Point 6-4. When returning the head to a neutral position, it is critical to stop the movement at the first sign of resistance, athlete apprehension, or increased pain; failure to do so may cause further damage to the cervical spinal column and/or spinal cord.*

Once neutral position or close to neutral has been accomplished, maintain manual stabilization until a mechanical device, such as a rigid cervical collar, can be placed on the athlete (Fig. 6-5). Manual stabilization should be maintained even after a cervical collar is in place. Athletes involved in collision sports (e.g., football, ice hockey, lacrosse) will be wearing protective equipment that will not allow effective application of a cervical collar while the equipment is in place. *(See later section on equipment removal.)* If a neutral or near-neutral cervical spine position cannot be achieved, the athlete should be immobilized to the spine board in the final cervical spine position.

Continue to monitor respiratory efforts and level of consciousness throughout the remainder of your assessment. A well-organized head-to-toe evaluation is the next step. *(See Chapter 2 for more information.)* The examination should be focused and easily repeated for continuity purposes. Performing a rapid trauma assessment is an effective way to achieve this. Begin by palpating the spine for pain, deformity, crepitus, muscle spasm, or warmth of the skin (Box 6-4).

Move on to inspecting the distal extremities and evaluate for both motor and sensory function. When assessing for **motor function,** perform all tests bilaterally, looking for resistance to be equal (Fig. 6-6). First, test grip strength by having the athlete squeeze your index and middle finger as hard as possible. Then, test finger abduction and adduction by having the athlete spread his or her fingers while you attempt to squeeze the second, third, and fourth fingers

---

Box 6-4   On-Field Secondary Assessment

1. **Palpation of neck: pain, obvious deformity, bleeding, spasm?**

2. **Motor testing of upper extremities**

3. **Sensory testing of upper extremities**

4. **Motor testing of lower extremities**

5. **Sensory testing of lower extremities**

6. **Reassessment of vital signs**

7. **Continued reassurance of injured athlete**

---

together. Finally, test wrist and finger extension. To do this, have the athlete extend his or her wrist against resistance. Repeat with the fingers extended. To assess the **sensory function** of the upper extremity, first question the athlete regarding any sense of numbness, tingling, paralysis, and pain. To test for sensation, have the athlete close his or her eyes and attempt to distinguish between sharp and dull touch. This can be accomplished by using a ball point pen or a safety pin to lightly touch the athlete with either the pointed or the rounded ends (Fig. 6-7). The athlete should be able to identify the difference over all dermatomes.

Motor and sensory function should next be assessed in the lower extremities. To perform these assessments, place your hands against the bottoms of the feet and have the athlete attempt to "push on the gas pedal" (Fig. 6-8A). Next, place your hands on the top of the toes and have the individual attempt to pull the toes toward the head (Fig. 6-8B). The sensory function can then be evaluated in the same manner as the upper extremity with the athlete attempting to note sharp from dull sensation.

If during the examination you are able to determine areas where sensation is diminished or absent, it may be helpful to mark this area for further reference. Care should

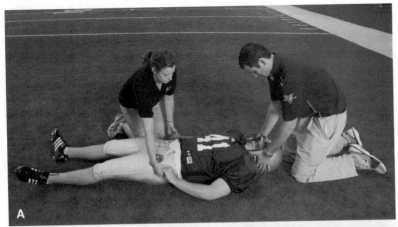

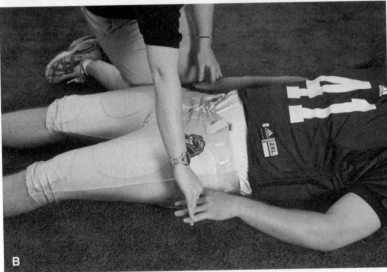

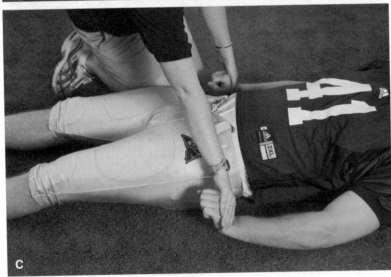

Figure 6-6. Upper-extremity motor function testing. **A:** Bilateral comparison of grip strength. **B:** Finger abduction/adduction. **C:** Wrist extension.

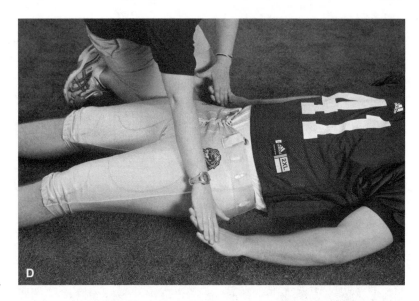

Figure 6-6. cont'd **D:** Finger extension.

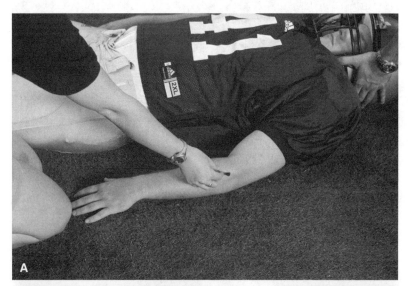

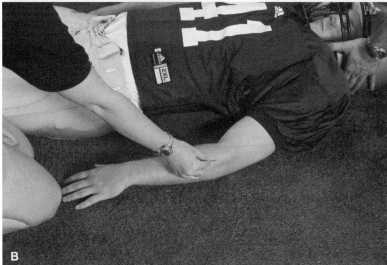

Figure 6-7. Upper-extremity sensory testing.
A: Soft brush, repeated over as many dermatomes as possible. **B:** Sharp pin, repeated over as many dermatomes as possible.

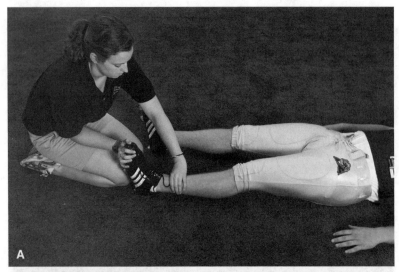

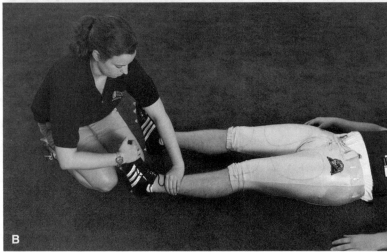

Figure 6-8. Lower-extremity motor function testing. **A:** "Pushing on the gas pedal" (ankle plantarflexion). **B:** Pulling toes toward the head (ankle dorsiflexion).

be taken not to alarm the athlete if it is recognized that sensation is not present. If the athlete recognizes a loss of sensation, be sure to keep him or her calm. Any positive finding in this examination should cause one to anticipate a spinal cord injury and lead one to treat the athlete appropriately.

Careful assessment of the vital signs should follow. Continually evaluating the vital signs is essential. The presence of shallow, diaphragmatic or absent respirations, hypotension, or bradycardia is a strong indication of injury to the spinal cord. Another important vital sign to watch carefully in an athlete with a potential spinal cord injury is body temperature. Individuals with spinal cord injuries lose their ability to maintain normal body temperature; therefore, one may note fluctuations, especially below the level of the injury.

✪ *STAT Point 6-5. Individuals with spinal cord injuries lose their ability to maintain normal body temperature; changes may be noted during evaluation, especially below the level of the injury.*

As in any traumatic injury, ongoing monitoring of vital signs is imperative. Recheck vital signs every 5 minutes and note any changes. Any change in level of consciousness, responsiveness, sensory, or motor function should be noted, keeping in mind that these findings may be improvements or deteriorations. Watch closely for a slowing pulse rate or the pulse rate staying the same while the blood pressure drops or a blood pressure that falls without any signs of shock. Any deterioration in vital signs is indicative of an emergent situation.

✪ *STAT Point 6-6. Deterioration of any vital signs is indicative of an emergent situation.*

Take particular care with the athlete who has a mechanism of injury that creates concern for the cervical spine without any other signs of spinal cord injury. Serious cervical spine injuries are not always apparent; in some cases, athletes with cervical spine fractures have walked off the field on their own before the medical staff was aware there had been an injury. Serious cervical spine injuries do not always exhibit measurable signs of neurological deficit or changing vital signs. Athletic trainers must keep in mind that if not managed appropriately, an otherwise stable injury may become unstable because of improper handling, thus placing the athlete at significant risk for a catastrophic outcome.

✪ *STAT Point 6-7. If not managed appropriately, an otherwise stable cervical spine injury may become unstable as a result of improper handling, thus placing the athlete at significant risk for a catastrophic outcome.*

Management

After completing the evaluation process and determining that the athlete needs to be immobilized, many things need to be accomplished. First, activation of the emergency action plan should be initiated if it hasn't already, including notification of the local EMS system. A rigid cervical collar should be applied if possible and the athlete should be stabilized by manual means, which should be maintained throughout the management process. Retrieval of the appropriate equipment—including a spine board, straps, head immobilization device, and airway control devices to carry out the necessary procedures—is also essential (Fig. 6-9). A flow chart of the decision-making process for suspected cervical spine injuries is shown in Figure 6-10.

The major goal of managing a suspected injury to the spinal cord is to maintain a neutral, in-line position. Beyond CPR, this is the single most important action that can be performed in these situations. Never overlook basic skills in order to apply more advanced skills.

In all cases where there is potential for a spinal cord injury, the athlete will be anxious. It is important that the athletic trainer continually calms, reassures, and communicates to the athlete what is being done and why. Immobilization on a long spine board can be uncomfortable and frightening.

This anxiety will only add to the athlete's discomfort and could negatively affect the outcome. It is also very important that scene control is addressed as part of the emergency action plan. Teammates, coaches, and parents can be emotional and also have a negative effect on the situation. Control of the scene should be maintained at all times.

If the athlete is found in the prone position, he or she should be log rolled to the supine position with the neck maintained in a neutral position *(more information on managing prone athletes later in this chapter)*. If the athlete is found in the supine position, then carefully move the neck into a neutral position as previously described. After moving the athlete, always reassess ABCs and sensory and motor function. Maintain a neutral cervical spine position by stabilizing the head and neck as described earlier. The person controlling the head will "lead" the spine boarding process by directing the other rescuers. This person should also maintain communication with the athlete, explaining each action and attempting to calm and reassure the athlete at all times, as previously discussed.

✪ *STAT Point 6-8. During the management process, after moving the athlete, always reassess ABCs and sensory and motor function.*

The decision as to how and when to move the athlete must be made based on the condition of the victim, the availability of adequate assistance, and proper equipment. Careful planning can eliminate unnecessary movement; this is important because each move increases the risk of causing further injury. Many methods are acceptable to move the athlete onto a long spine board, the most common being the log roll and straddle slide. Whatever method is chosen, it should be one in which all personnel are familiar and comfortable. The movement must be coordinated and smooth. The key factor throughout any procedure is to move the athlete as a unit, maintaining the head and neck in neutral alignment.

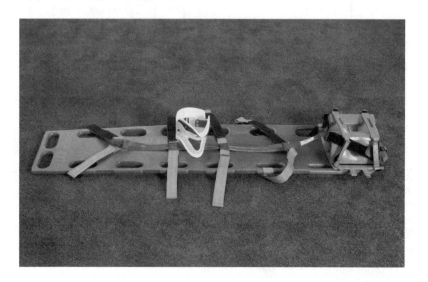

Figure 6-9. Specific equipment required for spine boarding procedure: long spine board with handles, rigid cervical collar, head immobilization device, straps.

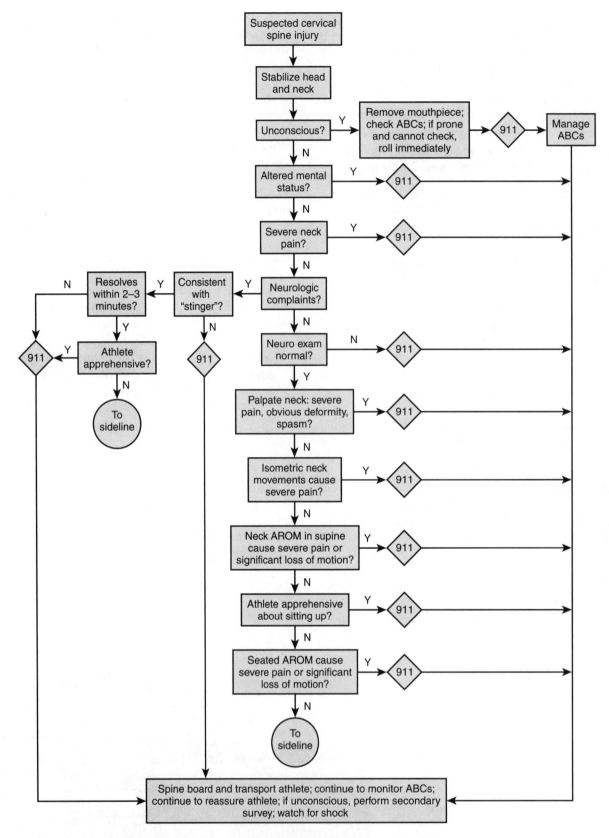

Figure 6-10. Decision-making flowchart for suspected cervical spine injury.

The Log Roll Method

The log roll can usually be accomplished with five people: one at the head, one controlling the board, and the other three spaced along the side of the athlete (Fig. 6-11). Larger athletes may require a sixth person. The lead rescuer will dictate the position of the other rescuers, keeping in mind that male athletes tend to carry more of their weight in the chest/shoulder area and females tend to carry more of their weight in the area of the pelvis. Stronger rescuers should be positioned accordingly. The three along the side of the athlete should position themselves equally spaced with their knees against the victim's side. To facilitate the roll, the arm of the athlete on the side of the direction of the roll should be carefully raised above the athlete's head; the legs of the athlete should be straightened with care, if necessary. The rescuers at the side should grasp the athlete on the opposite side, being sure to place their hands in a position in which they can maintain a grasp of the person. It is recommended that the body of the athlete, rather than just the clothing, be grasped because clothing held by itself is likely to shift and slide during the roll. On command of the person controlling the head, all three people should roll the athlete toward them, resting the athlete against their thighs when the command to stop is given. At this time the spine board should be placed behind the athlete with one edge anchored on the ground and the other edge angled up off the ground so that the flat surface of the board is close to the athlete. On command the athlete should be carefully rolled back to the board, and the athlete and board should be lowered carefully to the ground with the athlete now resting on the spine board in a supine position. The person controlling the head must be sure to maintain a neutral alignment by lining up the chin of the victim with the midline of the thorax and to not allow flexion or extension to occur; maintaining neutral alignment will require the person at the head to rotate the athlete's head as the athlete's body is rolled (Box 6-5).

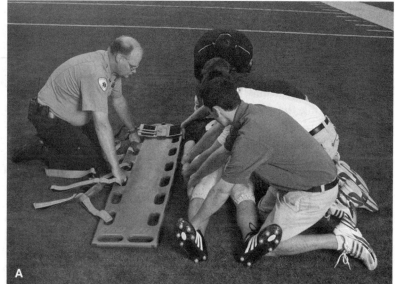
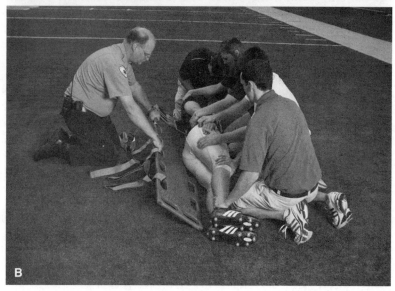

Figure 6-11. Log roll method. **A**: Five rescuers are involved: one at the head maintaining manual stabilization and directing the procedure, one controlling the spine board, and three positioned to roll the athlete. The rescuer controlling the spine board ensures that the straps are out of the way and will not be trapped under the athlete. The hands of the rescuers rolling the athlete are reaching under the athlete; clothing is not grasped because it tends to slip during the roll. The knees of the rescuers rolling the athlete will block the athlete from sliding toward the rescuers during the roll. The arm of the athlete on the side of the direction of the roll is abducted as high as possible. On command, the athlete is carefully rolled as a unit toward the three rescuers until the "stop" command is given. **B**: Once the athlete is rolled to one side, the spine board is pushed into position against the athlete, angled upward, and held firmly in that position. On command, the athlete is then carefully rolled back onto the spine board, which is lowered to the ground. The athlete is now supine on the spine board.

Box 6-5   Log Roll Method

1. **All commands will come from the rescuer controlling the head of the athlete.**

2. **The athlete is positioned with arm overhead, straight legs.**

3. **Rescuers and spine board are positioned.**

4. **The athlete is grasped by rescuers.**

5. **On command, the athlete is carefully rolled toward rescuers until the command to stop is given; the athlete is held against rescuers' thighs.**

6. **The spine board is positioned.**

7. **On command, the athlete is carefully rolled back to supine position.**

The Straddle Slide Method

The straddle slide method also incorporates five rescuers: one at the head, one controlling the board, and the other three straddling the victim with a foot on either side (Fig. 6-12). Extreme care must be taken not to step on or kick the athlete. Again, larger athletes may require the use of a sixth person. In this method, the athlete's arms and legs should be carefully straightened; both arms should be down at the athlete's side. The lead rescuer will position the other rescuers based on their relative physical strength, as described earlier. Each of the three rescuers straddling the athlete places their hands under the sides of the athlete at the shoulders, waist, and knees. On the command of the person at the head, the three rescuers lift the athlete until the person controlling the head instructs them to stop. At this point a long spine board is slid under the athlete from the feet and on command the athlete is lowered onto the spine board. Using this method the person at the head must lift the head as the athlete's body lifts, maintaining the head and neck in a neutral position. With this method the athlete's weight and the strength of the rescuers must be taken into account (Box 6-6).

Managing the Prone Athlete

Rescuers who are managing athletes in a prone position must consider this fact when applying manual stabilization to the head and neck. If a rescuer uses a standard hand placement, the rescuer's arms will be crossed after the athlete is rolled to the supine position. A crossed-arm position makes safe manual stabilization of the cervical spine difficult, and control of the head therefore may need to be transferred to

another rescuer. This is not recommended because unintended movement of the athlete's head and neck may occur during the transfer. The rescuer should instead use a crossed-arm technique when first reaching the athlete; this will allow for effective control of the athlete's head and neck after the roll to a supine position (Fig. 6-13).

⭐ *STAT Point 6-9. When applying manual stabilization to a prone athlete, the lead rescuer should initially use a crossed-arm technique.*

When an athlete is found in the prone position, it is best to log roll directly onto a spine board to avoid the necessity of a second log roll or lift for board placement. However, the first priority is still to check level of consciousness and ABCs. If ABCs cannot be effectively checked, or if they are not present, the athlete must immediately be log rolled, even if the spine board is not yet positioned (Box 6-7).

⭐ *STAT Point 6-10. If ABCs cannot be effectively checked in a prone athlete, or if they are not present, the athlete must immediately be log rolled.*

Immobilization

Once the athlete is correctly positioned on the spine board, he or she must be immobilized effectively. A person who is not secured to the spine board is not considered to be immobilized. The head of the athlete should be placed in an immobilizing device. A number of different products are available for immobilizing the head of an athlete on a spine board (Fig. 6-14). Alternately, tightly rolled towels can be used in combination with sturdy tape to secure the athlete's head to the board. Manual stabilization must be maintained until the head of the athlete is secured to the spine board. If satisfactory stabilization cannot be achieved for whatever reason, manual stabilization should be maintained until it is determined that there is no longer risk to the athlete's cervical spine.

The athlete should be strapped to the board in a manner that will not allow movement even in the event that the board needs to be turned to the side if vomiting were to occur. Special strapping techniques are also required if the athlete needs to be extricated up or down stairs or in tight corridors where the spine board may need to be stood up on end (Figs. 6-15 and 6-16).

The Lift and Transfer

Once the athlete is secured to the spine board, it is safe to lift and transfer the spine board. This transfer will most often be directly onto an ambulance gurney or onto a motorized cart for transport off the field. It is important that the medical staff continue to work in a coordinated, careful manner throughout the lift and transfer. Commands should

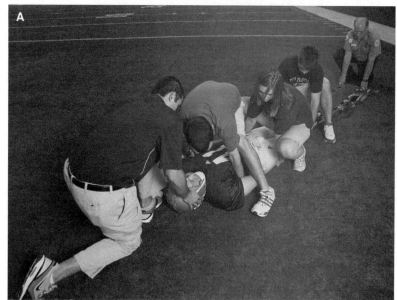

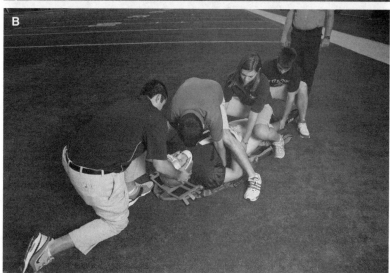

Figure 6-12. Straddle slide method. **A:** Five rescuers are involved: one at the head maintaining manual stabilization and directing the procedure, one controlling the spine board, and three positioned to lift the athlete. The hands of the rescuers lifting the athlete are reaching under the athlete; clothing is not grasped because it tends to slip during the lift. On command, the athlete is carefully lifted as a unit until the "stop" command is given. Notice in this photo that the face mask has been removed prior to placing the athlete on the spine board. **B:** Once the lift has stopped, the rescuer controlling the spine board quickly slides the spine board beneath the athlete until it is appropriately positioned under the athlete. At that point, the rescuer controlling the head will tell the rescuer controlling the spine board to stop. In this photo, the spine board is appropriately positioned under the athlete when the head immobilization device is centered beneath the athlete's helmet. Once the spine board is positioned, on command the athlete will be carefully lowered as a unit down to the spine board.

Box 6-6 Straddle Slide Method

1. **All commands will come from the rescuer controlling the head of the athlete.**

2. **The athlete is positioned with straight legs, arms at sides.**

3. **Rescuers and spine board are positioned.**

4. **The athlete is grasped by rescuers.**

5. **On command, the athlete is carefully lifted straight up until the command to stop is given.**

6. **The spine board is positioned.**

7. **On command, the athlete is carefully lowered back down to the spine board.**

continue to come from the same person who has control of the head. The spine board should have handles along its perimeter, and these handles should be easy to grasp even if the spine board is resting on a flat surface, such as a basketball court. Members of the medical staff should be evenly spaced along the perimeter of the spine board and there should be enough personnel to easily lift and carry the weight of the spine board and athlete. The lift must occur smoothly and on command. In some cases, the spine board will need to be walked a short distance, and this must also be carefully coordinated and occur on command so that everyone carrying the board is starting and stopping their movements simultaneously. Lifting and walking the loaded spine board should be part of regular practice sessions for the sports medicine staff. If the transfer is to a gurney, EMS personnel will be available to help direct the transfer. If the transfer is to a cart, the sports medicine staff should also include the transfer and securing of the spine board to the cart as part of regular practice sessions.

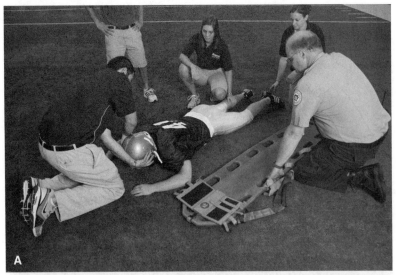

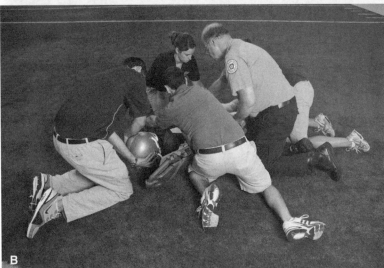

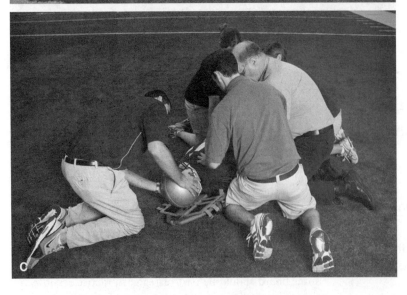

Figure 6-13. Placement on a spine board from a prone position. **A:** Lead rescuer initially uses a crossed-arm technique for manual stabilization. Once the athlete is rolled to supine, the lead rescuer's arms will have been uncrossed. **B:** One rescuer is positioned opposite the direction of the roll to help control the athlete's position and prevent sliding of the athlete and/or the spine board. The other three rescuers rest the spine board against their upper legs; this holds the spine board in an upwardly angled position and also allows the rescuers to use their knee and upper leg to hold the spine board tight against the athlete. The three rescuers reach across the athlete for a firm hold on the athlete's body (not the clothing). On command, the athlete is rolled toward the three rescuers and onto the spine board. **C:** Once the athlete is on the spine board, it is carefully lowered to the ground. During the roll and lowering of the spine board, the rescuer on the opposite side helps to control the roll and to prevent the athlete from sliding toward that edge of the spine board. Notice that the lead rescuers arms are now uncrossed, allowing for simplified manual stabilization.

Box 6-7 Log Rolling From a Prone Position

1. All commands come from the rescuer controlling the head of the athlete.

2. The athlete's arms and legs are carefully straightened as directed.

3. Three (or four) rescuers are positioned on the side of the direction of the roll with the spine board lying against their upper legs; one rescuer is positioned on the opposite side of the athlete to help control the roll and to help prevent the athlete from sliding as the board is lowered.

4. On command, the athlete is carefully rolled from prone to sidelying and then down onto the spine board; the position of the head in relation to the trunk is maintained throughout the roll.

5. The spine board is carefully lowered to the ground.

6. The head can then be slowly and incrementally returned to a neutral position as discussed earlier in this chapter.

7. A rigid cervical collar should then be applied. Or, in cases where the athlete is wearing a helmet, the face mask should be removed.

Managing Protective Equipment

Collision sports such as football, ice hockey, and lacrosse require players to wear protective equipment that presents an additional challenge to athletic trainers. Managing football equipment will be covered in the following sections. Considerations for managing the ice hockey player with a suspected cervical spine injury will be covered in Chapter 12.

If the decision has been made to spine board an injured football player, the player should be immobilized with all of the equipment on if possible. The face mask should always be completely removed to allow access to the athlete's airway in the event that respiratory distress or arrest occurs. Athletic training professionals currently universally support the theory that the helmet and shoulder pads should remain in place until definitive care can be achieved. Some controversy has existed with EMS professionals who have been taught to remove helmets prior to spine boarding a person. The most common reasons given for helmet removal include inability to obtain proper immobilization with the helmet in place, inability to visualize injuries to the skull, inability to control the airway, and hyperflexion of the neck with the helmet in place. These reasons certainly may apply to motorcycle and auto racing helmets but not to the football helmet.

⭐ *STAT Point 6-11. When managing an athlete wearing a helmet, the face mask should always be completely removed to allow access to the athlete's airway.*

The football helmets used today are designed to fit snugly and therefore do not allow the head to move inside

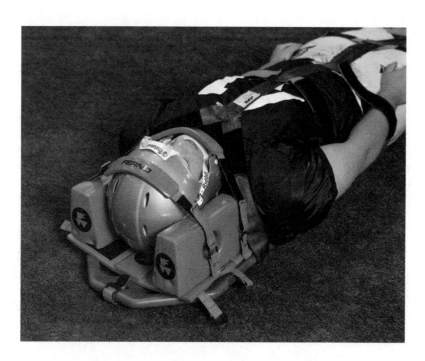

Figure 6-14. Head immobilization device. Firm blocks on either side of the head prevent motion in rotation or lateral flexion. These blocks are easily adjustable to provide for a tight fit against different sizes of head or helmet. Two straps across the forehead and chin of the athlete prevent movement in the direction of flexion. Instead of straps, strong tape can be used for this same purpose.

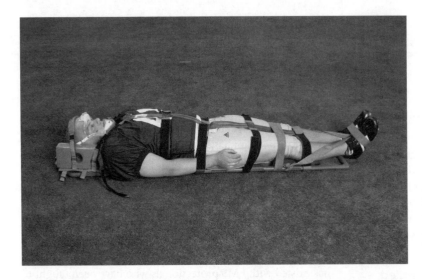

Figure 6-15. Strapping technique to secure the athlete to the spine board. Notice that the arms and feet of the athlete are also secured. The arm is easily accessible to EMS personnel in the event an IV is warranted.

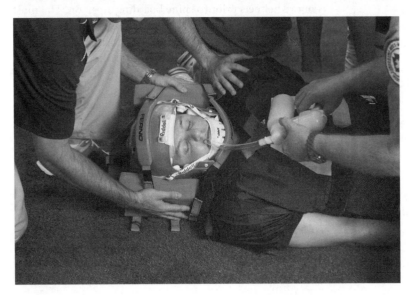

Figure 6-16. Turning the spine board to manage vomiting with manual suction. A properly secured athlete will not slide on the spine board even when it is turned to the side. Notice the large-bore tubing being used on the suction unit.

the shell. Therefore, immobilizing the helmet on the spine board will also effectively immobilize the head inside the helmet. The mechanism of injury in a football player is generally axial loading or an extreme motion in one direction, such as hyperextension. Traumatic injuries to the skull and soft tissues of the head and face are simply not seen as is frequently the case in motorcycle accidents, which involve exponentially higher forces than those experienced in collision sports such as football. The ears can be visualized through the ear holes, and the neck can be palpated and pupils checked without difficulty with the helmet in place. There is no need to remove a football helmet for this reason.

Removal of the face mask will allow the rescuer to effectively maintain control of the airway. The vast majority of cervical spine injuries in football players occur at the lower level of the cervical spine C5-C7. For this reason respiratory distress is rare. In the event that airway difficulties are present, all appropriate procedures can be carried out with little difficulty once the face mask is removed. There is no need to

remove the entire helmet to effectively manage the airway of an injured athlete.

A person wearing a motorcycle helmet or a football helmet *without* shoulder pads who is supine will be forced into a position of cervical hyperflexion because of the thickness of the back of the helmet. Shoulder pads elevate the thorax such that the spine will be in a neutral position when an athlete wearing a helmet is supine. Removing the helmet and not the shoulder pads would therefore allow the cervical spine of the athlete to fall into a position of hyperextension (Fig. 6-17).

Face Mask Removal

Face mask removal may be accomplished by either cutting or unscrewing the four plastic clips: two above the forehead and one by each cheek (Fig. 6-18). Clip designs may change from year to year; it is essential that the athletic trainer be aware of the type of clip design being used on the helmets of their athletes and that the athletic trainer has practiced

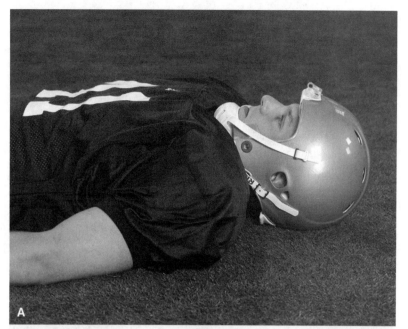

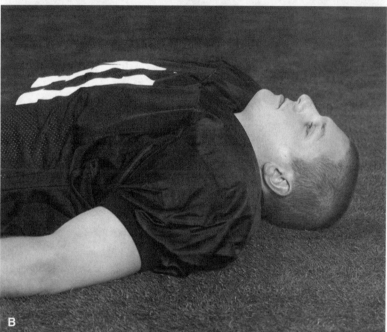

Figure 6-17. Relative cervical spine positions in a supine athlete wearing shoulder pads. **A:** With helmet in place, the position of the cervical spine is essentially neutral. **B:** With the helmet removed but shoulder pads remaining in place, significant cervical extension occurs.

removing those clips. Keep in mind that there may be several different models of helmets in use by the same team; in these instances, it is likely that the athletic trainer will need to be prepared to manage different types of clips. Whether to cut or to unscrew the clips will be determined by the athletic trainer based in part on the model of helmet worn and the type of fastener used for the face mask. Athletic trainers will also decide which removal tool they feel best suits them. Numerous tools have been developed specifically to aid in removing football helmet face masks (Fig. 6-19). The exact removal method should be predetermined by the sports medicine staff and practiced frequently to ensure efficiency and competency. It is generally accepted that the face mask

should be entirely removed, rather than just cutting the side clips and flipping the mask up (Fig. 6-20). In this position, the face mask presents an obstacle to efficient management and is a hazard for accidental bumping and subsequent head movement of the athlete. Athletic trainers should be prepared with at least two different tools for face mask removal in case the first choice of tool is ineffective for any reason.

Removing the Helmet and Shoulder Pads

If the athletic trainer cannot remove the face mask to access the airway in a relatively short amount of time, or if it appears that the helmet and/or shoulder pads fit loosely and

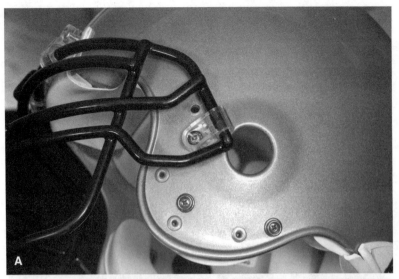

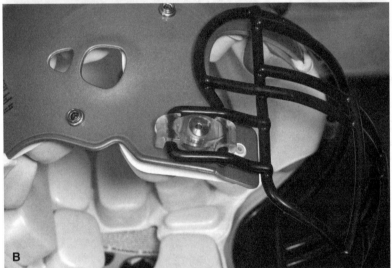

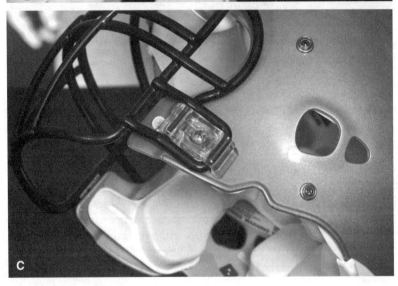

Figure 6-18. Face mask clips come in a variety of designs depending on the helmet manufacturer. **A:** Traditional "single bar" design using a traditional screw. **B:** "Double bar" design using a nontraditional screw. In this type of design, the side of the clip closest to the front of the helmet can be difficult to cut because of the proximity of the adjacent face mask bars. A power screwdriver with the appropriate tip may be the most efficient means of removing this clip. **C:** Another "double bar" design, this one with a traditional screw. Again, the side of the clip closest to the front of the helmet can be difficult to cut in this design.

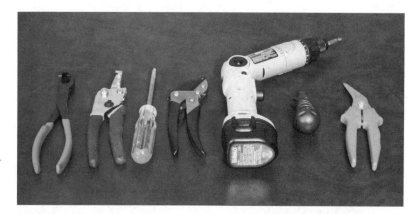

Figure 6-19. Various face mask removal tools. Athletic trainers should practice with several different types of removal tools to determine which tool they are most comfortable using.

therefore will not hold the athlete motionless once secured to the spine board, it is recommended that the helmet *and* shoulder pads be removed. Safe removal will involve transfer of control of the head and neck of the athlete twice during the procedure. It is therefore necessary that those involved be thoroughly competent and confident in what they are doing; the importance of frequent practice cannot be overstated (Box 6-8 and Fig. 6-21).

✪ *STAT Point 6-12: If the face mask cannot be removed in a relatively short amount of time, or if it appears that the helmet and/or shoulder pads fit loosely and therefore will not hold the athlete motionless once secured to the spine board, it is recommended that the helmet and shoulder pads be removed. Helmet and shoulder pads are always removed together, never one or the other.*

In summary, basic immobilization techniques are essential in the care of any individual with a suspected injury to the spinal cord. If these basic skills are not carefully applied, the potential for permanent disabilities, or even fatalities, exist. These skills must be practiced until complete competency is achieved by all who may be involved in the process. Without successful basic care and treatment, advanced techniques, which may include the use of medications to control secondary injury, are useless. These advanced techniques will be determined by local protocol and should be known by the athletic trainer and team physicians.

Steroids

In the event of a spinal cord injury, the secondary injury caused by inflammation may compound the damage. In the past, steroids have been used to limit the inflammatory process and therefore reduce the damage that could occur due to swelling. The most commonly used steroids for this purpose are methylprednisolone and dexamethasone. These medications are most effective if administered within the first eight hours of trauma. More recently, some physicians have questioned the efficacy of this treatment in mitigating

secondary injury. Protocols should be established by your team physician and/or local EMS service regarding the use of steroids to manage spinal cord injury.

Neurogenic Shock Management

Spinal cord injuries can result in neurogenic shock, as discussed earlier in this chapter. A direct consequence of the large-scale vasodilatation is pooling of blood throughout the body, resulting in essentially what is known as hypovolemia. Because of the lack of sympathetic response, heart rate does not increase adequately to overcome the loss of volume, and shock results. *(For more information on shock, see Chapter 2.)* To treat this, a **fluid challenge** is followed by the introduction of a vasopressor such as dopamine. The fluid challenge is accomplished by infusing 250 mL of IV fluid through a large-bore IV catheter. If the response to this infusion is that of increased blood pressure, slower heart rate, and better perfusion, then a second infusion should be considered. If there is not a positive response to the first bolus of fluid, then the administration of a **vasopressor** (dopamine) should be considered. If the bradycardia persists, then the use of atropine may be indicated to increase the heart rate. The dosages and indications will be set by local protocol.

The incidence of serious spinal cord injury in the athletic population is small, but the potential for permanent disability or death is always present. Appropriate evaluation and management of these injuries are only possible if careful planning and practice of these skills are carried out. The significance of the injury may not be immediately apparent, so a high level of suspicion should always be maintained in cases of potential cervical spine injury. A thorough and well-rehearsed emergency action plan will also allow for a more effective management of such injuries. All of the issues surrounding the care and treatment of individuals with potential cervical spine injuries must be discussed and evaluated by the sports medicine team as a whole, and protocols should be developed subsequently for the emergency action plan. Medical personnel outside the immediate sports medicine team should also be consulted during this planning, including local EMS personnel and emergency room personnel.

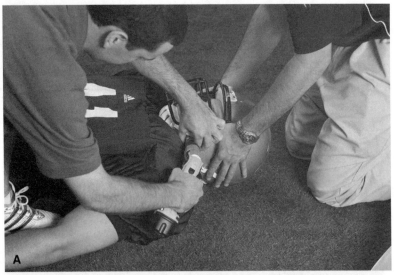

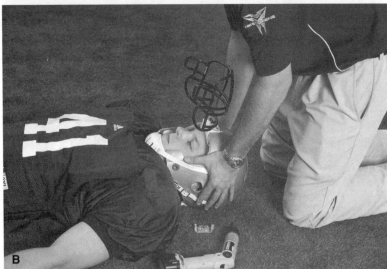

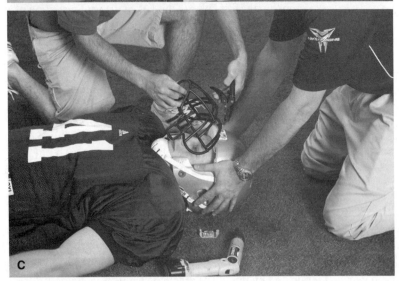

Figure 6-20. Face mask removal. **A:** While the lead rescuer maintains manual stabilization, the second rescuer uses a power screwdriver to carefully remove the face mask clip screw. During this process, the conscious athlete is continually reassured. The second rescuer will repeat this process on the other side of the athlete; alternately, a third rescuer could remove the clip on that side. **B:** Once the side clips are removed, the face mask will flip up, allowing easy access to the mouth and nose of the athlete. Notice that leaving the face mask in this position will present a serious hazard for rescuers to accidentally bump the face mask and impart a force to the head and neck of the athlete. **C:** In this photo, a cutting tool is being used to cut the top clips; the face mask can subsequently be completely removed from the helmet.

Box 6-8   Helmet and Shoulder Pad Removal

1. The athlete must be supine. It is understood that the face mask has either already been removed, cannot be removed, or a decision has been made to remove all equipment right away.

2. While lead rescuer maintains manual stabilization, the second rescuer:

   ■ Cuts the front of the jersey from waist to neck

   ■ Cuts the sleeves of the jersey from arm holes to neck

   ■ Removes the jersey

   ■ Cuts all shoulder pad straps and/or strings

   ■ Cuts any additional protective equipment that is attached to both the shoulder pads and helmet

   ■ Cuts the chinstrap

3. If the helmet uses an internal air bladder as part of the fitting system, the bladder should be deflated while the second rescuer works on the jersey and shoulder pads. Athletic trainers should be prepared with the correct tool to perform this procedure if the athletes in their care are using this type of helmet.

4. Cheek pads are removed from the helmet using a tongue blade or other flat, stiff object that will not cut the athlete's face to unsnap the pads.

5. The second rescuer positions his or her hands to take over manual stabilization: one hand at posterior cervical spine/occiput and the other at the jaw of the athlete.

6. Other rescuers position themselves to lift the torso of the injured athlete as a unit on command; these rescuers must be sure that their hand placement will not interfere with removal of the shoulder pads.

7. In an order predetermined and rehearsed by the medical staff: the second rescuer assumes primary control of manual stabilization and becomes command giver; the torso of the athlete is carefully lifted several inches and held still.

8. The first rescuer carefully removes the athlete's helmet by gently pulling and simultaneously rolling the helmet slightly forward as it is pulled off. It is not recommended that the sides of the helmet be pulled outward during helmet removal because this tends to tighten the helmet at the forehead and occiput.

9. The first rescuer quickly pulls the shoulder pads out from beneath the athlete.

10. On command, the athlete is carefully lowered back to the ground.

11. The first rescuer reassumes control of manual stabilization and management of the athlete's condition continues.

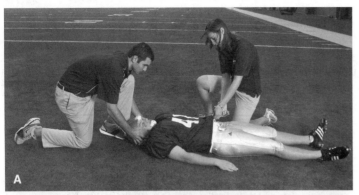

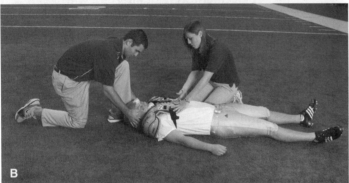

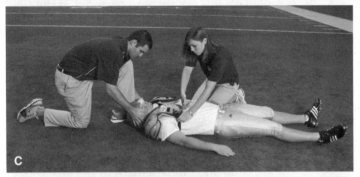

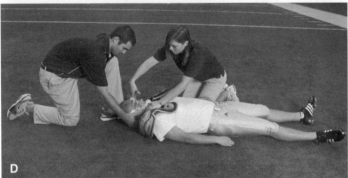

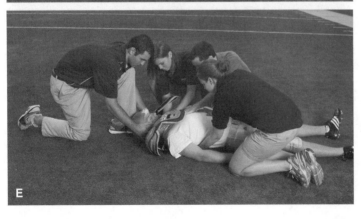

Figure 6-21. Equipment removal. **A:** While the first rescuer maintains manual stabilization, the second rescuer cuts and removes jersey. If the helmet contains an air bladder, this is an opportune time for a third rescuer to release the air for easier helmet removal. Note that in this photo the face mask has already been removed. It is not necessary to remove the face mask prior to removing the helmet and shoulder pads, but in some situations the decision to remove the equipment may come after the face mask has already been removed. **B:** Shoulder pad straps or strings are cut on the front of the pads. **C:** Shoulder pad straps on both sides are cut. **D:** The chinstrap is cut and removed. **E:** The second rescuer positions hands to take over manual stabilization. Other rescuers position hands to lift torso of athlete. As with rolling of the athlete, clothing should not be grasped because it tends to slip during the lift.

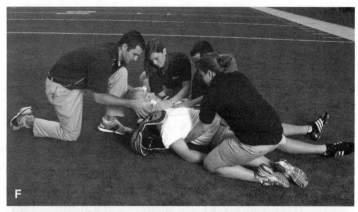

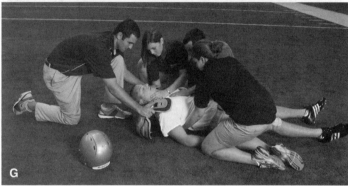

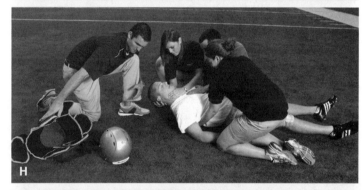

Figure 6-21. cont'd **F:** On command, the athlete's torso is lifted and held. The first rescuer carefully removes the helmet with a simultaneous pulling and slight forward rolling of the helmet. **G:** The first rescuer then quickly pulls shoulder pads off of the athlete. **H:** Notice that the helmet and shoulder pads are placed well out of the way. **I:** On command, the athlete is carefully lowered back to the ground. The first rescuer resumes manual stabilization.

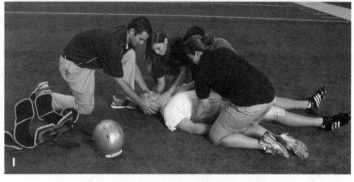

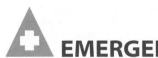 EMERGENCY ACTION

As you assess the athlete you are unable to awake him, so you establish manual stabilization. You then instruct meet officials to contact 911 while your athletic training student is sent to get your emergency care bag along with the spine board. The athletic trainer from the opposing team joins you. With the assistance of the visiting athletic trainer, your student, and the coach you prepare to log roll the athlete to the supine position. The team manager places the spine board next to the athlete, and you proceed to log roll the athlete onto the board and move the head and neck into a neutral position. A cervical collar is applied. The athlete remains unconscious but his vital signs are stable, and you instruct the others to strap the athlete to the spine board. As the final straps are tightened the EMS crew arrives, you give a complete report, and the athlete is transported to the local trauma center.

CHAPTER HIGHLIGHTS

- Injuries to the cervical spine can be devastating because of the potential for lifelong disability or even death.

- The spinal column is vulnerable to many types of injuries that in turn may lead to injury to the spinal cord. These injuries are typically the result of an excessive load through the cervical spine that causes disruption of soft tissues or fractures.

- Injuries to the spinal cord are characterized as either primary or secondary.

- Assessing an athlete with a potential spinal cord injury should begin with trying to determine the mechanism of injury. If the mechanism of injury is not known, then one should always assume the cervical spine is injured until proven otherwise, especially in athletes with a decreased level of consciousness or who are unconscious.

- When applying manual stabilization for the head and neck, care should be taken not to apply traction or compression to the spine.

- Prior to applying a rigid cervical collar, the head and neck of the athlete should be returned to a neutral position. If any resistance is felt during this movement, or the conscious athlete indicates significant apprehension and/or an increase in pain, immediately stop the movement and immobilize in that position. Failure to stop the movement immediately may cause further damage to the cervical spinal column and/or spinal cord.

- The major goal of managing a suspected injury to the spinal cord is to maintain a neutral, in-line position. Beyond CPR, this is the single most important action that can be performed in these situations. Never overlook basic skills in order to apply more advanced skills.

- In all cases where there is potential for a spinal cord injury the athlete will be very anxious. It is important that the athletic trainer continually calms, reassures, and communicates to the athlete what is being done and why.

- The log roll method and the straddle slide method are both effective techniques for moving an athlete onto a spine board.

- For athletes found in a prone position, the first priority is to establish level of consciousness and ABCs. If ABCs cannot be effectively checked with the athlete in the prone position, the athlete must quickly be rolled into a supine position.

● Protective equipment such as helmets and shoulder pads should not be removed unless absolutely necessary. The airway can be controlled and an AED can be applied with only the helmet face mask removed.

● Reasons for removing a helmet include inability to remove the face mask or situations in which the helmet does not hold the athlete's head securely.

● If the helmet is removed, the shoulder pads must also be removed to prevent potential hyperextension of the athlete's cervical spine.

● Secondary injury to the spinal cord can be limited with the appropriate use of steroid medications immediately following the traumatic event.

Chapter Questions

1. Which of the following is not a normal motion of the cervical spine?

   A. Flexion

   B. Extension

   C. Supination

   D. Lateral flexion

2. What can be the most important information regarding treatment decisions for the potentially injured cervical spine?

   A. Mechanism of injury

   B. Previous history

   C. Age

   D. Vital signs

3. Move the spine to a neutral position unless the following is/are noted:

   A. Bleeding

   B. Resistance

   C. Pain

   D. A and C

4. Injuries to the spinal cord may be categorized as:

   A. Primary or secondary

   B. Critical

   C. Mild or moderate

   D. None of the above

5. The major goal of spinal immobilization is to:

   A. Maintain neutral, in-line position

   B. Calm the athlete

   C. Make it easier to lift the athlete

   D. Meet federal guidelines

6. When a force is applied through the length of the spine it is known as:

   A. Subluxation

   B. Sagittal plane

   C. Axial loading

   D. Ischemia

7. An athlete found not breathing is:

   A. Deceased

   B. Tachycardic

   C. Stable

   D. Apneic

8. Central cord syndrome is most commonly seen with:

   A. Females

   B. Hyperextension

   C. Lateral flexion

   D. Males

9. A football player with shoulder pads and a helmet on should be immobilized:

   A. With both on

   B. With helmet off

   C. Quickly

   D. On his or her side

10. Administering corticosteroids to an athlete with a spinal cord injury will:

    A. Ease his or her pain

    B. Minimize swelling

    C. Calm the athlete down

    D. None of the above

■ *Case Study 1*

While covering a junior varsity football game you are notified by your athletic training student covering the varsity practice on an adjacent field that a player is down with a neck injury and no one knows what to do. You quickly leave the game field and report to the practice field and find the injured player lying supine with his shoulder pads on and helmet removed. He is complaining of severe neck pain, and the coach tells you the athlete tackled another player with his head down. The coach took the injured athlete's helmet off because the athlete was complaining that he was having difficulty breathing at the time.

Case Study 1 Questions

1. Has this situation been handled correctly? If not, what should have been done differently?

2. What would you do next?

3. What steps would you take to prevent this situation from happening again?

■ *Case Study 2*

An opposing player charging the net runs into the goalie for your ice hockey team, and the goalie lays motionless on the ice. When you get to him he is conscious and alert but complaining of not being able to move. He denies having any pain and is becoming very anxious and scared. He has no difficulty breathing. You complete your initial evaluation and find all vitals to be within normal limits, but the athlete does not respond to painful stimuli in his extremities and has no motor activity. You instruct the coach to contact the local EMS system and decide to wait for the assistance of the EMS personnel to stabilize the athlete on a spine board. While you are waiting, the athlete states he is beginning to feel some stinging in his feet and can now move his fingers slightly.

Case Study 2 Questions

1. What condition do you think this athlete is suffering from?

2. What do you expect to see happen over the next several minutes?

3. What would you do if by the time the ambulance arrives the athlete has fully recovered his sensation and motor function?

Suggested Readings

1. Allen BL, Ferguson RL, Lehman TR, et al. A mechanistic classification of closed indirect fractures and dislocations of the lower cervical spine. Spine. 1982;7:1–27.

2. Almquist JL. Spine injury management: A comprehensive plan for managing the cervical spine-injured football player. Sports Med Update. 1998;13:8–11.

3. Anderson JC, Courson RW, Kleiner DM, et al. National Athletic Trainer's Association position statement: Emergency planning in athletics. J Athl Train. 2002;37:99–104.

4. Bailes JE, Maroon JC. Management of cervical spine injuries in athletes. Clin Sports Med. 1989;8:43–57.

5. Burney RE, Waggoner R, Maynard FM. Stabilization of spinal injury for early transfer. J Trauma. 1989;29:1497–1499.

6. Denegar C, Saliba E. On the field management of the potential cervical spine injured football player. J Athl Train. 1989;24:108–111.

7. Domeier RM, Evans RA, Swor RA, et al. Prehospital clinical findings associated with spinal injury. Prehosp Emerg Care. 1997;1:11–15.

8. Donaldson WF, Lauerman WC, Heil B, et al. Helmet and shoulder pad removal from a player with a suspected cervical spine injury: A cadaveric model. Spine. 1998;23:1729–1733.

9. Feld F, Blanc R. Immobilizing the spine injured football player. J Emerg Med Serv. 1987;12:38–40.

10. Fourre M. On-site management of cervical spine injuries. Phys Sportsmed. 1991;19:53–56.

11. Gardner A, Grannum S, Porter KM. Cervical spine trauma. Trauma. 2005;7:109–121.

12. Haight RR, Shiple BJ. Sideline evaluation of neck pain: When is it time to transport? Phys Sportsmed. March 2001;29:45–62.

13. Kleiner DM, Almquist JL, Bailes J, et al. A document from the Inter-Association Task Force for Appropriate Care of the Spine-Injured Athlete. Dallas, TX: National Athletic Trainer's Association; March, 2001.

14. Neifeld GL, Keene JG, Hevesy G, et al. Cervical injury I: Head trauma. J Emerg Med. 1998;6:203–207.

15. Pre-Hospital Trauma Life Support, Third Edition. St. Louis: Mosby-Year Book; 1994:143.

16. Smith M, Bourn S, Larmon B. Ties that bind: Immobilizing the injured spine. J Emerg Med Serv. 1987;4:28–35.

17. Swenson TM, Lauerman WC, Donaldson WF, et al. Cervical spine alignment in the immobilized football player: Radiographic analysis before and after helmet removal. Am J Sports Med. 1997;25:226–230.

18. Vegso JJ, Lehman RC. Field evaluation and management of head and neck injuries. Clin Sports Med. 1987;6:1–15.

19. Waninger K. Management of the helmeted athlete with suspected spine injury. Am J Sports Med. 2004;32:1331.

20. White AA, Johnson RM, Panjabi MM, et al. Biomechanical analysis of clinical stability in the cervical spine. Clin Orthop. 1975;109:85–95.

Appendix 6-1

Lacrosse Equipment

Men's lacrosse is considered a collision sport and, as such, players wear protective equipment that includes a helmet and shoulder pads. In almost all respects, suspected cervical spine injuries in lacrosse players wearing a helmet and shoulder pads should be managed just as a suspected cervical spine injury in a football player. At least one study has shown that removal of only the helmet and not the shoulder pads in lacrosse players will result in significant cervical spine movement.[1] Therefore, just as with football players, if the helmet must be removed to effectively manage a lacrosse player with a suspected cervical spine injury, the shoulder pads should be removed as well.

Lacrosse helmets differ significantly from football and ice hockey helmets (see photo). One major difference is the inclusion in some models of the solid chinguard, which must be removed along with the face mask for effective management of the airway. The athletic trainer must be familiar with the specifics of the model of helmet that is being used because there are some variations between helmet brands in terms of exactly how the face mask/chinguard must be removed. In some models, the same screws that secure the face mask also attach the chinguard and the entire assembly can be removed using a only power screwdriver. In other models, however, both a power screwdriver *and* a cutting tool will be required for complete removal of the face mask and the chinguard. It is critical that the athletic trainer be aware of what tools will be required for timely removal of the face mask/chinguard assembly being used by their athletes.

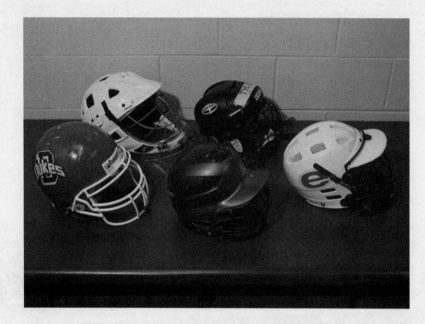

Helmets for collision sports: football, ice hockey, lacrosse. Notice the solid chinguard on the lacrosse helmet (top row, left).

Reference

1. Sherbondy P, Hertel J, Sebastianelli W. The effect of protective equipment on cervical spine alignment in collegiate lacrosse players. AJSM. 2006;34(10):1675–1679.

Chapter 7

Emergent General Medical Conditions

Tom Sisk, MD, and David Stone, MD

KEY TERMS

Aneurysm

Angiogram

Aortic dissection

Aortic stenosis

Arrhythmogenic right
    ventricular dysplasia

Asthma

Beta-2 agonists

Brugada syndrome

Cardiomyopathy

Cholinergic urticaria

Coronary artery
    anomalies

Diabetes mellitus

Diabetic ketoacidosis

Exercise-induced
    anaphylaxis

Hypercapnia

Hypertension

Hypertrophic
    cardiomyopathy

Hypoxemia

Kawasaki disease

Long QT syndrome

Lymphadenopathy

Lymphocytosis

Marfan's syndrome

Mitral valve prolapse

Mononucleosis

Nebulizer

Osmotic diuresis

Polydipsia

Polyuria

Pulsus paradoxus

Rhabdomyolysis

Sarcoidosis

Sickle cell trait

Ventricular ectopy

Viral myocarditis

Wolff-Parkinson-White
    (WPW) syndrome

 ### EMERGENCY SITUATION

A 15-year-old wrestler with insulin-dependant diabetes is brought to the athletic training room half-way through practice by a teammate who states that the wrestler appears to be confused and "out of it." He does not think that he had hit his head but has been saying things that don't make any sense. When you question the wrestler about what he had eaten and when he last took his insulin, he slurs his words and is not able to focus on what you are saying. What should you do next?

Emergencies in the care of athletes are uncommon. However, different sports present different risks for the athletes participating in those sports, and these differing risks increase the challenge for the athletic trainer who must prepare for a variety of sports injuries in a number of different sports (Box 7-1). In general, emergency preparation should begin with a plan to address issues with the facility; the arrangement of transportation; emergency equipment; the personnel involved in the decisions to transport and/or treat; and, ultimately, ongoing care after the initial management has been addressed. The sports medicine team should review and, ideally, practice emergency care prior to the season, so that each member of the team knows his or her role and can execute it without incident. Undoubtedly, preparation and practice for emergency care are the most important components of successful management in the emergency setting.

⊛ *STAT Point 7-1. Preparation and practice for emergency care are critical components of successful management of emergencies.*

Athletic trainers should be aware of field conditions, including possible hazards on or near the field. They should know where emergency transportation personnel are located, how easily an ambulance can get to a player on the field, and what issues with transportation can alter a basic emergency plan. A comprehensive plan should include who should be in charge when a catastrophic injury occurs, the closest and best-equipped hospital to transport the patient to, and the potential consultants to provide emergency care. *(See Chapter 1 for more information on emergency care planning.)*

Sudden Death

The majority of cases of sudden death are related to undiagnosed cardiac conditions, but pulmonary problems, hyperthermia, drug abuse, blunt chest trauma, **sarcoidosis**, and **exercise-induced anaphylaxis**, among others, have also been reported as causes.[1,2] Sudden cardiac death is defined as death within 24 hours of the onset of symptoms,[3] although some authors have used 1 hour as a definition.[1] It is extremely uncommon in athletes, with approximately 100 cases occurring during exertion per year among 25 million participants in competitive sports.[4] It is usually precipitated by activity, and the majority of cases occur in the late afternoon and the evening.[2] In Maron's series of high school and college athletes experiencing nontraumatic death,[2] 134 athletes died of cardiac causes, but only 12 experienced symptoms before their sudden death episode. In a second series,[5] only 8 of 29 athletes experienced symptoms prior to their episode.

The most common cause of sudden cardiac death varies from study to study,[5–8] but in athletes older than age 35 years, it is most commonly results from coronary artery disease.[5,6] The majority of these patients will have at least one risk factor for cardiovascular disease.[9] About half will experience some type of cardiac-related symptoms prior to the episode of sudden death. The incidence is low, generally about 6 per 100,000. No specific pattern of coronary artery disease correlates with the risk of sudden death.[10]

In athletes younger than 35 years of age, a variety of different conditions are responsible for sudden death, but the most common is **hypertrophic cardiomyopathy**, which is generally responsible for about one third of all cases (Box 7-2).[11] In older literature,[4] this condition is cited in almost one half the cases. Hypertrophic cardiomyopathy is a congenital condition with an incidence of about 1 in 500 persons in the general population.[12] The mechanism of sudden cardiac death is not clear, but primary arrhythmias, hemodynamic events associated with diminished stroke volume, and ischemia have all been implicated.[13] Hypertrophic cardiomyopathy is associated with impaired diastolic filling, decreased ventricular compliance, and impaired ventricular emptying resulting from hypertrophy of the interventricular septum and left ventricle (Fig. 7-1). Unfortunately, pre-participation physical examinations do not accurately predict sudden death,[1,2] with the characteristic murmur at the lower left sternal border that increases with standing and decreases with squatting not being a consistent finding. Electrocardiograms demonstrate ventricular hypertrophy and marked symmetrical T-wave inversion and can be an effective screening test, but an echocardiogram is a better test.

⊛ *STAT Point 7-2. Pre-participation physical examinations do not accurately predict those at risk for sudden cardiac death. Electrocardiograms and echocardiograms can be helpful in identifying those at risk but not in all cases.*

An increasingly diagnosed cause of sudden death is **arrhythmogenic right ventricular dysplasia**,[14,15] a genetic condition characterized by replacement of the myocardium by fat and fibrous tissue. The prevalence in the general population is estimated at 1:5000, but in certain regions of Italy the incidence is as high as 0.4 to 0.8%.[16] The disease is diagnosed

---

Box 7-1   Medical Emergencies

1. Sudden cardiac death

2. Exercise-induced anaphylaxis

3. Pulmonary issues

4. Diabetic emergencies

5. Mononucleosis and sickle cell trait

6. Hypertension

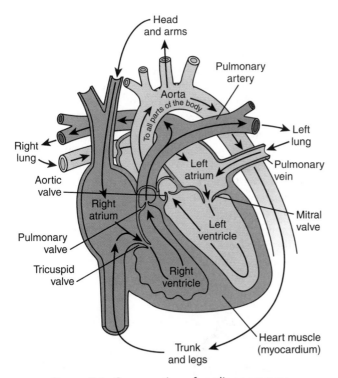

Figure 7-1. Cross section of cardiac anatomy.

in patients younger than 40 years 80% of the time.[17] There is a genetic predisposition, although the true prevalence of the disease is unknown. The areas of fibrosis result in right ventricular arrhythmias during exercise. In Italy, it has been shown to be the most common disease leading to exercise-induced cardiac death in athletes.[18]

Coronary artery anomalies are consistently seen as a cause of sudden death in young athletes, although they are less frequently diagnosed than hypertrophic cardiomyopathy and arrhythmogenic right ventricular dysplasia.[1] The majority of the recorded cases occurred in junior high school and high school athletes,[19] with basketball and soccer being the most common sports of occurrence. The majority will die without prior symptoms, but syncope and chest pain will occur in a minority of cases and clearly should be evaluated with an **angiogram** because echocardiogram and electrocardiogram findings will not typically be present. Stress test results are positive in a minority of the athletes in these cases.[19]

Primary electrophysiological abnormalities represent a group of athletes with structurally normal hearts but who are at increased risk of dying from cardiac arrhythmias (Box 7-3). Included in this group is **long QT syndrome**, **Wolff-Parkinson-White (WPW) syndrome**, and **Brugada syndrome**. Long QT syndrome can be acquired or inherited. It was initially thought that there were two inherited forms: autosomal dominant, the most common, and an autosomal recessive form associated with congenital deafness.[20] More recent data demonstrate that genetic heterogeneity is substantial, and the genetics are more complex than initially thought.[21] The acquired forms are most frequently related to medication use or electrolyte imbalances—in particular, potassium and magnesium. The common feature of long QT syndrome is prolongation of cardiac repolarization. Competitive sports are discouraged for patients with this syndrome, but recreational activities are considered acceptable.[22]

WPW syndrome is a congenital cardiac abnormality in which the ventricle of the heart receives electrical stimulation from accessory pathways from the atrium.[23] These pathways can result in "pre-excitation," a cardiac abnormality in which the ventricular myocardium receives electrical activation from the atrium prior to the normal conduction from the atrioventricular (AV) node. WPW syndrome has been associated with syncope and has been considered a potential cause of sudden death in athletes.[24,25] The diagnosis can be made on electrocardiogram. Atrial fibrillation occurs in 10% to 30% of patients with WPW and may be a risk factor for sudden death,[26] although no specific predictor of sudden death has been found.[26] Treatment is to ablate accessory pathways from the atrium to the ventricle.

Brugada syndrome was first described in 1992[27] and has a high risk for sudden death in young and otherwise-healthy adults. It is a genetic disease characterized by abnormal electrocardiogram findings and is fatal due to ventricular fibrillation. It has a high prevalence in Japan but a much lower prevalence in Europe and the United States.[28] Males appear at higher risk of sudden death. At present, the most accepted treatment is placement of an intracardiac defibrillator.

Valvular heart disease is associated with sudden death in a minority of athletes. **Mitral valve prolapse** has a low incidence of sudden cardiac death, especially if significant mitral regurgitation, **ventricular ectopy,** and a positive family history of sudden death are not present.[13] The condition affects 5% of the general population and is considered the most common cardiac valve disorder.[29] The diagnosis is made on physical examination, with auscultation of a mid systolic to late systolic click. Most physicians adopt a permissive attitude toward participation in sports.[30]

Aortic stenosis has been found in some[9] but not all[1,2] studies of sudden death in athletes (Fig. 7-2). The usual explanation for this is that it should be easily diagnosed on a pre-participation physical examination,[25] with identification of the presence of a harsh systolic murmur that increases on squatting and decreases with Valsalva maneuver.[24] Patients with mild aortic stenosis may participate in all competitive sports, but patients with moderate stenosis may participate in only low-intensity sports, and patients with severe stenosis are generally excluded from sports participation.

Commotio cordis, or cardiac concussion, is defined as sudden cardiac death as a result of blunt, nonpenetrating chest trauma. These athletes do not have antecedent heart disease. It is most common in children and adolescents,

with a mean age of occurrence of 13 years.[9] It is thought that this age group has a compliant chest wall that facilitates the transmission of the force from the blow through the chest to the myocardium. The most common scenario is in baseball, where a batter is hit with a pitched ball,[31] but a karate kick, a helmet-to-chest tackle, and a lacrosse ball were also mechanisms of commotio cordis[31] cited in the literature, and in no case was the force of the blow considered excessive. An animal model replicating the events of commotio cordis demonstrated that the blow must be directly over the heart and occur within 15 to 30 microseconds of the T-wave peak, which is the vulnerable phase of cardiac repolarization.[32,33]

Viral myocarditis with or without left ventricular dysfunction is associated with cardiac arrhythmias and sudden death.[34] These patients typically present with chest discomfort and dyspnea, in addition to a variety of symptoms associated with viral infections.[35] Although coxsackie viruses have been thought to be responsible for most of these infections,[36] a variety of viruses are now considered to cause this condition.[35] Diagnosis can be difficult, with a variety of studies, including myocardial biopsy, and polymerase chain reaction/reverse transcriptase-polymerase studies failing to demonstrate an infectious agent in some cases.[35]

Myocarditis has also been associated with sudden death in **Kawasaki disease** secondary to coronary arteritis, leading to **aneurysm** formation,[37] and sarcoidosis[2,38] (Fig. 7-3). In sarcoidosis, sudden death may be the presenting manifestation of the disease because sarcoidosis is known to have an affinity for the conduction system of the heart.[39]

Ruptured aortic aneurysm is associated with **Marfan's syndrome**, a genetic disorder of connective tissue with an incidence as high as 1 in 3000.[40] Blood pressure increases during sports stress the aortic walls and may result in increased risk of aortic aneurysm rupture. The diagnosis of Marfan's syndrome should occur during the pre-participation examination and is often seen in volleyball and basketball players where the prevalence of aortic root dilation was 10 times that of other sports.[40] Athletes with Marfan's syndrome should be restricted from intense athletic competition; if the diagnosis

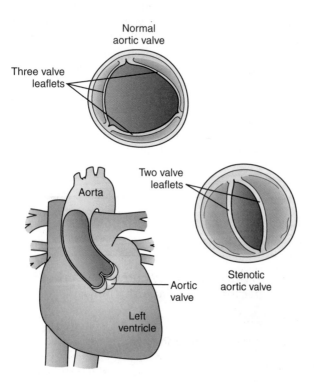

Figure 7-2. Aortic stenosis.

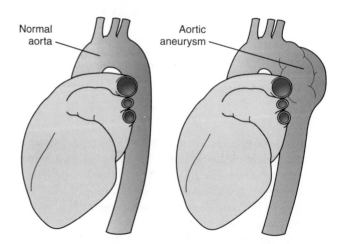

Figure 7-3. Aneurysm in vessel wall.

is missed, the rate of aortic dilatation and ruptured aortic aneurysm is thought to increase.[41] Diagnosis of aortic aneurysm can be challenging because the condition can present with a variety of signs and symptoms, including chest pain, back pain, syncope, heart failure, limb ischemia, pulse deficits, and cerebrovascular manifestations.[42]

A small number of deaths in athletes has been related to use of supplements such as ephedra or drugs such as anabolic steroids or cocaine.[9] Theses deaths are thought to be largely inferential because of the time between ingestion and the episode of sudden death.[9] Cocaine use is associated with a wide range of arrhythmias (benign and malignant), **aortic dissection**, and **cardiomyopathy.**[43] *(For more information on sudden cardiac death, see Chapter 4.)*

Management of Victims of Sudden Cardiac Death

Management of sudden cardiac death begins with basic life support. Major management errors were uncovered by research in the science of resuscitation after guidelines for basic life support were changed in the year 2000. To correct these errors, guidelines were altered again in 2005.[44] The most important of these errors were the long pauses that occurred without chest compressions and the suboptimal compressions that typically occur during basic life support. Animal models have demonstrated that these result in inadequate blood flow during cardiac arrest and reduce chances of restoring spontaneous circulation and survival.[45] At the same time, ventilation during cardiac arrest is frequently excessive and potentially harmful, producing adverse effects on coronary perfusion pressure as a result of impaired venous return from high intrathoracic pressures.[46] These findings have resulted in recommendations for a ratio of chest compressions to ventilation of 30:2, a compression rate of 100 per minute, and pauses for 2 ventilations limited to 1 second per ventilation.

Automated External Defibrillators

The development and use of automated external defibrillators (AEDs) has shifted emphasis from basic life support to the delivery of electric current when indicated.[47] Use of external defibrillators has been associated with two issues. First, if used early in the resuscitation, a period of blood flow with cardiopulmonary resuscitation (CPR) preceding defibrillation may improve fibrillation success. Second, analyzing the rhythm before and after defibrillation increases the period where chest compressions are not being performed and should be avoided.[48,49] It is now recommended that a period of cardiopulmonary resuscitation of 90 to 120 seconds precedes use of an AED if resuscitation is started more than 5 minutes after the athlete collapses. It is also recommended that chest compressions begin immediately after use of an AED. Finally, if the AED the athletic trainer is using has adjustable energy outputs, the trainer should know if the AED being used is

monophasic, biphasic truncated exponential (BTE), or rectilinear biphasic (RB). Monophasic defibrillator waveforms are being phased out, but if the AED used is monophasic, it is recommended that the highest energy output of 360 joules be used for the first shock. If a BTE waveform is being used, 150 to 200 joules can be utilized for the first shock. For an RB waveform, 120 joules is recommended for the first shock.[47]

Exercise-Induced Anaphylaxis

Exercise-induced anaphylaxis is a rare form of physical allergy that occurs during physical activity. It has become increasingly recognized in the past 30 years as more people participate in sports.[50] Three major types of the condition are described: (1) **cholinergic urticaria,** (2) classic exercise-induced anaphylaxis, and (3) variant type exercise-induced anaphylaxis. These may occur separately or together. Cholinergic urticaria is a skin condition manifested by small (2–5 mm) punctate papules surrounded by an erythematous base usually occurring about 6 minutes into exercise. Lesions come on in response to exercise, warming, or emotional stress and generally begin on the chest and neck but may occur anywhere on the body. Increased lacrimation, salivation, and diarrhea may occur from cholinergic stimulation, and if the inciting stress persists, hives and angioedema may occur but vascular collapse is uncommon. Symptoms typically resolve in 2 to 4 hours. Onset typically occurs between 10 and 30 years of age.[51] Diagnosis of exercise-induced urticaria can be made with the results of a methacholine skin test challenge.

Exercise-induced anaphylaxis is most commonly precipitated by running, but a variety of activities have been associated with its occurrence. Symptoms last from 30 minutes to 4 hours after cessation of activity. Symptoms are not consistently reproducible,[50] even in a laboratory situation. These patients present with systemic symptoms often in a sequence beginning with fatigue, generalized warmth, pruritus, and erythema that progresses to an urticarial eruption. Transient periods of lost consciousness occur in some patients, and a completely developed attack includes choking, stridor, and gastrointestinal colic, with nausea and vomiting. Skin manifestations will include hives (erythematous lesions) 10 to 15 mm in size. The diagnosis is most commonly made by history, but passive warming may help differentiate cholinergic urticaria from exercise-induced anaphylaxis,[52] and exercise challenge testing under controlled conditions also is used. Exercise challenge testing can be difficult because of variability of symptom occurrence.

Variant type exercise-induced anaphylaxis is the least common form of exercise-induced anaphylaxis. It is characterized by punctuate urticaria (2–4 mm) associated with exercise-induced vascular collapse. It is precipitated only by exercise and not by vascular warming.[53] Choking and stridor resulting from upper airway edema occur in some patients with exercise-induced anaphylaxis, but changes in pulmonary function are uncommon.[53]

Treatment of exercise-induced anaphylaxis consists of subcutaneous epinephrine, intravenous (IV) fluid, oxygen, antihistamines, and airway maintenance. Once the athlete is stabilized, prophylactic use of antihistamines and anticholinergic medications and a search for precipitating causes should be initiated. Exercising with a partner, quick availability of an autoinjector of epinephrine (such as an EpiPen), and patient education are highly advisable; patient education about the disease will also help to reduce the rate of recurrences. In the literature, only one death has been attributed to this disorder.[53]

Pulmonary Problems: Acute Asthma

Asthma is a chronic inflammatory disorder of the airways associated with hyperresponsiveness of the inflammatory system, reversible airflow limitation, and respiratory symptoms.[54] It is the most common chronic lung disease in both the developed and developing worlds. Overall, 6% of children in the United States younger than age 19 have asthma, the highest prevalence in any age group.[55] From 1980 to 1994, a 160% increase in asthma prevalence for children up to age 4 has been observed.[56] Among all children, asthma prevalence is greatest in urban areas, with some parts of inner cities reporting rates as high as 14%. Of this percentage, the prevalence is highest among African Americans and those living in households with low family income.[56] All patients with asthma are at risk of having exacerbations, characterized by a progressive increase in shortness of breath, cough, wheezing, or chest tightness and by a decrease in expiratory airflow that can be quantified by simple measures of pulmonary function such as peak expiratory flow rate (PEFR).[57]

✪ *STAT Point 7-3. Asthma is the most common chronic lung disease.*

✪ *STAT Point 7-4. The prevalence of asthma is highest among African Americans and those living in low-income households.*

✪ *STAT Point 7-5. Signs and symptoms of an asthma attack include progressive increase in shortness of breath, coughing, wheezing, or chest tightness and a decrease in peak expiratory flow rate.*

With this in mind, asthma presents a special challenge to athletic trainers and sports medicine physicians alike. Not only must these health care workers be proficient in assessment and management of sports-related injuries, but they also must be particularly adept at recognizing the features of an impending or ongoing asthma attack. Early treatment of asthma is essential.

Asthma triggers cause exacerbations by inducing airway inflammation, provoking acute bronchospasm, or

both (Fig. 7-4). The most frequently identified triggers include allergen exposure, air pollutants, respiratory tract infections, exercise, weather changes, foods, additives, drugs, and extreme emotional responses (Box 7-4). The mechanisms of airflow limitation vary according to the stimulus. Allergen-induced bronchoconstriction results from the release from airway mast cells of mediators, including histamine, prostaglandins, and leukotrienes, that contract the smooth muscle. Acute airflow limitation may also occur because airways in asthma are hyperresponsive to a wide variety of stimuli. In this case, the mechanisms for causing bronchoconstriction consist in combinations of release of mediators from inflammatory cells and stimulation of local and central neural reflexes. Finally, airflow limitation results from edematous swelling of the airway wall with or without smooth muscle contraction. The increase in microvascular permeability and leakage leads to mucosal thickening and swelling of the airway outside the smooth muscle (Box 7-5).[57]

Progressive airway narrowing resulting from airway inflammation and/or increased bronchiolar smooth muscle tone is the hallmark of an asthma attack and leads to increased flow resistance, pulmonary hyperinflation, and ventilation/perfusion mismatching. Without correction of airway obstruction, respiratory failure is a consequence of increased work of breathing, gas exchange inefficiency, and respiratory muscle exhaustion.[57]

Two different scenarios are involved in the progression of an asthma attack.[58] When airway inflammation is predominant, patients show a progressive (over many hours, days, or even weeks) clinical and functional deterioration.

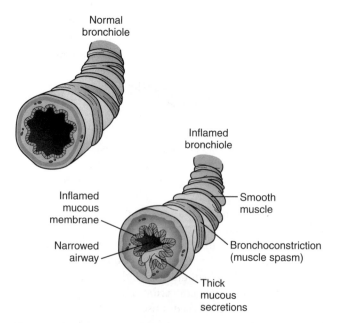

Figure 7-4. Normal airway and constricted airway. In the constricted airway, the muscles around the bronchial tubes are contracted, narrowing the passageway. In addition, an inflammatory response results in increased mucous production, further obstructing airflow.

Box 7-4 Common Asthma Triggers

- **Allergen exposure**
- **Air pollutants**
- **Respiratory tract infections**
- **Exercise**
- **Weather changes**
- **Foods**
- **Additives**
- **Drugs**
- **Extreme emotional responses**

Box 7-5 Mechanisms of Airway Constriction

- **Release of mast cell mediators that contract smooth muscle**
- **Constriction of smooth muscle secondary to stimulation of central neural reflexes**
- **Swelling of airway wall secondary to microvascular permeability and leakage**

Box 7-6 Common Signs and Symptoms of Worsening Asthma

- **Coughing**
- **Shortness of breath**
- **Wheezing**
- **Tightness in the chest**

---

symptoms.[60] Severe symptoms include **pulsus paradoxus** (a decrease in systolic blood pressure by at least 12 mmHg during inspiration), use of accessory muscles of inspiration (sternocleidomastoid muscles), diaphoresis, and inability to lie supine because of breathlessness.[62] If an athlete presents with any of these symptoms, it is the athletic trainer's responsibility to quickly assess the severity of the attack.

✪ *STAT Point 7-6. An important sign that an athlete's asthma is worsening is use of a quick-relief rescue inhaler more than twice a week because of symptoms.*

Disease severity is determined by clinical examination, pulmonary function measurements, asthma symptoms, and the need for rescue medication. Several factors complicate the assessment of asthma severity. Disease classification is based on the symptoms the patient had before starting treatment. In addition, asthma is a variable disease. Studies have shown that patients with asthma rarely remain in the same category over time and that patients themselves often underestimate their symptoms.[61,63]

Particular attention should be given to the athlete's general appearance. Those with the most severe conditions will be sitting upright.[62] The use of accessory muscles can also be used as an indicator of severe obstruction.[57] The presence of sternocleidomastoid retractions or suprasternal retractions correlates well with severe impairment in lung function.[57,64]

Wheeze and dyspnea are present in virtually all patients with acute asthma, and they correlate poorly with the degree of airflow limitation.[65] Respiratory rate (RR) >30 breaths per minute, tachycardia >120 beats per minute, or pulsus paradoxus >12 mm Hg have also been described as vital signs of acute severe asthma. Of importance, in a series of patients with near-fatal attacks, few arrhythmias other than sinus tachycardia or bradycardias were found.[57]

When an acute asthma attack begins, athletic trainers should perform a peak expiratory flow measurement to aid in guiding initial management (Box 7-7). Athletes may not be able to perform a complete peak flow measurement, and this should be interpreted as an indicator of a severe exacerbation. Once one to three measurements have been performed, the readings can be compared to the athlete's

Data from multiple cohort studies show that the prevalence of this type of asthma progression is between 80% and 90% of all adults with acute asthma who present to the emergency department.[57] In the second scenario, bronchospasm is predominant and patients present with a sudden-onset asthma attack. It is characterized by rapid development of airway obstruction in less than 3 to 6 hours after the onset of the attack. These patients show a more rapid and complete response to treatment.[58,59]

Prior to evaluating the severity of an asthma exacerbation, athletes and athletic trainers must be proficient in recognizing all of the possible symptoms that encompass an exacerbation. Common symptoms are coughing, shortness of breath, wheezing, and a feeling of tightness in the chest (Box 7-6).[60] Other symptoms include night cough, worsening symptoms at night, fast breathing and symptoms occurring or worsening with exercise, viral infections, changes in weather, strong emotions, or menses. Symptoms that occur in the presence of animals, dust mites, mold, smoke, pollen, or chemicals may also be present.[61] Another clue that an athlete's asthma is flaring up is requiring extra doses of quick-relief rescue inhaler more than twice a week because of

Box 7-7   Use of Peak Flow Meter

1. Reset the indicator of the peak flow meter by shaking or swinging the meter until the colored indicator is resting within the diamond shape near the mouthpiece.

2. The patient should take as deep a breath as possible.

3. The patient should put the mouthpiece in his or her mouth, sealing lips around it.

4. The patient should blow out as hard and as fast as possible.

5. Read the peak expiratory flow as the number indicated by the new position of the colored indicator.

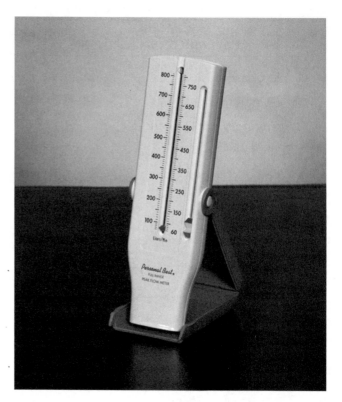

Figure 7-5. Peak flow meter.

personal best, a value that both the athlete and athletic trainer should be aware of. Peak flow readings can then be applied to an athlete's asthma action plan to guide appropriate management (Fig. 7-5). During mild exacerbations, athletes may notice shortness of breath with walking or exercise but feel normal at rest. They can usually breathe well enough to talk in complete sentences. Wheezing may be audible, but it is mostly at the end of expiration. Peak flow readings will be 80% to 100% of the athlete's personal best (Table 7-1). During moderate exacerbations, athletes may feel short of breath with talking or lying supine. Communication is in a few words rather than whole sentences, which worsen the feeling of shortness of breath. Athletes may be anxious or tense. Neck musculature may be used to help take deeper breaths. Loud wheezing is audible, in particular with exhalation. Peak flow readings will range from 50% to 80% of personal best. During severe exacerbations, breathing will be very labored and faster than usual. Athletes will feel short of breath even at rest. Dyspnea limits speech to a few words at a time, often punctuated with forced inspiration. Peak flow readings will be less than 50% of personal best. As severe exacerbations progress, the athlete may become sleepy and confused, and the work of breathing will make them increasingly fatigued.[61]

⭐ *STAT Point 7-7. Athletic trainers and team physicians should be aware of an asthmatic athlete's personal best peak expiratory flow readings.*

The primary goals of therapy for acute asthma are the rapid reversal of airflow obstruction and the correction, if necessary, of severe **hypercapnia** or **hypoxemia**.[66] Doctors do not consistently teach patients the appropriate steps to take in response to an asthma attack. Patients were likely to administer rescue medication at the onset of the exacerbation or just before an emergency department visit but were nonadherent with all other National Heart Lung and Blood Institute (NHLBI) recommendations.[56]

Inhaled short-acting **beta-2 agonists** are the mainstay of emergent treatment of acute asthma exacerbations.[67] Albuterol is the most widely used short-acting beta-2 agonist in the acute setting.[68] Their onset of action is rapid, and their side effects are well tolerated. Albuterol has an onset of action of 5 minutes and duration of action of 6 hours. Other used drugs are metaproterenol, terbutaline, and fenoterol. Long-acting beta-2 agonists cannot be recommended for emergency treatment because of their longer onset time for effectiveness. The inhaled route has a faster onset and fewer adverse effects and is more effective than systemic routes (IV, oral medication in pill form, injection).[57] Doses and dosing intervals should be individualized using objective measures of airflow obstruction (i.e., peak flow meters) as guides. A substantial body of evidence supports the use of high and repeated doses. The aim of treatment is to induce maximal stimulation of beta-2 receptors without causing significant side effects.[57] Treatment should be individualized for the patient by his or her doctor and documented for the athletic trainer, who should have access to the medications at practice and competition for ready use.

Approximately two thirds of patients will be sensitive to inhaled albuterol, and the optimal treatment for this group is for the medication to be delivered by metered dose inhaler (MDI) with spacer (Fig. 7-6) or by **nebulizer**

Table 7-1   **Peak Expiratory Flow Readings**

Percentage of Athlete Personal Best	Category of Exacerbation	Signs and Symptoms	Action*
80%–100%	Mild	Shortness of breath during activity but normal at rest; wheezing with expiration; able to talk in complete sentences	
50%–80%	Moderate	Shortness of breath while talking; not using complete sentences; loud wheezing; athlete anxious; accessory muscles may be used during inspiration	
<50%	Severe	Breathing rapid and very labored; shortness of breath at rest; difficulty speaking; use of accessory muscles for inspiration; athlete very anxious; athlete may become sleepy and/or confused	

*Management actions for each category will be dictated by team physician. Athletes should always be educated on proper management actions. Severe exacerbations should always be considered an emergency requiring immediate transfer.

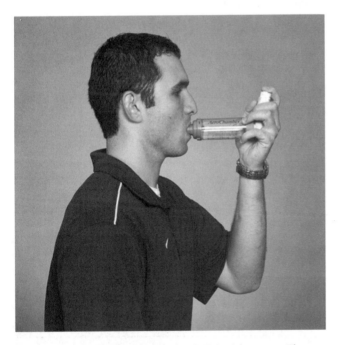

Figure 7-6. Metered dose inhaler (MDI) with spacer. The spacer increases the effectiveness of the MDI in delivering the medication efficiently.

(Fig. 7-7).[69,70] For the remainder of patients, albuterol even in high doses has little effect. A more slowly resolving asthma attack is likely demonstrative of significant airway inflammation.[57]

Administration of inhaled beta-2 agonists may be performed using small-volume nebulizers or MDIs. Studies show these methods appear to be equally effective for children and adults of all ages and with a wide range of illness severity.[68] Each beta-2 agonist treatment with an MDI and spacer takes 1 to 2 minutes as compared with 15 to 20 minutes for each treatment with a nebulizer. It seems reasonable to conclude that the MDI plus spacer is the most efficient way to deliver high doses of bronchodilators to a patient with acute severe asthma.[57] Nebulizers generate a relatively large particle size in which up to 90% of the medication remains in the machine or is lost to the atmosphere from the expiratory port.[66,68] Although portable battery-operated nebulizers are now available, many still remain constrained by the need for an external power source.

Side effects of beta-2 agonists are dose dependent and can occur with all routes of administration. Inhaled administration is associated with the least frequency of side effects. Receptors on vascular smooth muscle result in tachycardia and tachyarrhythmia. Those on skeletal muscle generate tremor and hypokalemia (as a result of potassium entry into muscle cells). Lastly, cells involved in lipid and carbohydrate metabolism cause an increase in blood-free fatty acids, insulin, glucose, and pyruvate.[57] The most common side effect seen after administration of beta-2 agonists is a fine tremor.

Managing Asthma Attacks

When confronted with an evolving asthma attack, athletic trainers should begin therapy with albuterol delivered via MDI and spacer. The usual dosing is 2 to 4 puffs delivered every 15 to 20 minutes for a total maximum of 3 doses. No studies describing optimal dosing for albuterol by MDIs have been performed. The 1997 NHLBI guidelines state that studies show that equivalent bronchodilation can be

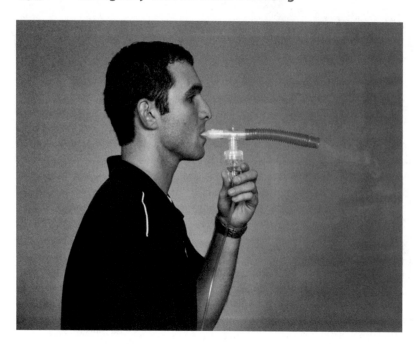

Figure 7-7. Nebulizers turn a liquid beta-2 agonist into an easily inhaled aerosol using pressurized oxygen. This is helpful for patients with asthma who have difficulty using an MDI. Note the tubing delivering oxygen from the nebulizer.

achieved by high doses (6–12 puffs) of a beta-2 agonist by MDI with a spacer.[68] The athlete's peak flow should be measured just before and a few minutes following administration of each dosing.

Current guidelines encourage institution of systemic corticosteroids as soon as insufficient improvement with beta agonist bronchodilators is identified. Patients in this category include those with the following: (1) less than 10% improvement in peak flow rates after the first dose of inhaled beta agonists, (2) an asthma attack that has developed despite daily or alternate day oral corticosteroids, and (3) a peak flow rate less than 70% of personal best after the initial hour of treatment.

It is important to point out that the onset of action of systemic corticosteroids is not clinically apparent until as long as 6 hours after administration. Thus, the beneficial effect is not likely to be observed during the few hours an athlete spends in the presence of an athletic trainer. Early administration helps to minimize the delay in improvement anticipated with systemic steroids.[66]

The dose of corticosteroids depends on the agent and route of administration. Prednisone, the most common oral corticosteroid in the United States used for asthma exacerbations in adults and teenagers, is generally dosed according to the patient's weight. The dosing regimen should be outlined by the athlete's team physician. The most common initial dose range given for teenagers and adults in an acute asthma exacerbation is 5 to 60 mg.

Studies comparing the use of oral versus inhaled corticosteroids in the emergency department are inconclusive at the present time. Several studies have found benefits of inhaled corticosteroids compared to oral corticosteroids in regard to earlier discharge, less vomiting, decreased relapse rate, improved clinical parameters, and improved pulmonary function.[68,71] Other studies have found equivalent outcomes between oral and inhaled corticosteroids.[68,72] Another study found improved pulmonary function and a lower relapse rate with oral prednisone compared to inhaled fluticasone.[68,73] The routine use of inhaled corticosteroids in addition to or instead of systemic corticosteroids in the management of acute asthma exacerbation in children cannot be recommended.[68]

Short-term side effects associated with oral and inhaled corticosteroids include, but are not limited to, blurry vision, abdominal pain, gastric irritation, nausea, vomiting, frequent urination, increased thirst, numbness, confusion, excitement, depression, hallucinations, and skin redness. Long-term side effects include increased fat deposition, headache, irregular heartbeat, menstrual problems, muscle cramping, pain, nausea, growth impairment, skin changes, edema, weakness, and vomiting (Box 7-8).[74]

Box 7-8   Side Effects of Oral and Inhaled Corticosteroids

Short term: blurred vision, abdominal pain, gastric irritation, nausea, vomiting, frequent urination, increased thirst, numbness, confusion, excitement, depression, hallucinations, and skin redness

Long term: increased fat deposition, headache, irregular heartbeat, menstrual problems, muscle cramping, pain, nausea, growth impairment, skin changes, edema, weakness, and vomiting

Indications for Referral to the Emergency Department

An athletic trainer with appropriate asthma education, proficiency in peak flow measurements, and a good understanding of appropriate management options will be well equipped to initially manage an impending asthma exacerbation. Even with appropriate management, an athlete's decline or lack of improvement in respiratory status may warrant emergency department referral. Indications for seeking emergency treatment are as follows: (1) peak flows of less than 50% of personal best; (2) peak flows of 50% to 80% of personal best that are unresponsive to bronchodilator therapy and have a decline in flow rate; (3) rapid decline of lung function evidenced by increasing symptoms of uncontrolled cough, breathlessness, or wheezing; (4) failure of peak expiratory flow to exceed 60% of personal best after inhaled bronchodilator therapy has been initiated or <2 hours duration of bronchodilation; (5) suprasternal retraction and/or use of accessory muscles; (6) cyanosis or pallor of nailbeds; and (7) speaking in words or phrases rather than sentences (Box 7-9).[75]

Risk Factors for Death

The National Asthma and Education Prevention Program's Expert Panel Report 2 provides a detailed list of risk factors for death from asthma (Box 7-10). These risk factors should

---

Box 7-10   Risk Factors for Death Secondary to Asthma

- Past history of sudden severe exacerbations
- Prior intubation or intensive care unit admission for asthma
- Two or more hospitalizations for asthma in the past year
- Three or more emergency care visits for asthma in the past year
- Hospitalization or an emergency care visit for asthma within the past month
- Use of two or more canisters per month of inhaled short-acting beta-2 agonist
- Current use of systemic corticosteroids or recent withdrawal from systemic corticosteroids
- Difficulty perceiving airflow obstruction or its severity
- Comorbidity as from cardiovascular disease or chronic obstructive pulmonary disease
- Serious psychiatric disease, psychological problems, or illicit drug use
- Low socioeconomic status and urban residence
- Sensitivity to the mold *Alternaria.*

Box 7-9   Indications for Immediate Referral to Emergency Department

- Peak flows of less than 50% of personal best
- Peak flows of 50% to 80% of personal best that are unresponsive to bronchodilator therapy and have a decline in flow rate
- Rapid decline of lung function evidenced by increasing symptoms of uncontrolled cough, breathlessness, or wheezing
- Failure of peak expiratory flow to exceed 60% of personal best after inhaled bronchodilator therapy has been initiated, or <2 hours duration of bronchodilation
- Suprasternal retraction and/or use of accessory muscles
- Cyanosis or pallor of nailbeds
- Speaking in words or phrases rather than sentences

---

be considered when confronted with an asthma exacerbation that warrants transport to an emergency room:

1. Past history of sudden severe exacerbations
2. Prior intubation or intensive care unit admission for asthma
3. Two or more hospitalizations for asthma in the past year
4. Three or more emergency care visits for asthma in the past year
5. Hospitalization or an emergency care visit for asthma within the past month
6. Use of two or more canisters per month of inhaled short-acting beta-2 agonist
7. Current use of systemic corticosteroids or recent withdrawal from systemic corticosteroids
8. Difficulty perceiving airflow obstruction or its severity

9. Comorbidity as from cardiovascular disease or chronic obstructive pulmonary disease

10. Serious psychiatric disease, psychological problems, or illicit drug use

11. Low socioeconomic status and urban residence

12. Sensitivity to the mold *Alternaria*[75]

Athletes with risk factors for death from asthma may require closer monitoring by athletic trainers, parents, and physicians. Athletic trainers should be proactive in coordinating this relationship among all members involved. In addition to a more detailed history, patients should be categorized according to the NHLBI asthma severity classification scheme.

Athletes who have positive risk factors for death from asthma, live a long distance from the emergency department, have poor social support, experience rapid decline, or are unresponsive to bronchodilator therapy should activate emergency medical services (EMS) for timely treatment and transport to the emergency department.[75] As a fail-safe, athletes, parents, and athletic trainers should be taught, if in doubt, to err on the side of caution and activate EMS for help.

⭐ *STAT Point 7-8. Athletes, parents, coaches, and athletic trainers should be taught that if in doubt about the proper management for an asthma attack to err on the side of caution and activate EMS.*

Diabetes Mellitus

Diabetes mellitus is a group of metabolic disorders resulting from defects in insulin secretion, action, or both. It is generally divided into four separate groups: (1) absolute insulin deficiency; (2) impaired insulin secretion and peripheral insulin resistance; (3) secondary to metabolic disorders, drugs, or other diseases; and (4) gestational diabetes. Historically, about 80% of patients have impaired insulin secretion and peripheral insulin resistance (type 2 diabetes), and about 15% have insulin deficiency (type 1 diabetes).[76] However, in children, only 2% to 3% of all diabetes was a result of impaired insulin secretion.[77] In the past 10 years, a 10-fold increase in the incidence of impaired insulin secretion has been reported in children.[78,79] These children are predisposed to diabetes by being obese, leading a sedentary lifestyle, and eating a high-fat and low-fiber diet[80]—risk factors not generally associated with athletics. However, a genetic predisposition exists for some individuals. The average age of onset of these children is 12 to 14 years of age,[80] and women are more often affected than men.

The development of type 2 diabetes is generally thought of as a gradual process, and many adolescents will not have undergone screening, so the athletic trainer may see these patients before the diagnosis is established and may have to manage the initial difficulties with hypoglycemia, hyperglycemia, dehydration, and electrolyte imbalances with exercise when the disease first occurs. These athletes will often present with hyperglycemia; dehydration; and, in most cases, electrolyte imbalances. In almost all cases, they will require transport to an emergency room. Both the team physician and athletic trainer will want these athletes to be transferred to an emergency room for proper laboratory work, including glucose, electrolyte, blood urea nitrogen, and complete blood count levels. Appropriate management of uncontrolled diabetes requires transfer.

⭐ *STAT Point 7-9. Appropriate management of uncontrolled diabetes requires transfer to an emergency department.*

To guard against noncompliance with medication dosage, both athletic trainers and physicians may need to constantly supervise athletes with established diabetes.[81] Older athletes with diabetes are at risk for cardiac disease,[82] foot fractures,[83] and ocular complications.[82]

For all athletes with diabetes, the main risk of exercise is hypoglycemia, which can occur during and after exercise.[84] The intensity of exercise, the duration of exercise, and the level of training can predispose to hypoglycemia; at higher intensities and longer durations, poorly conditioned athletes will present the greatest risk. Planning pre-practice meals; providing carbohydrates during practices; and carefully monitoring glucose levels before, during, and after practice and games can prevent episodes. When episodes of hypoglycemia occur, having a ready source of carbohydrate minimizes complications.

⭐ *STAT Point 7-10. For all athletes with diabetes, the main risk of exercise is hypoglycemia during or following exercise. Paying attention to meal planning, providing carbohydrates during practices, and monitoring of glucose levels can prevent episodes. When episodes of hypoglycemia occur, having a ready source of carbohydrate minimizes complications.*

Athletes who do not adequately dose themselves with insulin are at risk of developing hyperglycemia, and potentially **diabetic ketoacidosis**, provoking a medical emergency. Hyperglycemia predisposes the athlete to **osmotic diuresis** and dehydration. The exact blood glucose levels at which exercise is contraindicated is controversial, and many athletes may try to practice and compete when they should not. The underlying insulin deficiency produces activation of cortisol, catecholamines, and growth hormone, resulting in breakdown of triglycerides and release of free fatty acids. These are released into the circulation and are taken up by the liver where they are converted into ketone bodies and released into the circulation. Diabetic ketoacidosis is a true medical emergency[85] and requires hospital admission.[85]

✪ *STAT Point 7-11. Diabetic ketoacidosis is a medical emergency and requires hospital admission for appropriate management.*

Clinically, diabetic ketoacidosis is most often seen in type 1 diabetes and often develops over a day or two. It often presents with **polydipsia** and **polyuria** and is associated with abdominal pain, nausea, and vomiting. Weight loss, weakness, and drowsiness are less frequent symptoms. Deep rapid breathing is also typical.[85] Dehydration is common and often difficult to assess.[86] Laboratory studies are required to establish the diagnosis of diabetic ketoacidosis and to assess the severity, although a patient with diabetes and a change in mental status is likely to have at least a moderate if not severe case.[86]

The management of diabetic ketoacidosis requires fluid and electrolyte therapy; insulin therapy; treatment of the precipitating causes; and a period of monitoring urine output, blood pressure, mental status, electrolytes, glucose, ketones, and potential complications. The most common complications include cerebral edema, pulmonary edema, electrolyte imbalances, hyperchloremic metabolic acidosis, vascular thrombosis, and renal failure. Any athlete with suspected diabetic ketoacidosis requires immediate transport to an emergency room.

The hyperglycemic hyperosmolar state is the other extreme in the spectrum of diabetic decompensation. Insulin deficiency results in hyperglycemia but not in ketone body production, and hyperglycemia and dehydration result. The reason for the absence of ketosis remains unknown.[87] The approach to diagnosis and treatment is similar to diabetic ketoacidosis, but there is a higher mortality rate.[88] The hyperglycemic hyperosmolar state is more often seen in older patients with type 2 diabetes and often develops over weeks.[89] Management with insulin, fluids, and frequent monitoring is similar to diabetic ketoacidosis.

Mononucleosis

The Epstein-Barr virus is the infectious agent in **mononucleosis**. Although most Epstein-Barr infections are asymptomatic,[90] mononucleosis syndrome is most commonly seen in adolescents and young adults. Infectious mononucleosis is characterized by a prolonged incubation period of 30 to 50 days[91] and an extremely wide array of clinical manifestations,[92] with nearly every organ system in the body potentially being involved. Diagnosis of mononucleosis syndrome is usually made clinically by the presence of sore throat, fever, headache, **lymphadenopathy,** and malaise, associated with a complete blood count demonstrating a **lymphocytosis** and the presence of atypical lymphocytes making up greater than 10% of the total white blood cell count. The heterophil antibody test, also known as the monospot, is positive in about 90% of older children and young adults with the syndrome,[92] but the test is positive in only 60% at 2 weeks and 90% at 4 weeks after

---

Box 7-11	**Signs and Symptoms of Mononucleosis**

- ■ Sore throat
- ■ Fever
- ■ Headache
- ■ Fatigue
- ■ Enlarged, tender lymph nodes
- ■ Enlarge spleen
- ■ Positive laboratory results
- ■ Positive monospot test (not 100% diagnostic)

---

symptoms are noted (Box 7-11). Because mononucleosis is associated with spontaneous rupture of the spleen,[93] it is imperative that the diagnosis be made quickly and efficiently, so the athlete is not put at unnecessary risk. In some cases, serologic testing should be performed. The majority of splenic ruptures occur between day 4 and 21 of symptoms; holding the athlete until spleen size is normal is recommended.[94]

Sickle Cell Trait

Although **sickle cell trait** is generally considered benign,[95] it has been associated with an increased risk of sudden death during exercise.[96] Risk factors for athletes with sickle trait include heat, dehydration, altitude, and asthma. There is also increased risk of splenic infarction and **rhabdomyolysis.**[97] Although screening is not recommended and high-level athletic activity is clearly possible, athletes with a history of collapse with exercise and sickle cell trait should be well hydrated and well monitored. Players may complain of cramplike pain in the legs and/or back when sickling occurs.[95]

Hypertension

More than 58 million people older than age 18 years are affected by **hypertension** (HTN) in the United States, and the prevalence of HTN increases with age. Recent research shows an increased lifetime risk of developing HTN and cardiovascular complications associated with blood pressure (BP) levels previously considered in the normal range. In an attempt to increase awareness of this major public health concern, the Joint National Committee (JNC-7) has introduced a new classification system for HTN:

- ■ Prehypertension: Systolic blood pressure (SBP) 120 to 139 or diastolic blood pressure (DBP) 80 to 89

- Stage I HTN: SBP 140 to 159 or DBP 90 to 99
- Stage II HTN: SBP >160 or DBP >100

Lifestyle modifications are advocated for the prevention, treatment, and control of HTN, with exercise being an integral component. The sports medicine community needs to be aware of a potentially life-threatening spectrum of clinical presentations where uncontrolled BP can lead to progressive or impending target organ dysfunction (TOD) known as hypertensive crises. The key clinical distinction between hypertensive emergency and hypertensive urgency is the presence of acute TOD and not on the absolute level of the BP.

Hypertensive Emergency

Hypertensive emergencies represent severe HTN *with* acute impairment of the central nervous system (CNS), cardiovascular system, or the renal system. These are considered target organ systems because they are most directly affected by changes in BP. To prevent permanent damage to target organs, the BP should be lowered aggressively over minutes to hours.

Hypertensive Urgency

Hypertensive urgency is defined as a severe elevation of BP *without* evidence of progressive TOD. These patients require BP control over several days to weeks.

Epidemiology

Hypertensive crises affect about 500,000 Americans or approximately 1% of adults with hypertension. They are more common in African Americans when compared with other races. Similarly, HTN develops at an earlier age, leads to more clinical manifestations, and is more common and severe in African Americans compared with age-matched non-Hispanic whites. Hypertensive crises are two times more frequent in males than in females, and the overall prevalence and incidence of HTN is slightly higher in men than in women. Both are more common with advancing age.

Mortality and Morbidity

The morbidity and mortality of hypertensive emergencies depend on the extent of initial TOD and the degree to which BP is controlled subsequently. With BP control and medication compliance, the 10-year survival rate of patients with hypertensive crises approaches 70%.

- One-year mortality rate for an untreated hypertensive emergency is greater than 90%.
- Five-year survival rate among all patients presenting with a hypertensive crisis is 74%.
- Median survival is 144 months for all patients presenting to the emergency department with a hypertensive crisis.

Death rates from both ischemic heart disease and stroke increase progressively as the BP increases. For every 20 mm Hg systolic or 10 mm diastolic increase in BP, the mortality rate from both ischemic heart disease and stroke doubles.

Acute Treatment Considerations

Optimal control of hypertensive situations balances the benefits of immediate decreases in BP against the risk of a significant decrease in target organ blood flow. The certified athletic trainer must be capable of the following:

- Appropriately evaluating patients with an elevated BP
- Determining the aggressiveness and timing of therapeutic interventions
- Making disposition decisions about obtaining further evaluation and treatment for the athlete

An important point to remember in the management of the patient with any degree of BP elevation is to "treat the patient and not the number."

Clinical Evaluation

History

The history should focus on the presence of TOD, the circumstances surrounding the HTN, and any identifiable cause. The history and physical examination determine the nature, severity, and management of the hypertensive event.

- Medications
  - Details of antihypertensive drug therapy and compliance
  - Intake of over-the-counter preparations such as stimulants or decongestants
  - Use of illicit drugs such as cocaine
- Duration and severity of preexisting HTN
- Degree of BP control
- Presence of previous TOD, particularly renal and cerebrovascular disease
- Date of last menstrual period
- History of other medical problems such as thyroid or endocrine diseases, lupus or autoimmune diseases, or prior renal disease
- Assess whether specific symptoms suggesting TOD are present.
  - Chest pain: myocardial ischemia or infarction
  - Back pain: aortic dissection
  - Dyspnea: pulmonary edema, congestive heart failure
  - Neurological symptoms: headache, nausea, vomiting, visual disturbances, altered level of consciousness (hypertensive encephalopathy), seizures

Physical Examination

The physical examination should assess whether TOD is present. More specific aspects of the physical examination can be done in the emergency department.

- Vitals: levels >180/120 mm Hg usually associated with hypertensive crises.
  - BP should be measured in both the supine position and the standing position (assess volume depletion)
  - BP should also be measured in both arms (a significant difference suggests an aortic dissection)
- Cardiovascular: evaluate for the presence of heart failure
  - Jugular venous distension
  - Crackles
  - Peripheral edema
- Abdomen: abdominal masses or bruits
- CNS
  - Level of consciousness
  - Visual fields
  - Focal neurological signs
- Ear, nose, and throat: presence of new retinal hemorrhages, exudates, or papilledema suggests a hypertensive emergency

Differential Diagnosis

The most common hypertensive emergency is a rapid unexplained increase in BP in a patient with chronic HTN. Other common causes include the following:

- Renal disease
- Cardiac disease
- Systemic disorders
- Endocrine disorders
- Drugs
- Drug interactions

Treatment

If the patient is in need of acute care, address the manifestations of a hypertensive emergency, such as chest pain or heart failure. Reduction of BP may not be indicated before getting the patient to the emergency department because rapid lowering of BP can critically decrease target organ blood flow and worsen TOD.

Emergency Department Care

- The fundamental principle in determining the necessary emergency department care of the patient with hypertension is the presence or absence of TOD.

- Initial considerations (if the patient is not in distress):
  - Place patient who is not in distress in a quiet room and reevaluate after an initial interview.
  - Consider the context of the elevated BP (e.g., severe pain often causes increase in BP).
- Screen for TOD: The patient's history, physical examination, laboratory studies, and diagnostic tests should be used to determine if TOD exists.
- Patients without evidence of TOD may be discharged with follow-up.
  - The misconception remains that a patient never should be discharged from the emergency department with an elevated BP. As a result of this belief, patients are given oral medicines, such as nifedipine, in an effort to lower BP rapidly before discharge. This is not indicated and may be dangerous.
  - Attempts to temporarily lower BP by using these medicines may result in a precipitous and difficult-to-correct drop in BP. Should this occur, target organ hypoperfusion may result. Furthermore, patients who present with high BP may have had this elevation for some time and may need chronic BP control but may not tolerate rapid return of BP to a "normal" level.
  - Acute lowering of BP in the narrow window of time in the emergency department visit does not necessarily improve long-term morbidity and mortality rates. The follow-up recommended for these situations by the Joint National Committee on High Blood Pressure is outlined in the Follow-up section.
- Patients with TOD usually require admission and rapid lowering of BP using intravenous (IV) medications. Suggested medication depends on the affected organ system.
  - Even in cases of hypertensive emergencies, the BP should not be lowered to normal levels.
  - Rapid reduction in BP will result in marked reduction in organ blood flow, possibly leading to ischemia and infarction.
  - In general, the MAP should be reduced by no more than 20% to 25% in the first hour of treatment. If the patient remains stable, the BP should then be lowered to 160/100 to 110 in the next 2 to 6 hours.
  - These BP goals are best achieved by a continuous infusion of a short-acting IV antihypertensive agent that can be titrated, along with constant, intensive patient monitoring.

Once the diagnosis of a true hypertensive emergency is established and TOD is confirmed, BP should be lowered by up to 20% to 25% of the MAP or the DBP should be decreased to 100 to 110 mm Hg over minutes to hours. More rapid reduction in BP should be avoided because it may worsen target organ function.

Follow-Up

Further Inpatient Care

- Patients with a true hypertensive emergency require the careful titration of IV medications for good control and a smooth reduction of their BP.

- Close monitoring is required; therefore, an intensive care unit is the most suitable place for admission.

- Other problems or comorbid conditions need to be addressed appropriately (i.e., surgery for aortic dissection).

Further Outpatient Care

- Hypertension is a chronic problem. The most important factor in a patient's overall risks of morbidity and mortality is appropriate long-term care.

- If a patient presents with a high BP but emergency department evaluation reveals no evidence of TOD, the patient does not need immediate treatment in the emergency department. The patient does require proper follow-up.

- The Joint National Committee on High Blood Pressure has published a series of recommendations for appropriate follow-up, assuming no TOD.

  - Prehypertension (SBP 120–139, DBP 80–89: BP should be rechecked within 1 year.

  - Stage I HTN (SBP 140–159, DBP 90–99): BP should be rechecked within 2 months.

  - Stage II HTN (SBP >160 or DBP >100): Refer to source of care within 1 month.

  - If BP is >180/110, patient should be evaluated and treated within 1 week.

Prognosis

- The 1-year mortality rate is higher than 90% for patients with untreated hypertensive emergencies.

- Median survival duration is 144 months for all patients presenting to the emergency department with a hypertensive emergency.

- Five-year survival rate among all patients presenting with hypertensive crisis is 74%.

Deterrence/Prevention

- Good long-term control of HTN is the best method for prevention of acute hypertensive emergencies.

- Patient education and close follow-up in patients who have had a hypertensive crisis are essential to prevent recurrent hypertensive emergencies.

- Proper use of antihypertensive medications by primary care physicians is the major tool in avoiding development of hypertensive emergencies.

 EMERGENCY ACTION

While you prepare your glucometer to obtain a blood glucose reading, you give the athlete a tube of glucose gel that you keep on hand for him. The blood glucose reading is 58. The athlete is beginning to become more coherent and requests another tube of gel. After ingesting the second tube, the athlete explains that he was unable to eat prior to practice and has been cutting weight for the past week. You send the athlete to the team physician for further evaluation and possible nutritional counseling.

CHAPTER HIGHLIGHTS

- The majority of cases of sudden death are related to undiagnosed cardiac conditions, but pulmonary problems, hyperthermia, drug abuse, blunt chest trauma, sarcoidosis, and exercise-induced anaphylaxis have been reported.

- In athletes younger than 35 years of age, a variety of different conditions are responsible for sudden death, but the most common is hypertrophic cardiomyopathy, which is generally responsible for about one third of all cases.

- Hypertrophic cardiomyopathy is associated with impaired diastolic filling, decreased ventricular compliance, and impaired ventricular emptying as a result of hypertrophy of the interventricular septum and left ventricle.

- The most frequently identified asthma triggers include allergen exposure, air pollutants, respiratory tract infections, exercise, weather changes, foods, additives, drugs, and extreme emotional responses.

- Mechanisms for bronchoconstriction consist of combinations of release of mediators from inflammatory cells and stimulation of local and central neural reflexes. Airflow limitation results from edematous swelling of the airway wall with or without smooth muscle contraction. The increase in microvascular permeability and leakage leads to mucosal thickening and swelling of the airway outside the smooth muscle.

- One indication that an athlete's asthma is flaring up is requiring extra doses of quick-relief rescue inhaler more than twice a week because of symptoms.

- When confronted with an evolving asthma attack, athletic trainers should begin therapy with albuterol delivered via metered dose inhaler and spacer. The usual dosing is 2 to 4 puffs delivered every 15 to 20 minutes for a total maximum of 3 doses.

- For athletes who have positive risk factors for death from asthma, live a long distance from the emergency department, have poor social support, experience rapid decline, or are unresponsive to bronchodilator therapy, EMS should be activated for timely treatment and transport to the emergency department.

- In the past 10 years, a 10-fold increase in the incidence of impaired insulin secretion has been reported in children.[78,79] These children are predisposed to diabetes by being obese, leading a sedentary lifestyle, and eating a high-fat and low-fiber diet.

- Clinically, diabetic ketoacidosis is most often seen in type I diabetes and often develops over a day or two.

- Laboratory studies are required to establish the diagnosis of diabetic ketoacidosis and to assess the severity, although a diabetic with a change in mental status is likely to have at least a moderate, if not severe, case.

- Diagnosis of mononucleosis syndrome is usually made clinically by the presence of sore throat, fever, headache, lymphadenopathy, and malaise, along with positive laboratory results.

- Because mononucleosis is associated with spontaneous rupture of the spleen,[93] it is imperative that the diagnosis be made quickly and efficiently, so the athlete is not put at unnecessary risk.

Chapter Questions

1. What is the most common cause of death in athletes younger than age 35 years?
   A. Diabetes
   B. Hypertrophic cardiomyopathy
   C. Hypertension
   D. Sickle cell trait

2. Wolf-Parkinson-White syndrome is a congenital problem that affects the:
   A. Coronary arteries
   B. Atrium
   C. Ventricles
   D. Lungs

3. Commotio cordis is the result of:
   A. Genetics
   B. Hypertension
   C. Diabetes
   D. Blunt chest trauma

4. Marfan's syndrome is most often seen in what sports?
   A. Volleyball
   B. Baseball
   C. Swimming
   D. Wrestling

5. Treatment of exercise-induced anaphylaxis includes which of the following?
   A. Oxygen administration
   B. Subcutaneous epinephrine
   C. IV fluids
   D. All of the above

6. A chronic inflammatory disease of the airway is:
   A. Asthma
   B. Bronchitis
   C. Exercise-induced anaphylaxis
   D. Mononucleosis

7. The common symptoms of asthma include:
   A. Cough
   B. Shortness of breath
   C. Wheezing
   D. All of the above

8. Dyspnea is:
   A. High blood pressure
   B. Low blood sugar
   C. A side effect of mononucleosis
   D. Difficulty breathing

9. The biggest risk for athletes with diabetes is:
   A. Hyperglycemia
   B. Hypoglycemia
   C. Diabetic coma
   D. Unconsciousness

10. The most serious side effect of mononucleosis is:
    A. Liver failure
    B. Contagiousness
    C. Spleen rupture
    D. There is no side effect

■ *Case Study 1*

A 16-year-old basketball player complains of lightheadedness at practice. He tells you he feels as if sometimes his chest is "fluttering." His blood pressure is 120/78 and his pulse is 60 and regular. He tells you he has no family history of unexplained deaths at a young age.

Case Study 1 Questions

1. What are the immediate dangers of his return to play?
2. What other information would be helpful?
3. Could this be deemed a true emergency?

■ *Case Study 2*

A 14-year-old girl swimmer who has been out of school for 6 days comes to the athletic training room and reports that she has been out sick with mononucleosis but her mom says it is okay for her to go back to practice. She is feeling much better and thinks that the exercise will help her get back to "normal."

Case Study 2 Questions

1. What are the contraindications to participating in sports with mononucleosis?
2. What possible complications could arise if she returns to practice?
3. What diagnostic tests could help you determine when and if it is safe for her to return?

References

1. Van Camp SP, Bloor CM, Mueller FO, et al. Non-traumatic sports death in high school and college athletes. MSSE. 1993;27:641–647.

2. Maron BJ, Shirani J, Poliac LC, et al. Sudden death in young competitive athletes clinical, demographic and pathological profiles. JAMA. 1996;276:199–204.

3. Wingel JF, Capeless MA, Ades PA. Sudden death in athletes. Sports Med. 1994;18:375–383.

4. Ades PA. Preventing sudden death: Cardiovascular screening of young athletes. Phys Sports Med. 1992;20:75–89.

5. Maron BJ, Epstein SE, Roberts WC. Causes of sudden death in competitive athletes. J Am Coll Cardiol. 1986;7:204–214.

6. Northcote RJ, Flannigan C, Ballantyne D. Sudden death and vigorous exercise: A study of 60 deaths associated with squash. Br Heart J. 1986;55:198–203.

7. Corrado D, Thiene G, Nava A, et al. Sudden death in young competitive athletes: Clinicopathologic correlations in 22 cases. Am J Med. 1990;89:588–596.

8. Wisten A, Forsberg J, Krantz P, et al. Sudden cardiac death in 15–35 year olds in Sweden during 1992–1999. J Int Med. 2002;252:529–536.

9. Maron BJ. Sudden death in young athletes. New Engl J Med. 2003;349:1064–1075.

10. Weaver WD, Lurch GS, Alvarez HA, et al. Angiographic findings and prognostic indicators in patients resuscitated from sudden cardiac death. Circulation. 1976;54:895–900.

11. Maron BJ, Epstein SE. Causes of sudden death in competitive athletes. JACC. 1986;7: 204–214.

12. Maron BJ. Hypertrophic cardiomyopathy: A systematic review. JAMA. 2002;287:1308–1320.

13. Antezano ES, Hong M. Sudden cardiac death. J Intensive Care Med. 2003;18:313–329.

14. Zipes DP, Wellens HJJ. Sudden cardiac death. Circulation. 1998;98:2334–2351.

15. Corrado D, Basso C, Thiene G, et al. Spectrum of clinicopathologic manifestations of arrhythmogenic right ventricular cardiomyopathy/dysplasia: A multicenter study. J Am Coll Cardiol. 1997;30:1512–1520.

16. Thiene G, Basso C. Arrhythmogenic right ventricular cardiomyopathy: An update. Cardiovasc Pathol. 2001;10:109–117.

17. Kies P, Bootsma M, Bax J, et al. Arrhythmogenic right ventricular dysplasia/cardiomyopathy: Screening diagnosis, and treatment. Heart Rhythm. 2006;3:225–234.

18. Pennell DJ, Sechtem UP, Higgins CB, et al. Clinical indications for cardiovascular magnetic resonance (CMR): Consensus Panel report. Eur Heart J. 2004;25: 1940–1965.

19. Basso C, Maron BJ, Corrado D, et al. Clinical profile of congenital coronary artery anomalies with origin from the wrong aortic sinus leading to sudden death in young competitive athletes. J Am Col Cardiol. 2000;35: 1493–1501.

20. Keating MT. The long QT syndrome: A review of recent molecular genetic and physiologic discoveries. Medicine. 1996;75:1–5.

21. Vincent GM. The molecular genetics of the long QT syndrome: Genes causing fainting and sudden death. Annu Rev Med. 1998;49:263–274.

22. Vincent GM, Timothy KW, Zhang L, et al. High prevalence of normal QT interval in patients with the inherited long QT syndrome: Important implications for diagnosis. Pacing Clin Electrophysiol. 1996;19:588.

23. Wagner GS. Marriott's practical electrocardiography, 9th ed. Philadelphia: Williams and Wilkins; 1994:104–114.

24. Rich BSE. Sudden death screening. Med Clin North Am. 1994;78:267–288.

25. Epstein SE, Maron BJ. Sudden death and the competitive athlete: Perspectives on preparticipation screening studies. JACC. 1986;7:220–230.

26. Grogin HR, Scheinman MM. Advances in evaluating and treating Wolff-Parkinson-White Syndrome. Curr Opin Cardiol. 1992;7:30–36.

27. Brugada P, Brugada J. Right bundle branch block, persistent ST segment elevation, and sudden cardiac death: A distinct clinical and electrocardiographic syndrome. A multicenter report. J Am Coll Cardiol. 1992;20: 1391–1396.

28. Antzelevitch C, Brugada P, Borggrefe M, et al. Brugada syndrome: Report of the Second Consensus Conference. Circulation 2005;111:659–670.

29. Jeresaty RM. Mitral valve prolapse: Definition and implications in athletes. J Am Coll Cardiol. 1986;7: 231–236.

30. Lieberthson RR. Sudden death from cardiac causes in children and young adults. New Engl J Med. 1996;334: 1039–1043.

31. Maron BJ, Poliac LC, Kaplan JA, et al. Blunt impact to the chest leading to sudden death from cardiac arrest during sports activities. New Engl J Med. 333: 337–342 1995.

32. Link MS, Wang PJ, Pandian NG, et al. An experimental model of sudden death due to low-energy chest wall impact (commotio cordis). New Engl J Med. 1998;338: 1805–1811.

33. Link MS, Maron BJ, VanderBrink BA, et al. Impact directly over the cardiac silhouette is necessary to produce ventricular fibrillation in an experimental model of commotio cordis. J Am Coll Cardiol. 2001;37:649–654.

34. Theleman KP, Kuiper JJ, Roberts WC. acute myocarditis (predominantly lymphocytic) causing sudden death without heart failure. Am J Cardiol. 2001;88: 1078–1083.

35. Mahrholdt H, Wagner A, Deluigi CC, et al. Presentation, patterns of myocardial damage, and clinical course of viral myocarditis. Circulation. 2006;114:1581–1590.

36. Friman G, Ilbäck N-G. Acute infection: Metabolic responses, effects on performance, interaction with exercise, and myocarditis. Int J Sports Med. 1998;19(Suppl 3):S172–S182.

37. Kato H, Ichinose E, Yoshioka F, et al. Fate of coronary aneurysms in Kawasaki disease: Serial coronary angiography and long-term follow-up study. Am J Cardiol. 1982;49:1758–1766.

38. Duke C, Rosenthal E. Sudden death caused by cardiac sarcoidosis in childhood. J Cardovasc Electrophysiol. 2002;13:939–942.

39. Sekiguschi M, Numao Y, Imai M, et al. Clinical and histopathological profile of sarcoidosis of the heart and acute idiopathic myocarditis. Concepts through a study employing endomyocardial biopsy. I. Sarcoidosis Jpn Circ J. 1980;44:249–263.

40. Kinoshita N, Mimura J, Obayashi C, et al. Aortic root dilatation among young competitive athletes: Echocardiographic screening of 1929 athletes between 15 and 34 years of age. Am Heart J. 2000;139:723–728.

41. Braverman AC. Exercise and the Marfan syndrome. Med Sci Sports Exerc. 1998;30:S387–S395.

42. Nienaber CA, Eagle KA. Aortic dissection: New frontiers in diagnosis and management. Part I: From etiology to diagnostic strategies. Circulation. 2003;108:628–635.

43. Egred M, Davis GK. Cocaine and the heart. Postgrad Med J. 2005;81:568–571.

44. Proceeding of the 2005 International Consensus on Cardiopulmonary Resuscitation and Emergency Cardiovascular Care Science with Treatment Recommendations. Resuscitation. 2005;67:157–341.

45. Sanders AB, Kern KB, Berg RA, et al. Survival and neurologic outcome after cardiopulmonary resuscitation with four different chest compression-ventilation ratios. Ann Emerg Med. 2002;40:553–562.

46. Aufderheide TP, Sigurdsson G, Pirrallo RG, et al. Hyperventilation-induced hypotension during cardiopulmonary resuscitation. Circulation. 2004;109: 1960–1965.

47. White RD. 2005 American Heart Association guidelines for cardiopulmonary resuscitation: Physiologic and educational rationale for changes. Mayo Clin Proc. 2006;81:736–740.

48. Berg RA, Hilwig RW, Kern KB, et al. Precountershock cardiopulmonary resuscitation improves ventricular fibrillation median frequency and myocardial readiness for successful defibrillation from prolonged ventricular fibrillation: A randomized, controlled swine study. Ann Emerg Med. 2002;40:563–570.

49. Eftestol T, Sunde K, Steen PA. Effects of interrupting precordial compressions on the calculated probability of defibrillation success during out-of-hospital cardiac arrest. Circulation. 2002;105:2270–2273.

50. Volcheck GW, Li JTC. Exercise-induced urticaria and anaphylaxis. Mayo Clin Proc. 1997;72:140–147.

51. Hirschmann JV, Lawlor F, English JS, et al. Cholinergic urticaria: A clinical and histologic study. Arch Dermatol. 1987;123:462–467.

52. Hosey RG, Carek PJ, Goo A. Exercise-induced anaphylaxis and urticaria. Am Fam Phys. 2001;64:1367–1372.

53. Sheffer AL, Austen KF. Exercise-induced anaphylaxis. J Allergy Clin Immunol. 1984;73:699–703.

54. Global strategy for asthma management and prevention. NIH Publication 02-3659; 2002.

55. Grant EN, Wagner R, Weiss KB. Observations on emerging patterns of asthma in our society. J Allergy Clin Immunol. 1999;104:1–9.

56. Scarfone RJ, Zorc JJ, Capraro GA. Patient self-management of acute asthma: Adherence to national guidelines a decade later. Pediatrics. 2001;108: 1332–1338.

57. Rodrigo GJ, Rodrigo C, Hall JB. Acute asthma in adults, a review. Chest. 2004;125:1081–1102.

58. Sur S, Hunt LW, Grotty TB, et al. Sudden-onset fatal asthma. Mayo Clinic Proc. 1994;69:495–496.

59. Sur S, Crotty TB, Kephart GM, et al. Sudden-onset fatal asthma: A distinct entity with few eosinophils and more neutrophils in the airway mucosa? Am Rev Respir Dis. 1993;148:713–719.

60. Managing your asthma flare-ups. Information from your family doctor. Am Fam Phys. 1998:58:1

61. Mintz M. Asthma update: Part I. Diagnosis, monitoring, and prevention of disease progression. Am Fam Phys. 2004;70:894–898.

62. Brenner BE, Abraham E, Simon RR. Position and diaphoresis in acute asthma. Am J Med. 1983;74:1005.

63. Calhoun WJ, Sutton LB, Emmett A, et al. Asthma variability in patients previously treated with beta-agonists alone. J Allergy Clin Immunol. 2003;112:1088–1094.

64. Smith DH, Weiss K, Sullivan SD. Epidemiology and costs of acute asthma. In Hadd JF, Corbridge T, Rodrigo C, et al, eds. Acute asthma: Assessment and management. New York: McGraw-Hill; 2000:1–10.

65. Shim CS, Williams MH. Relationship of wheezing to the severity of obstruction in asthma. Arch Intern Med. 1983:143: 890–892.

66. Fanta CH. Treatment of acute exacerbations of asthma in adults. Up To Date Search. September 2006:1–16.

67. Ben-Zvi Z, Lam C, Hoffman J, et al. An evaluation of the initial treatment of acute asthma. Pediatrics. 1982;70:348.

68. Scarfone RJ. Management of acute asthma exacerbations in children. Up To Date search. September 2006: 11–24.

69. Cydulka RK, McFadden ER, Sarver JA, et al. Comparison of single 7.5 mg dose treatment vs. sequential multidose 2.5 mg treatments with nebulized albuterol in the treatment of acute asthma. Chest. 2002;122:1982–1987.

70. Abramson MJ, Bailey MJ, Couper FJ, et al. Are asthma medication and management related to deaths from asthma? Am J Respir Crit Care Med. 2001:12–18.

71. Scarfone RJ, Loiselle JM, Willey JF II, et al. Nebulized dexamethasone vs. oral prednisone in the emergency department treatment of acute asthma in children. Ann Emerg Med. 1995;26:480.

72. Volovitz B, Bentur L, Finkelstain Y, et al. Effectiveness and safety of inhaled corticosteroids in controlling acute asthma attacks in children who were treated in the emergency department: A controlled comparative study with oral prednisolone. J Allergy Clin Immunol. 1998;102:605.

73. Schuh S, Dick PT, Stephens D, et al. High-dose inhaled fluticasone does not replace oral prednisolone in children with mild to moderate acute asthma. Pediatrics. 2006;118:644.

74. Medline Plus Drug Information. Corticosteroids glucocorticoid effects. http://www.nlm.nih.gov/medlineplus/druginformation.html

75. Smaha DA. Asthma emergency care: National guidelines summary. Heart Lung. 2001;20:472–474.

76. Gerch JE. Oral hypoglycemic agents. New Engl J Med. 1986;321:1231–1245.

77. Callahan ST, Mansfield MJ. Type 2 diabetes mellitus in adolescents. Curr Opin Pediatr. 2000;12:310–315.

78. Pinhas-Hamiel O, Dolan LM, Daniels SR, et al. Increased incidence of non-insulin-dependent diabetes mellitus among adolescents. J Pediatr. 1996;128:608–616.

79. Neufeld N, Raffiel L, Landon C, et al. Early presentation of Type 2 diabetes in Mexican-American youth. Diabetes Care. 1998;21:80–86.

80. Glaser NS. Non-insulin dependent diabetes mellitus in childhood and adolescence. Pediatr Clin North Am. 1997;44:307–337.

81. Ebeling P, Tuominen JA, Bourey R, et al. Athletes with IDDM exhibit impaired metabolic control and increased lipid utilization with no increase in insulin sensitivity. Diabetes. 1995;44:471–477.

82. Fahey PJ, Stallkamp ET, Kwatra S. The athlete with Type I diabetes: Managing insulin, diet and exercise. Am Fam Phys. 1996;53:1611–1617.

83. Wolf SK. Diabetes mellitus and predisposition to athletic pedal fracture. J Foot Ankle Surg. 1998;37:16–22.

84. Horton ES. Exercise and diabetes mellitus. Med Clin North Am. 1988;72:1301–1321.

85. Chiasson JL, Aris-Jilwan N, Belanger R, et al. Diagnosis and treatment of diabetic ketoacidosis and the hyperglycemic hyperosmolar state. CMAJ. 2003;168:859–866.

86. Eledrisis MS, Alshanti MS, Shah MF, et al. Overview of the diagnosis and management of diabetic ketoacidosis. Am J Med Sci. 2006;331:243–251.

87. Ennis Ed, Stahl E, Kreisberg RA. The hyperosmolar hyperglycemic syndrome. Diabetes Rev. 1994;2: 115–126.

88. Fishbein H, Palumbo PJ. Acute metabolic complications in diabetes. In: National Diabetes Data Group. Diabetes in America. Bethesda, MD: National Institute

of Health, National Institute of Diabetes and Digestive and Kidney Diseases; 1995;283–291.

89. Braaten JT. Hyperosmolar nonketotic diabetic coma: Diagnosis and management. Geriatrics. 1987;42:83–92.

90. Tynell E, Aurelius E, Brndell A, et al. Acyclovir and prednisolone treatment of acute infectious mononucleosis: A multicenter, double-blind, placebo-controlled study. J Infect Dis. 1996;174:324–331.

91. Maki DG, Reich RM. Infectious mononucleosis in the athlete: Diagnosis, complications, and management. Am J Sports Med. 1982;10:162–173.

92. Pochedly C. Laboratory testing for infectious mononucleosis: Cautions to observe in interpreting results. Postgrad Med. 1987;81:335–342.

93. Rutkow IM. Rupture of the spleen in infectious mononucleosis: A critical review. Arch Surg. 1978;113: 718–720.

94. Haines JD. When to resume sports after infectious mononucleosis: How soon is safe? Postgrad Med. 1987;81:331–333.

95. Bergeron MF, McKeag DB, Casa DJ, et al. Youth football: Heat stress and injury risk. Roundtable Consensus Statement. Med Sci Sports Exerc. 2005;37:1421–1430.

96. Kark JA, Posey DM, Schumacher HR, et al. Sickle cell trait as a risk factor for sudden death in physical training. New Engl J Med. 1987:317:781–787.

97. Shamsky DJ, Green GA. Sports haematology. Sports Med. 2000;29:27–38.

Suggested Readings

1. Aggarwal M, Khan IA. Hypertensive crisis: Hypertensive emergencies and urgencies. Cardiol Clin. 2006;24:135–146.

2. Bennett NM, Shea S. Hypertensive emergency: Case criteria, sociodemographic profile, and previous care of 100 cases. Am J Public Health. 1988;78(6):636–640.

3. Calhoun DA, Oparil S. Treatment of hypertensive crisis. N Engl J Med. 1990;323(17):1177–1183.

4. Chobanian AV, Bakris GL, Black HR, et al. JNC 7 report: The seventh report of the Joint National Committee on detection, evaluation, and treatment of high blood pressure. JAMA. 2003;289:2560.

5. Frohlich ED. Target organ involvement in hypertension: A realistic promise of prevention and reversal. Med Clin N Am. 2004;88(1):209–221.

6. Gallagher EJ: Hypertensive urgencies: Treating the mercury? Ann Emerg Med. 2003;41(4):530–531.

7. Hall WD. Resistant hypertension, secondary hypertension, and hypertensive crises. Cardiol Clin. 2002;20(2): 281–289.

8. Lip GY, Beevers M, Beevers DG. Complications and survival of 315 patients with malignant-phase hypertension. J Hypertens. 1995;13(8):915–924.

9. Murphy C. Hypertensive emergencies. Emerg Med Clin North Am. 1995;13(4):973–1007.

10. Panacek E. Controlling hypertensive emergencies: Strategies for prompt, effective therapeutic intervention. Emergency Medicine Reports. 1992;13: 53–61.

11. Patel R, Ansari A, Grim CE. Prognosis and predisposing factors for essential malignant hypertension in predominantly black patients. Am J Cardiol. 1990;66:868.

12. Pescatello LS, Franklin BA, Fagard R, et al. Exercise and hypertension. Medicine & Science in Sports & Exercise 2004 Special Communications Position Stand; 2004: 533–553.

13. Varon J, Marik PE. Clinical review: The management of hypertensive crises. Crit Care. 2003;7(5):374–384.

14. Vaughan CJ, Delanty N. Hypertensive emergencies. Lancet. 2000;356(9227):411–417.

15. Vidt DG. Hypertensive crises: Emergencies and urgencies. J Clin Hypertens. 2004;6(9):520–525.

Chapter 8

Environment-Related Conditions

Keith M. Gorse, MEd, ATC

KEY TERMS

Acute mountain
  sickness
Ataxia
Cold exposure
  and illness
Frostbite
Heat cramps

Heat exhaustion
Heat exposure
  and illness
Heat index
Heat stroke
High-altitude cerebral
  edema

High-altitude pulmonary
  edema
Hyperthermia
Hypothermia
Wind chill factor

 EMERGENCY SITUATION

A college football team is practicing in the early evening on their outdoor practice field right next to the locker room facility. Without much warning a thunderstorm begins near the facility. The athletic trainer on duty does not have a lightning warning device but decides to speak with the head football coach to warn him about the impending danger. The athletic trainer decides to have the entire team leave the playing field and go into the locker room. As the team is leaving the field, a bolt of lightning strikes the field area and knocks down two football players. Both players fall in the middle of the field and appear to be unconscious. What should the athletic trainer do to help the stricken football players? What should the athletic trainer do to prevent the possibility of this dangerous situation from occurring again?

As more physically active individuals participate in outdoor athletic activities, the frequency of environmentally related illnesses will increase. Participants in sporting events of long duration and those requiring particularly inclement weather and adverse conditions are especially prone to developing injury or illness. Heat-related illness, **hypothermia,** lightning strikes, and high-altitude illnesses are multisystem emergencies that require immediate, specific therapeutic treatments. Athletic trainers must be able to recognize the signs and symptoms of these medical emergencies and institute definitive care.

Areas of interest for the proper recognition of emergency environmental conditions to be discussed in this chapter will include the following:

1. **Heat exposure and illness** including **heat exhaustion** and **heat stroke**
2. **Cold exposure and illness** including hypothermia and **frostbite**
3. Severe thunderstorms and lightning emergencies
4. Altitude illness including **acute mountain sickness**
5. Prevention and care of environmental emergencies in athletics

Severe environmental conditions can cause injury to or illness in the athlete and may even cause death. For proper care to take place, specific intervention for environmental emergencies depends not only on the athlete's physical condition, but also on the safety of the scene. The athletic trainer must educate the athletes, coaches, and administrators on basic preventive measures if they are going to participate in outdoor sporting activities. The athletic trainer must also be prepared and equipped with the means necessary to reduce injury and illness risk and carefully treat cases of athlete collapse as a result of severe environmental conditions.

Heat-Related Emergenices

Heat-related emergencies such as heat stroke claim the lives of athletes every year despite being among the most preventable of sports-related health problems. Although heat-related deaths have decreased in recent years, just one death is far too many when most of these problems can be controlled by simple measures and the proper education of health-care professionals and coaching staffs.

Body Temperature Regulation

Because the body depends on water for normal function, long duration of sweating or excessive sweating without fluid replacement could be dangerous to the athlete. Efficient function of many of the body's various organs and systems require that core temperature be maintained within a narrow range. As the muscles work during exercise, a tremendous amount of heat is generated. The body relies on a number of different methods to help dissipate this heat and maintain core temperature within a desirable range. These include convection, conduction, evaporation, and radiation (Box 8-1). Of these, evaporation is the most efficient method for the body to lose excess heat. However, the rate of sweat evaporation from an athlete's skin is highly dependent on the amount of heat and humidity already present in the air. The warmer and more humid the air is, the harder it will be for sweat to evaporate and the higher an athlete's core temperature will become. As water is lost though sweating, electrolytes and other chemicals are also lost from the body. This loss of electrolytes can also contribute to an imbalance of the cooling system.[1] and lead to **hyperthermia**. It is important for the athlete to replace both fluids and electrolytes as they are lost through sweating associated with exercise.

As the body's core temperature rises and water and electrolytes deplete, heat illnesses can become a reality if immediate proper care does not take place.[2] Recognition of the early stages of heat illness in an athlete is vital. Although heat illnesses in athletics can appear in a progressive manner, dangerous situations such as heat exhaustion and heat stroke may arise with little or no warning (Box 8-2).

Box 8-1   Methods of Core Temperature Regulation

■ *Convection:* the body will gain or lose heat depending on the temperature of the surrounding air or water. Example: an athlete in cold water will have a decrease in body temperature.

■ *Conduction:* the body will gain or lose heat depending on the temperature of whatever surface it is in contact with. Example: an athlete lying on hot artificial turf will have an increase in body temperature.

■ *Evaporation:* water on a surface dissipates into the atmosphere, releasing heat. Example: sweat evaporating from the skin of an athlete results in a loss of heat and a lower body temperature.

■ *Radiation:* heat is transferred from areas of high temperature to areas of lower temperature. Example: blood from working muscles travels close to the surface of the skin. If the blood is warmer than the air temperature surrounding the skin, heat will be transferred from the warmer blood to the cooler atmosphere.

Box 8-2   Types of Heat Illnesses

- Heat cramps
- Heat exhaustion
- Heat stroke*

---

*Medical emergency

Heat Cramps

Heat cramps are common in athletics and should not be overlooked because they can be considered as the first stage of heat-related emergencies. Heat cramps tend to occur mainly in the leg area such as the calf and hamstring muscles. They are usually recognized by intense pain with persistent muscle spasms in the working muscle during prolonged exercise.[3]

Heat cramps are generally thought to be caused by muscle fatigue with rapid water and electrolyte loss via the sweating mechanism. Other factors may include lack of acclimatization, resulting in a less-efficient sweat mechanism and excessive sweating; irregular meals, resulting in less than optimal electrolyte stores; and a history of cramping.[2] Treatment for cramping includes removing the athlete from activity and incorporating gentle passive stretching of the involved muscle group in combination with ice massage (Box 8-3). It is vital that immediate water and electrolyte replacement take place to prevent further muscle cramping and the possible progression to more serious forms of heat illness.[1]

✪ *STAT Point 8-1. Heat cramps are generally thought to be caused by muscle fatigue with rapid water and electrolyte loss via the sweating mechanism.*

Heat Exhaustion

Heat exhaustion is a condition when the body is near to total collapse because of dehydration and a dangerously elevated core temperature. Heat exhaustion is not considered a medical emergency, although it is a serious condition and is considered to be a precursor to heat stroke. In an athlete suffering from heat exhaustion, the body's cooling mechanisms are intact but are no longer functioning efficiently.[2] The signs and symptoms of heat exhaustion are progressive in nature, and health-care professionals should take notice of them as soon as the athlete exhibits any of the signs (Box 8-4).[4]

✪ *STAT Point 8-2. An athlete suffering from heat exhaustion will experience difficulty losing heat, but the body's cooling mechanism will remain intact.*

Treatment for heat exhaustion should begin immediately. Fluid replacement and gradual cooling by getting the athlete out of the heat and sun and into a shaded or air-conditioned area is of major importance (Box 8-5). The athlete suffering from heat exhaustion should not return to sport activity until all vital signs return to normal and the athlete has been cleared by the team physician.[5]

Box 8-4   Signs and Symptoms of Heat Exhaustion

- Athlete has elevated core body temperature.
- Athlete may feel generally weak or fatigued.
- Athlete may feel nauseated.
- Athlete has sweaty/wet skin.
- Athlete's skin is pale.
- Athlete's breathing is rapid and shallow.
- Athlete's pulse is weak.

Box 8-3   Treatment of Heat Cramps

- Remove athlete from activity.
- Rehydrate and replace electrolyte losses.
- Try gentle passive stretching of involved muscle.
- Try light massage with ice to reduce the muscle spasm.

Box 8-5   Treatment of Heat Exhaustion

- Check all vital signs.
- Measure core body temperature (rectal).
- Remove excess clothing.
- Cool athlete with ice towels/ice bags.
- Place athlete in a cool or shaded area.
- Start fluid replacement.
- Alert team physician or transfer athlete to local emergency care facility.

Weight loss between practice sessions should be kept to only 2% to 3% of the athlete's pre-practice bodyweight, or less if at all possible. Of course, this assumes the athlete's original weight is reflective of a well-hydrated state. Team physicians should establish guidelines for weight loss between sessions. Excessive weight loss of approximately 5% or more of an athlete's body weight during one practice session should be closely monitored by the team physician; activity limits should be strongly considered for these athletes until they have replaced their fluid losses. Before and after athletic events, including practices, during warm weather months the athletic trainer should use weight charts to track weight changes (Fig. 8-1).[6] It is commonly recommended that athletes drink approximately 15 ounces of fluid for every pound of body weight lost during a practice session. These fluids should also contain some electrolytes.

Heat Stroke

The most severe heat-related condition is heat stroke. This condition involves a breakdown of the body's heat regulation mechanism resulting in a dangerously high core temperature. The most notable symptoms of heat stroke are hot and red-colored skin.[4] Commonly a strong and rapid pulse is present, with a high chance of unconsciousness or mental confusion (Box 8-6). It is a common misconception that an athlete will first suffer from heat exhaustion before heat stroke. Although this can occur, it is not always the case and the sports medicine staff should always be looking for the signs and symptoms of heat stroke in any athlete exercising in the heat.

✪ *STAT Point 8-3. The most notable symptoms of heat stroke are hot and red-colored skin.*

When heat stroke develops, it is critical that the body be cooled down immediately. The athlete should be moved out of the sun, and excessive clothing should be removed at once (Box 8-7). Cooling may be initiated with fans or ice towels, although a more effective and faster means of cooling is to place the athlete in a pool or tub of cool water (Fig. 8-2). Heat stroke is a true medical emergency that can result in death if not treated with urgency. Athletes suffering from heat stroke should be immediately cooled down, then transported to an emergency care facility via ambulance.[7]

Prevention of Heat-Related Emergenices

Initial prevention measures when considering heat illness emergencies involve the recognition of all environmental factors and being able to implement an on-site emergency action plan (EAP). The EAP should address the prevention and recognition of heat-related emergencies and then a plan of action to evaluate and treat the affected athlete.[2]

Weigh-In Chart

PLAYER NAME	IN	OUT	IN	OUT	IN	OUT	IN	OUT	IN	OUT
Adams, Harry A.										
Arn, John										
Barrett, Bo										
Boyer, Jeff										
Boyer, Michael										
Bunger, Jon										
Coley, Matt										
Cotter, Mark										
Dalton, Jake										
Danielowski, Ben										
Demus, Nate										
Demus, Ron										
Dimond, Nate										
Engelson, Blake										

Figure 8-1. Weight chart for pre- and post-practice weigh-ins.

Box 8-6 Signs and Symptoms of Heat Stroke

- Athlete has an increased core body temperature of more than 104°F.
- Athlete has hot and dry/wet skin.
- Athlete's skin is red.
- Athlete's pulse is strong and rapid (110–120 bpm).
- Athlete may be weak and nauseated.
- Athlete's mental status is altered or athlete exhibits irrational behavior.
- Athlete may be unconscious.

Box 8-7 Treatment of Heat Stroke

- Move the athlete out of the sun.
- Check and monitor all vital signs.
- Measure core body temperature (rectal is most accurate).
- Assess cognitive function.
- Activate emergency action plan.
- Remove all excess clothing.
- Lower the core body temperature as quickly as possible.
- Immerse body in pool or tub of cool water.
- Manage airway if athlete is unconscious.
- Transport to emergency care facility as quickly as possible.

Athletic trainers and other health-care providers must be prepared to respond in a quick and appropriate manner to alleviate symptoms and minimize the chance of heat-related death. The EAP will prepare all involved in the proper management of all heat-related emergencies.[2,6]

Ways to prevent heat-related emergencies in athletics include the following[2,6,8–11]:

1. Ensure that appropriate medical personnel (athletic trainers) are present at all sporting events. This includes practices and games.

2. Conduct an approved pre-participation physical examination on all athletes to acquire information about those athletes that may be predisposed to heat illness.

3. Educate athletes and coaches regarding recognition and care of heat illness and the risks associated with playing in the heat and humidity.

4. Develop practice and game guidelines for hot and humid weather using the **heat index** table (Table 8-1).

5. Measure factors of heat and humidity by determining the wet-bulb globe temperature (WBGT) using a sling psychrometer before and during all outdoor sporting events (Table 8-2).

6. Consider adjusting practice and game times with respect to heat and humidity factors. An example is to move an afternoon practice to the evening when the air temperature has decreased. Plan on rest breaks to match the conditions and intensity of activity.

7. Acclimatize properly before the season begins, making sure that the athlete is in proper condition for the heat and humidity.

8. Ensure sufficient fluid replacement is available and consumed before, during, and after athletic activities. There should be an unlimited access to water and sports drinks, and they should be consumed freely.

9. Minimize the amount of equipment and clothing worn by the athlete during athletic activity.

10. Weigh athletes before and after athletic activities when the weather is hot and humid. This is done to estimate amount of body water lost during activity and therefore determine what should be replenished before the next activity.

Recovery and return to activity from heat-related emergencies are entirely based on physician assessment and clearance.[6] Severity of the heat-related incident should dictate the length of recovery time. The athlete should carefully begin gradual return to physical activity to regain fitness and acclimatization under the supervision of a physician, athletic trainer, or other qualified health-care professional.[9]

Heat-related emergencies are potentially critical medical conditions that are common in outdoor athletics. It must also be stressed that heat-related emergencies are highly preventable. Environmental factors such as high temperature, high humidity, and lack of wind contribute to the potential of an athlete to suffer any type of heat illness.[11] It cannot be stressed enough that fluids should be consumed liberally before, during, and after practices and competitions.[8]

Cold-Related Emergencies

Serious health conditions can result from prolonged exposure to cold weather. The most common cold-related emergencies are hypothermia and frostbite.[12] Signs and symptoms

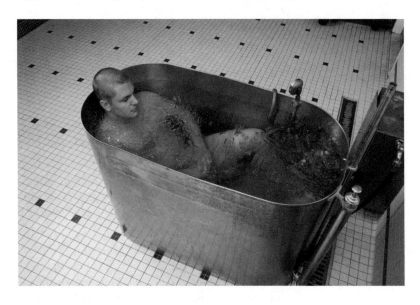

Figure 8-2. Athlete in tub of cold water.

Table 8-1 Heat Index Table

°F	5%	10%	15%	20%	25%	30%	35%	40%	45%	50%	55%	60%	65%	70%	75%	80%	85%	90%	95%	100%
80	74	75	76	77	77	78	79	79	80	81	81	82	83	85	86	86	87	88	89	91
85	79	80	81	82	83	84	85	86	87	88	89	90	91	93	95	97	99	102	105	108
90	84	85	86	87	88	90	91	93	95	96	98	100	102	106	109	113	117	122		
95	88	90	91	93	94	96	98	101	104	107	110	114	119	124	130	136				
100	93	95	97	99	101	104	107	110	114	119	124	130	136							
105	97	100	102	105	109	113	118	123	129	135	142	149				**DANGER ZONE**				
110	102	105	108	112	117	123	130	137	143	150										

Table 8-2 Wet-Bulb Globe Temperature (WBGT) Risk Table

°F	°C	Risk Hazard	Flag Color
<64	<18	Low	Green
64–73	18–23	Moderate	Yellow
73–82	23–28	High	Red
>82	>28	Hazardous	Black

The WBGT guide takes into account air temperature, relative humidity, and solar radiation by measuring three temperatures. Air temperature is measured using a standard dry-bulb thermometer (DBT). Relative humidity is assessed with a wet-bulb thermometer (WBT). WBGT = 0.3 × DBT + 0.7 × WBT

for cold-related emergencies, especially hypothermia, can be subtle, and an accurate diagnosis often is difficult because they can occur even when temperatures outside are not considered very low.

Cold-related emergencies occur when the body is unable to protect itself from the outdoor environment. Inadequately clothed athletes are at risk for accidental cold injuries caused by prolonged exposure to low air temperature, humidity, and wind.[13] Clothing made wet as a result of perspiration from activity or from wet weather conditions may also contribute to an athlete's risk. Exposed body parts not protected by clothing are particularly susceptible to freezing in frigid temperatures.

✪ *STAT Point 8-4. Inadequately clothed athletes are at risk for accidental cold injuries caused by prolonged exposure to air temperature, humidity, and wind.*

Athletic trainers, emergency medical services personnel, physicians, officials, and coaches should be aware of the many signs and symptoms associated with the various classifications of cold-related emergencies such as hypothermia and frostbite. Immediate care must be instituted to protect the exposed athlete from potential serious injury and possible death.

Hypothermia

Hypothermia is a condition in which the body's temperature becomes dangerously low. Many of the body's organs can be damaged by hypothermia. Normal body temperature ranges between 97.2°F and 99.5°F. If the body temperature is just a few degrees lower than this, bodily functions tend to slow down and become less efficient. If the body temperature drops too low and stays low for more than a couple of hours, the body's organs can begin to shut down, and death will ultimately result.[14]

Body temperature can drop gradually as the body is continually exposed to cold temperatures. This could happen when an athlete is outside in the cold weather without proper protection against the cold, wind, rain, or snow. Hypothermia can also occur when an athlete is out in the cold wearing wet clothing for an extended period. The signs and symptoms of hypothermia usually appear gradually (Box 8-8).[15] They progress from relatively mild conditions to extreme catastrophic events that could result in death if not treated promptly. An athlete with hypothermia needs immediate attention. Steps for immediate treatment are listed in Box 8-9. Take the athlete to an emergency care facility as soon as possible for continued or advanced care if necessary. The extent of care will depend on how low the body temperature has dropped. Health-care providers may use warm oxygen, warm intravenous fluids, and warming blankets. Specific treatments for affected organs may also be given in the emergency care facility.[14]

Rewarming the athlete must be done slowly to prevent a rush of blood to the surface of the body away from the vital

---

Box 8-8 Signs and Symptoms of Hypothermia

Progressively:

- Individual feels cold and begins to shiver.
- Individual has difficulty thinking and becomes mentally confused.
- Individual loses the ability to shiver.
- Individual's heart starts beating irregularly.
- Individual falls into a coma and death may occur.

Box 8-9 Treatment of Hypothermia

1. Monitor/maintain airway, breathing, and circulation.
2. Move the athlete out of the cold.
3. Take off cold and wet clothing.
4. Wrap the athlete in warm blankets and cover the head.
5. Do not try to warm cold skin by rubbing or massage.
6. Do not allow the athlete to walk.
7. Do not give anything by mouth if the athlete is not alert.
8. Transport to an emergency care facility as soon as possible.

---

organs that need blood.[16] It is important to rewarm the athlete in a gradual way that includes the use of dry clothes and blankets. The most important aspect is to get the athlete into a dry and warm environment as soon as possible.

⭐ *STAT Point 8-5. Rewarming the athlete must be done slowly to prevent a rush of blood to the surface of the body away from the vital organs that need blood.*

The duration of the effects of hypothermia depends on how badly the athlete's organs have been damaged. In many cases the athlete will recover in 3 to 12 hours with treatment.[16] In some cases, hypothermia can result in permanent disability or death.

Frostbite

Frostbite is a medical condition in which the nerves, blood vessels, and other cells of the body are temporarily frozen by exposure to cold temperature. In frostbite, intracellular water actually freezes and blood supply to the affected areas is compromised or even stopped altogether, resulting in a skin injury. Frostbite commonly occurs at the extremities: toes, fingers, tip of the nose, earlobes, and cheeks.[17] In most circumstances, the **wind chill factor** determines how quickly frostbite occurs.[18] Frostbite can also be much worse if the skin or clothing is wet at the time of the cold exposure.

⭐ *STAT Point 8-6. Frostbite commonly occurs at the extremities: the toes, fingers, tip of the nose, earlobes, and cheeks.*

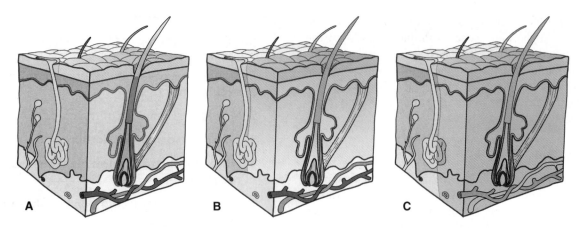

Figure 8-3. **A:** Frostnip. **B:** Superficial frostbite. **C:** Deep frostbite.

Frostbite comes in three different levels of severity (Fig. 8-3)[18]:

1. Frostnip: skin appears white and waxy. There is possible numbness or pain in affected areas. No skin blistering occurs.

2. Superficial frostbite: skin appears white, blue, or gray. Superficial skin feels hard but deeper tissue is soft and insensitive to touch. This is a serious medical condition; permanent damage is imminent. Skin blistering to affected areas is possible.

3. Deep frostbite: skin is white or blue and has a hard, wooden feel. The tissue underneath is hard and cold to touch. The entire area is numb. Skin blistering occurs to affected areas. It is a life-threatening emergency because of probable hypothermia and later risk of infection to affected body parts.

If frostbite is suspected, the damaged area should be protected from any further freezing until rewarming can safely begin. The freeze-thaw process causes more damage than leaving the tissue frozen until proper medical direction is available.[18] All wet clothing should be removed, and the damaged tissue should be covered with a dry dressing. The affected tissue should never be rubbed because this may cause further damage to the frostbite area as a result of the intracellular ice crystals.[17]

The athlete should be taken to an emergency care facility as soon as possible to be checked for possible hypothermia.[18] If an athlete is also suffering from hypothermia, the first concern is core rewarming. When frostbite alone is the problem, the best way to rewarm the tissue is by immersion in water at temperatures between 98°F and 102°F for 20 to 30 minutes (Box 8-10).[17]

A common error is to apply snow to a frostbitten area or to massage it; both can cause serious damage to the thawing tissues.[18] Do not rewarm an area with dry heat, such as a heat lamp, because frostbitten skin is easily burned as a result of the numb condition.

Athletes suffering from frostbite may experience increased skin sensitivity or permanent tissue damage.[17] It is

---

Box 8-10   Treatment for Frostbite

■ **Do not rub area.**

■ **Remove all wet clothing.**

■ **Cover area with dry bandage and/or clothing.**

■ **Gently rewarm the area by blowing warm air on area.**

■ **Place the area against a warm body part.**

■ **Place the area into warm (98°F –102°F) water for several minutes.**

■ **If not certain that the area will stay warm after rewarming, do not rewarm it. Refreezing thawed frostbitten tissue can cause more extensive tissue damage.**

■ **If an athlete is also suffering from hypothermia, the first concern is core rewarming.**

■ **Transport athlete to an emergency care facility as soon as possible.**

---

strongly advised that the athlete keep frostbitten areas covered with clothing during the winter to prevent further damage to the affected body tissues that have not recovered.

Prevention of Cold-Related Emergencies

The initial prevention measure when considering cold-related emergencies involves recognizing all environmental factors and being able to implement an on-site EAP. The EAP should address the prevention and recognition of cold-related emergencies and then provide a plan of action to evaluate and treat the affected athlete.[14]

Athletic trainers and other health care providers must be prepared to respond in a quick and appropriate manner to alleviate symptoms and minimize the chance of cold-related injuries or even death. The EAP will help prepare all involved for the proper management of all cold-related emergencies.

Prevention of cold-related emergencies in athletics includes the following[12–18]:

1. Have a wind chill chart on hand to determine the possibility of hypothermia or frostbite (Table 8-3).

2. Dress in layers.

3. Cover the head to prevent excessive heat loss.

4. Stay dry by wearing breathable and water-repellent clothing materials.

5. Stay adequately hydrated before and during activity.

6. Eat regular and nutritious meals so the body is well-fueled and therefore more efficient; this also ensures adequate calories available for shivering.

7. Avoid alcohol and nicotine because they accelerate heat loss.

8. Educate athletes, coaches, officials, and parents to recognize cold-related emergencies.

9. If unsure whether an athlete is suffering from hypothermia and/or frostbite, always stay on the side of caution and treat accordingly.

Cold-related emergencies may occur in most parts of the country, but it is a major concern for the athletes who participate in cold weather sports. Prompt recognition by an athletic trainer on the field is important for all cold-related emergencies.

Preparation is the key to protecting athletes from the effects of the cold weather, and hypothermia and frostbite should always be taken seriously. Proper treatment and immediate transportation to an emergency care facility can mean the difference between life and death for an athlete.

Lightning

Lightning is the most consistent and significant weather hazard that may affect athletics. According to the United States Weather Service, the annual number of lightning-related injuries in this country has been estimated to vary between 200 to 1000 people.[19] Also, approximately 100 fatalities as a result of lightning strikes in the United States occur each year.[20] Although the chance of being struck by lightning is very low, the odds are significantly greater when a storm is in the area of athletic events and the proper safety precautions are not followed.

Few people really understand the dangers of thunderstorms. Many people do not act promptly to protect their life and the lives of others because they do not understand how lighting strikes occur and how to reduce their risk. The most important step in solving this problem is for athletic trainers, who make decisions regarding health and safety issues, to educate coaches, athletes, and parents about the risk of lightning strikes during outdoor athletic activities.

Mechanisms of Lightning Injury

Injury from lightning can occur via five mechanisms[21,22]:

1. *Direct strike:* most commonly occurs to the head, and lightning current enters the orifices.

Table 8-3   Wind Chill Table

Wind Chill Chart: °F, wind in knots; 1 knot = 1.151 mph

Wind (knt)	Temperature (°F)													
	40	35	30	25	20	15	10	5	0	−5	−10	−15	−20	−25	−30
5	36	30	25	19	14	8	3	−2	−8	−13	−19	−24	−30	−35	−40
10	26	20	13	7	1	−6	−12	−18	−25	−31	−37	−44	−50	−56	−63
15	20	13	6	−1	−7	−14	−21	−28	−35	−42	−49	−56	−63	−70	−77
20	16	9	2	−6	−13	−20	−28	−35	−42	−50	−57	−64	−72	−79	−86
25	13	6	−2	−9	−17	−25	−32	−40	−47	−55	−63	−70	−78	−85	−93
30	11	4	−4	−12	−20	−28	−35	−43	−51	−59	−66	−74	−82	−90	−98
35	10	2	−6	−14	−22	−30	−37	−45	−53	−61	−69	−77	−85	−93	−101
40	9	1	−7	−15	−23	−31	−39	−47	−55	−63	−71	−79	−87	−95	−103

2. *Contact strike:* most commonly occurs when the lightning victim is touching an object that is in the pathway of the lightning current.

3. *Side flash:* most commonly occurs when the lightning strikes an object near the victim and then jumps from the object to the victim.

4. *Ground current:* most commonly occurs when the lightning current flowing in the ground radiates outward in waves from the strike point.

5. *Blunt injury:* most commonly occurs when the lightning current causes violent muscular contractions that throw victims a distance from strike point.

Guidelines on Lightning Safety

The following guidelines on lightning safety were developed as part of a position statement from the National Athletic Trainers' Association[22]:

1. Establish a chain of command that identifies who is to make the call to remove individuals from the athletic field.

2. Name a designated weather watcher to consider and then communicate possible threatening weather to the chain of command.

3. Have a means of subscribing to a weather monitoring system to receive forecasts and warnings. This is best done through a lightning detection device, a computer link to weather radar, or television or radio announcements from the National Weather Service.

4. Designate a safe shelter for each outdoor venue. A safe shelter should be a building with four solid walls, electrical wiring, and plumbing, all of which aid in the grounding of the structure. A secondary shelter would be an enclosed vehicle with a metal roof and windows completely closed.

5. Use the flash-to-bang count to determine when to go to safety. By the time the flash-to-bang count approaches 30 seconds, all individuals should already be inside a safe shelter (Box 8-11).

⭐ *STAT Point 8-7. Use the flash-to-bang count to determine when to go to safety.*

6. Once the activities have been suspended, wait at least 30 minutes after the last lightning flash before resuming an activity.

7. Avoid being, or being near, the highest point in an open field. Do not take shelter under or near trees, flagpoles, or light poles.

8. For those individuals who are caught in the open and who feel their hair stand on end, feel their skin tingle, or hear "crackling" noises, assume the lightning safety position. This position includes crouching on the ground, with weight on the balls of the feet, feet

Box 8-11	Thunderstorm Flash-to-Bang Method

Begin counting after seeing a lightning flash. Counting is stopped when the associated bang of thunder is heard. Divide this count by five to determine the distance to the lightning flash in miles. *Example:* a flash-to-bang count of 30 seconds equates to a distance of 6 miles.

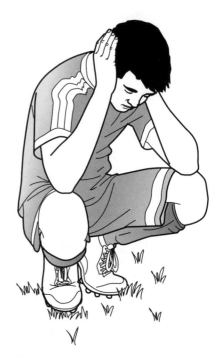

Figure 8-4. Lightning safety position.

together, head lowered, and ears covered (Fig. 8-4). An individual should never lie flat on the ground.

9. Observe the emergency first aid procedures in managing victims of a lightning strike (Box 8-12).

10. All individuals have the right to leave an athletic site to seek a safe shelter if the person feels in danger of impending lightning activity—without fear of penalty from anyone.

11. Blue sky and the absence of rain are not protection from lightning. Lightning can, and does, strike as far as 10 miles away from the rain shaft. It does not have to be raining for lightning to strike.

Lightning is the most consistent and significant environmental hazard that may affect athletics. There is no absolute protection against lightning. However, the risk of being struck by lightning can be substantially reduced by following general safety rules that apply to athletic events.

Box 8-12 Emergency First Aid Procedures: Lightning Strike

■ Activate local emergency medical service.

■ Lightning victims do not "carry a charge" and are safe to touch.

■ Move the victim with care to a safer location.

■ Evaluate airway, breathing, and circulation.

■ Begin cardiopulmonary resuscitation (CPR) or rescue breathing if necessary.

■ Evaluate for apnea and asystole.

■ Evaluate and treat for shock and hypothermia.

■ Evaluate and treat for fractures and/or burns.

■ Transport to emergency care facility.

Because of the risks associated with thunderstorms and lightning strikes, athletic trainers should develop and implement appropriate lightning safety procedures through the organization's EAPs for all of their outdoor facilities. Because the location, terrain, climate, and outdoor playing venue vary with different sports, lightning safety procedures may have distinct elements for different athletic activities. It is important that all EAPs and lightning safety procedures are regularly evaluated and modified when necessary.

Altitude-Related Emergencies

Athletic competition in the high-altitude environment continues to increase in popularity for amateur and professional athletes (Box 8-13). As a result of this growing popularity, the athletic trainer will have increasing opportunity and responsibility to serve the needs of the athlete performing in the high-altitude environment. Sports activities that are related to high-altitude performance can be individual or

Box 8-13 What Is High Altitude?

Some medically defined examples of high altitude[31,35]:

High altitude: 1500–3500 m (5000–11,500 ft)
Very high altitude: 3500–5500 m (11,599–18,000 ft)
Extreme altitude: above 5500 m (18,000 ft)

team activities. The scope of sports medicine practice by the athletic trainer ranges from pre-event prevention of common medical conditions that are unique to the high-altitude environment to the on-site event coverage and care requiring skills in outdoor medical care.

In high-altitude sports participation, the most obvious change is an increase in pulmonary ventilation, which can give the feeling of being out of breath. The response is highly variable among athletes and may not be felt for a few days. Because there is less oxygen in the atmosphere at altitude, the heart rate in an athlete may be elevated to increase cardiac output and maintain an adequate oxygen supply to the body, both at rest and during exercise.

The term "high-altitude emergencies" is used to describe illnesses or syndromes that can develop in athletes that are not acclimated to the high altitude. Because many athletes travel to high-altitude locations each year to participate in sports activity, acute mountain sickness is a health problem that must be taken seriously by health professionals. High-altitude pulmonary and cerebral edema, although uncommon in athletics, can be potentially fatal.

Acute Mountain Sickness

Acute mountain sickness is common in athletes who ascend from near sea level to altitudes higher than approximately 3000 m, but it may occur in altitudes as low as 2000 m. General symptoms for acute mountain sickness are characterized by headache, lightheadedness, breathlessness, fatigue, insomnia, loss of appetite, and nausea.[23] Usually, these symptoms will begin 2 to 3 hours after the athlete has reached peak ascent, but the condition is generally self-limiting and most of the symptoms disappear after 2 to 3 days (Fig. 8-5).

✪ *STAT Point 8-8. General symptoms for acute mountain sickness are characterized by headache, lightheadedness, breathlessness, fatigue, insomnia, anorexia, and nausea.*

The best way to prevent acute mountain sickness is by ascending gradually and allowing for acclimatization. Acclimatization is the process of the body adjusting to the decreasing availability of oxygen. Some authors suggest that with any ascent to an altitude above 3000 m, there should be a 2- to 3-day rest before further heavy athletic activity occurs.[23,24] Treatment of acute mountain sickness by oxygen or descent is not usually required; aspirin, acetaminophen, or ibuprofen may relieve most headaches. Other medications such as acetazolamide and dexamethazone may be given by a physician if the symptoms are severe.[25] Severe prolonged acute mountain sickness responds to descent to a more normal altitude for the athlete.

High-Altitude Pulmonary Edema

Another form of altitude illness is **high-altitude pulmonary edema,** or fluid in the lungs. Although it often occurs with acute mountain sickness, it is not felt to be related and the

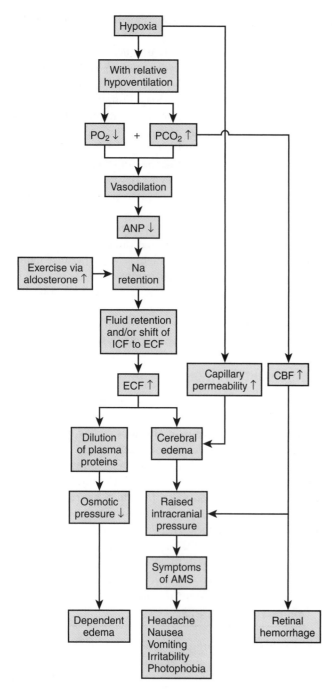

Figure 8-5. Mechanisms underlying acute mountain sickness. (Reproduced with permission from Ward MP, Milledge JS, West JB. High altitude medicine and physiology, 2nd ed. London: Chapman & Hall; 1995:372.)

symptoms for acute mountain sickness may be absent. Causes of the edema are not clearly understood; it may have to do with changes in cellular permeability in some people at altitude. Signs and symptoms of high-altitude pulmonary edema may include extreme fatigue, breathlessness at rest, severe cough with sputum, gurgling breaths, chest tightness, and blue- or gray-colored lips and fingernails.[24]

★ *STAT Point 8-9. Signs and symptoms of high-altitude pulmonary edema may include extreme fatigue, breathlessness at rest, severe cough with sputum, gurgling breaths, chest tightness, and blue- or gray-colored lips and fingernails.*

The treatment for high-altitude pulmonary edema is immediate descent to a safe altitude level. This must be done with the utmost urgency. Delay may be fatal. A safe altitude is usually described as the last elevation where the athlete felt well on awakening from a restful sleep. Oxygen should be administered if available. Medications such as nifediphine, salmeterol, and sildenafil may be given by a physician to help relieve the symptoms of high-altitude pulmonary edema.[26]

High-Altitude Cerebral Edema

High-altitude cerebral edema is rare but potentially serious, even fatal. The condition often follows acute mountain sickness, and many people think that the two are closely related and that high-altitude cerebral edema is the extreme end of the spectrum. It is defined as a condition in which the brain swells and ceases to function properly.[26,27] Like high-altitude pulmonary edema, the cause of high-altitude cerebral edema is poorly understood but is again likely related to changes in cellular permeability. Once high-altitude cerebral edema is present, it can progress rapidly and can be fatal within a few hours. Athletes with this illness are often confused and may not recognize that they are ill.

The classic sign of high-altitude cerebral edema is a change in mental status. Signs and symptoms may include confusion, changes in behavior, unusual or irrational behavior, and lethargy.[23] It may be easier to recognize a characteristic loss of coordination called **ataxia.** This is a staggering walk that resembles the way a person walks while intoxicated on alcohol. The most extreme cases of high-altitude cerebral edema may involve the athlete going into a coma with death occurring within hours.

★ *STAT Point 8-10. The classic sign of high-altitude cerebral edema is a change in the ability to think.*

The treatment for high-altitude cerebral edema is descent to a lower altitude as quickly as possible. Oxygen should be administered if available. Medications such as dexamethasone can be given by a physician to decrease the severity of the symptoms.[26] Athletes with high-altitude cerebral edema sometimes recover rapidly after descent to a lower and safer altitude.

Practicing sports medicine in high-altitude environments can be challenging for the athletic trainer. Medical conditions related to the altitude require additional training and experience because they can be unique to the standard practice setting. As sport medicine knowledge progresses, the athletic trainer will have increasing resources to better serve the athlete at high altitudes.

EMERGENCY ACTION

The athletic trainer should activate the EAP for that facility. This includes surveying the scene for safety, then checking the athlete's vital signs, calling for the local emergency medical service, and implementing immediate first aid care. Because of the storm being present around the outdoor field, the athletic trainer should first survey the scene to determine if it would be safe to reach the stricken athletes without putting their own life in peril. Once the scene is determined to be safe, the athletic trainer should stabilize the athletes quickly and carefully and then remove them to a safe indoor area until emergency medical services arrive. The athletic trainer should monitor the vitals throughout the entire transfer process.

The athletic trainer should have within his or her EAP a system to take care of potentially dangerous situations such as lightning. This includes the implementation of the flash-to-bang method of determining the distance of the last lightning strike. The athletic trainer should always check local weather reports to see if there are any weather watches or warnings. Proper weather checks should then be communicated with the head coach to let him or her know that there can be a potentially dangerous storm arriving during the team event.

CHAPTER HIGHLIGHTS

- Environmental conditions that can affect the athlete include heat illness disorders, cold injuries, lightning strikes, and altitude disorders.

- Heat illness disorders are classified as heat cramps, heat exhaustion, and heat stroke.

- Heat disorders are preventable with appropriate acclimatization, modified coaching techniques, improved equipment and clothing, and adequate fluid replacement.

- Treatment for heat illness disorders includes the rapid cooling and rehydration of the athlete.

- Cold injuries are classified as hypothermia and frostbite.

- The treatment for cold injuries includes rapid rewarming of the body or affected body part.

- Injuries and deaths as a result of lightning strikes are rare, but because many athletes practice and compete outdoors, they must be a concern for athletic trainers.

- Written policies that are understood and adhered to by the sports medicine and coaching staffs can help to prevent lightning injuries and deaths.

- Altitude disorders occur at altitudes more than 3000 meters above sea level. These disorders are classified as acute mountain sickness, high-altitude pulmonary edema, and high-altitude cerebral edema. All are treated with rapid descent from high altitude.

Chapter Questions

1. Which one of the following is a symptom of heat exhaustion?

   A. Red and dry skin

   B. Strong and rapid pulse

   C. Pale and wet skin

   D. Athlete is unconscious

2. Which one of the following is considered treatment for heat stroke?

   A. Activate emergency action plan

   B. Transport to hospital

   C. Remove excess clothing

   D. All of the above

3. What factors are measured to determine the heat index?

   A. Percent relative humidity

   B. Temperature

   C. Wind velocity

   D. Both a and b

4. A symptom of hypothermia in an athlete is when:

   A. The athlete loses the ability to shiver

   B. The athlete feels cold

   C. The athlete's body temperature rises

   D. Both A and C

5. What is the best treatment for hypothermia?

   A. Keep athlete outside until EMS arrives

   B. Remove athlete from outdoors

   C. Massage body parts with vigor

   D. Let athlete eat and drink anything

6. What is the best treatment for frostbite to a body part?

   A. Gentle and gradual rewarming

   B. Do not rub area

   C. Cover area with dry bandage

   D. All of the above

7. The thunderstorm flash-to-bang method is best described as:

   A. Count seconds between lightning and thunder and divide by 5

   B. Count seconds between lightning and thunder and multiply by 5

   C. Count seconds between lightning and thunder and multiply by 2

   D. Count seconds between lightning and thunder and divide by 2

8. The first thing an athletic trainer must do when aiding a lightning victim is:

   A. Move victim to a safe location

   B. Evaluate victim for shock

   C. Survey the scene for safety

   D. Evaluate victim for burns

9. High altitude is medically defined as (above sea level):

   A. 1500–2000 ft.

   B. 5000–11,500 ft

   C. 2500–3000 ft

   D. None of the above

10. Treatment for acute high-altitude illness is usually:

    A. Descending to a safer altitude

    B. Providing oxygen to athlete

    C. Administering medications

    D. All of the above

...otball practice on a 95°F afternoon began to develop dizzi-
...pisode of vomiting. After alerting the football coach and
...athlete was taken to the emergency department via a
...n practicing football two times a day for the previous
...al was at 9:00 p.m. the night before, when he ate a small bag
of potato... ...can of carbonated soda. He stated that at football practice the
coach only allo... ...nletes to stop for water once every hour. He denied any chest pain,
abdominal sympto...s, or shortness of breath. He said that he had been feeling out of shape
from the summer and that the twice-daily football practices had been strenuous and had
taken their toll on his body. He denied any sick contacts or recent illnesses.

Case Study 1 Questions

1. What are injury prevention issues in this case?
2. What injury prevention strategies can be applied here?
3. What is the role of the athletic trainer in this situation?

■ *Case Study 2*

A 20-year-old female cross-country runner was jogging the college course just outside of her
campus in early February. The air temperature was 25°F, and the wind speed was 25 to 40 mph.
Just prior to dusk, she staggered into the athletic training room at the football stadium. Her
warm-up jacket and pants were wet, and she was not wearing a hat or gloves. She said she "felt
like a slug"; when the athletic trainer asked what she meant by this, she became agitated and
upset. The runner was an All-American athlete with a lean body weight and low percentage of
body fat. She was not shivering. The skin on her face was erythematous. Her lips demonstrated
a bluish hue; otherwise, the initial examination by the athletic trainer was near normal.

Case Study 2 Questions

1. What are injury prevention issues in this case?
2. What injury prevention strategies can be applied here?
3. What is the role of the athletic trainer in this situation?

References

1. Casa DJ, Armstrong LE, Hillman SK, et al. National
   Athletic Trainers' Association position statement:
   Fluid replacement for athletes. J Athl Train.
   2000;35:212–224.

2. Binkley HM, Beckett J, Casa DJ, et al. National Athletic
   Trainers' Association position statement: Exertional
   heat illnesses. J Athl Train. 2002;37:329–343.

3. Hubbard R, Gaffin S, Squire D. Heat-related illness. In:
   Auerbach PS, ed. Wilderness medicine. 3rd ed. St Louis:
   Mosby-Year Book; 1995:167–212.

4. Armstrong LE, Hubbard RW, Kraemer WJ, et al. Signs
   and symptoms of heat exhaustion during strenuous
   exercise. Ann Sports Med. 1987;3:182–189.

5. Casa DJ. Exercise in the heat, II: Critical concepts in
   rehydration, exertional heat illnesses, and maximizing
   athletic performance. J Athl Train. 1999;34:253–262.

6. Casa DJ, Roberts WO. Considerations for the medical
   staff: Preventing, identifying, and treating exertional
   heat illnesses. In: Armstrong LE, ed. Exertional heat illnesses. Champaign, IL: Human Kinetics; 2003:169–196.

7. Casa DJ, Armstrong LE. Heatstroke: A medical emergency. In: Armstrong LE, ed. Exertional heat illnesses. Champaign, IL: Human Kinetics; 2003.

8. Casa DJ, Armstrong LE, Hillman SK, et al. National Athletic Trainers' Association position statement: Fluid replacement for athletes. J Athl Train. 2000;35:212–224.

9. Czerkawski JT, Meintod A, Kleiner DM. Exertional heat illness: Teaching patients when to cool it. Your Patient Fitness. 1996;10:13–20.

10. Armstrong LE, De Luca JP, Hubbard RW. Time course of recovery and heat acclimation ability of prior exertional heatstroke patients. Med Sci Sports Exerc. 1990;22:36–48.

11. Rich B. Environmental concerns: Heat. In: Sallis RE, Massimino F, eds. Essentials of sports medicine. St Louis: Mosby-Year Book; 1997:129–133.

12. NCAA Sports Medicine Handbook. 2003–2004. Indianapolis: National Collegiate Athletic Association; 2003.

13. Murray R. Practical advice for exercising in cold weather. In: Murray R. Endurance training for performance. Barrington, IL: Gatorade Sports Medicine Institute; 1995.

14. Bodine KL. Avoiding hypothermia: Caution, forethought, and preparation. Sports Med Alert. 2000; 6(1):6.

15. Thein L. Environmental conditions affecting the athlete. J Orthop Sports Phys Ther. 1995;21(3):158.

16. Thompson RL, Haywood JS. Wet-cold exposure and hypothermia: Thermal and metabolic responses to prolonged exercise in rain. J App Physiol. 1996;81(3):1128.

17. Centers for Disease Control and Prevention. Preventing injuries associated with extreme cold. Int J Trauma Nurs. 2001;7:26–30.

18. Kanzanbach TL, Dexter WW. Cold injuries: Protecting your patients from dangers of hypothermia and frostbite. Post Grad Med. 1999;105(1):72.

19. Andrews CJ, Cooper MA, Darveniza M. Lightning injuries: Electrical, medical, and legal aspects. Boca Raton, FL: CRC Press; 1992.

20. Walsh KM, Hanley MJ, Graner SJ, et al. A survey of lightning policy in selected Division I colleges. J Athl Train. 1997;32:206–210.

21. Craig SR. When lightning strikes: Pathophysiology and treatment of lightning injuries. Postgrad Med. 1986;79:109–112, 121–123.

22. Walsh KM, Bennett B, Cooper MA, et al. National Athletic Trainers' Association position statement: Lightning safety for athletics and recreation. J Athl Train. 2000;35(4):471–477.

23. Hacket PH, Roach RC. Current concepts: High altitude illness. New Engl J Med. 2001;345(2)107.

24. Basnyat B. High altitude illness. Lancet. 2003;361: 1967–1974.

25. Bovard R, Schroene RB, Wappers JR. Don't let altitude sickness bring you down. Phys Sports Med. 1995; 23(2):87.

26. West JB. The physiologic basis of high—Altitude diseases. Ann Intern Med. 2004;141(10):789.

27. Coote JH. Medicine and mechanisms in altitude sickness: Recommendations. Sports Med. 1995;20(3):148.

Suggested Readings

1. The National Athletic Trainers' Association: www.nata.org

2. The National Collegiate Athletic Association: www.ncaa.org

3. National Lightning Safety Institute: www.lightningsafety.com

4. The Weather Channel: www.weather.com

5. The National Center for Sports Safety: www.sportssafety.org

6. United States and Local Weather: www.uslocalweather.com

7. Maps with weather information: www.mapnation.com

8. Weather with heat and altitude information: www.weatherbug.com

Chapter 9

Orthopedic Injuries

Giampietro L. Vairo, MS, ATC, ACI

KEY TERMS

Acute compartment
   syndrome
Alignment
Apposition
Avascular necrosis
Colles' fracture
Destot sign
Dysphagia
Essex-Lopresti
   fracture

Excursion
Gravity (modified
   Stimson's) method
Iatrogenic
Lisfranc fracture
Myositis ossificans
Osteomyelitis
Ottawa rules
Paresis
Radial palsy

Roux sign
Self-reduction technique
Smith's fracture
Traction/external rotation
   procedure
Volkman's ischemic
   contracture

 EMERGENCY SITUATION

As an athletic trainer covering a football game, you are called onto the field after an athlete remains grounded after a violent tackle. It appears as if the athlete has suffered a serious arm or shoulder injury. He complains of severe pain in his injured shoulder and upper arm but denies previous pathology to the involved extremity. An examination of the involved upper extremity reveals significant swelling at the proximal humerus with pain on palpation. There is no evidence of an obvious anatomical deformity or open fracture. The athlete is unable to actively move his injured shoulder, and he cannot extend the wrist. However, he is able to actively flex and extend his elbow. Assessments of brachial and radial pulses find them within normal limits. From this on-field evaluation you suspect the athlete has sustained a proximal humerus fracture and associated radial nerve injury. What would proper emergency medical care of this traumatic orthopedic sports injury entail?

Regardless of sex, age, activity, and competitive level, athletes participating in sports are potentially more susceptible to traumatic orthopedic injuries than are sedentary individuals. Orthopedic sports injuries range from capsuloligamentous sprains, musculotendinous strains, or skeletal fractures to joint subluxations or dislocations. On-site emergency care of traumatic orthopedic injuries may present diverse examination and treatment challenges for the athletic trainer. It is pertinent that athletic trainers be aware of inherent traumatic risk potential for specific athletic activities typically encountered in orthopedic sports medicine. As frequent first-responders, athletic trainers must also formulate effective protocols for successfully managing these types of traumatic sports injuries. As such, an initial response to a traumatic orthopedic sports injury comprises determining if a true emergency exists. If indeed an orthopedic medical emergency transpires, athletic trainers must be properly prepared to implement appropriate treatment and transport of the injured athlete. This chapter introduces the essential principles of emergency medical care for the athletic trainer to properly manage traumatic skeletal fractures and joint dislocations commonly encountered in sports.

Basic Emergency Medical Care

The athletic trainer must be well versed in examining life- and limb-threatening circumstances and determining appropriate interventions for successfully managing such injuries. Sound didactic and practical instruction is vital in preparing athletic trainers to manage traumatic orthopedic injuries so as to avoid catastrophic consequences. Examination and treatment of traumatic orthopedic injury during athletic events are unique and may be challenging at times. Ambient noise and spectators can pose a hindrance to the efficient delivery of appropriate emergency medical care. Furthermore, despite the aggressive dynamic of sports, the health and well-being of injured athletes must remain the athletic trainer's foremost priority. This is true regardless of challenges to an athletic trainer's interventions by unqualified individuals such as the injured athlete's teammates or members of the coaching staff.

Management of traumatic orthopedic injury should always involve the athletic trainer's awareness of the action unfolding in a sporting event. This greatly assists athletic trainers in assessing a situation by increasing the clinician's awareness for particular events leading to an injury. When a traumatic event occurs, examination of the injured athlete starts with a sound primary survey, as presented in Chapter 2. Once a thorough primary survey is completed, a focused orthopedic secondary survey is performed. This consists of obtaining a history and screening the torso and extremities for obvious deformities, open wounds, and adequate circulation. Fundamental issues to address when providing emergency care for traumatic orthopedic injuries include establishing the degree of injury, evaluating neurovascular

function, determining appropriate management for optimal outcomes, and providing correct splinting for immediate protection.

Fundamentals of Skeletal Fractures

Fractures of the human skeletal system result when a bone is cracked or broken as a result of a single large force applied all at once (macrotrauma) or many small forces that accrue over a long period (microtrauma). General clinical symptoms of fractures involve the disruption to correct osseous anatomical integrity, significant focal pain, edema, and ecchymosis.[3,29] Skeletal fractures are often classified based on anatomical location of pathology and structures involved and are typically referred to as the distal segment relative to a proximal segment.[29] Orthopedic sports medicine literature uses standardized terminology to properly describe skeletal fractures. Box 9-1 displays a classification of skeletal fractures frequently referred to in orthopedic sports medicine.

⭐ *STAT Point 9-1. Skeletal fractures are often classified based on anatomical location of pathology and structures involved and are typically referred to as the distal segment relative to a proximal segment.*

Skeletal fracture classification is also based on the orientation of fragments and may be described as transverse, spiral, oblique, comminuted, compound, and greenstick (Fig. 9-1). Additional parameters of skeletal fracture

---

Box 9-1 Fracture Categorization Relative to Soft Tissue Pathology

- *Closed:* Skin is not disrupted at fracture site [*simple* — handwritten]
- *Open:* Skin is disrupted at fracture site [*Compound* — handwritten]
- *Complete:* Fracture produces discontinuity between two or greater fragments of bone [*all the way through* — handwritten]
- *Incomplete:* Fracture results in partial discontinuity of bone [*half way* — handwritten]
- *Complicated:* Fracture fragments induce injury to muscular, ligamentous, intraarticular, neurovascular, and visceral tissues [*fragments cause other injuries* — handwritten]
- *Uncomplicated:* Fracture causes minor soft tissue pathology
- *Occult:* Fracture is not identifiably demonstrated but is suspected on clinical examination

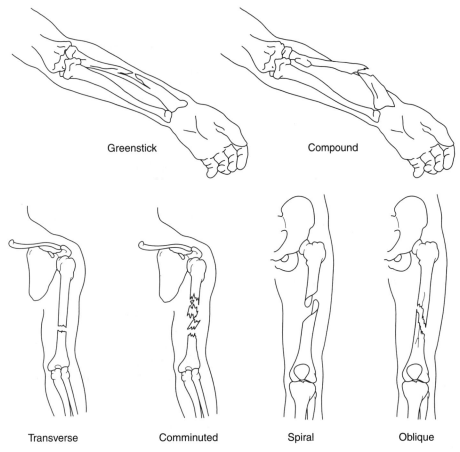

Figure 9-1. Fracture types.

shattered

specificity include alignment and **apposition.** Alignment refers to the association of long-bone fragment axes to one another and is measured in degrees of angulation from the distal fragment in relation to the proximal fragment. Apposition is referred to as the contact of skeletal fracture fragments and may be expressed as a partial, bayonet, or distraction. Bayonet apposition presents as displaced fragments overlapping one another, whereas distraction occurs as fragments are displaced along a longitudinal axis.

Fractures to the skeletally immature athlete are of special concern because injury to the epiphysis or growth plate may result in abnormal future bone development. The epiphysis is located near the end of long bones and influences mature skeletal length and morphology.

Management

Management of skeletal fractures includes a thorough history for determining mechanism of injury with vigilant attention given to position of the injured extremity. Athletic equipment covering an injured extremity should be safely removed to permit direct visualization of the affected anatomy.[29] Assessing a possible fracture also includes inspecting the extremities bilaterally to gain a detailed appreciation of individual skeletal structure and composition. A thorough observation of the skin at the injury site is

crucial to rule out an open fracture. Any break in the skin should be considered an open fracture. Palpation of potentially fractured bone typically elicits point tenderness, significant pain, and crepitus. Joints proximal and distal to a fractured site should be consistently evaluated for associated injury (Box 9-2).

Open fractures increase the incidence of infection and are deemed true traumatic orthopedic emergencies. Hence, any bleeding noted in the vicinity of a skeletal fracture should be considered open and managed as such. Soft tissue wounds and exposed bone should be thoroughly irrigated with sterile saline solution to remove debris and should be immediately dressed with ample sterile materials to decrease the risk of infection and **osteomyelitis.** Careful, direct pressure should be maintained on the open wound with sterile materials to limit blood loss (Box 9-3).[10,19]

⭐ *STAT Point 9-2. Open fractures increase the incidence of infection and are deemed true traumatic orthopedic emergencies.*

Significant vascular compromise that leads to profuse bleeding or absent pulses jeopardizes not only integrity of the associated extremity, but also may raise concern for a life-threatening scenario.[3] Significant bleeding should be controlled with direct pressure initially and then with

Box 9-2 Fundamentals of Initial Fracture Management

- Activate EMS when appropriate.
- Remove clothing and protective equipment from site of injury.
- Carefully visually inspect area bilaterally.
- Carefully inspect skin in the area for breaks.
- Carefully palpate area for pain and crepitus.
- Evaluate neurovascular function distal to injury.
- Evaluate joint integrity proximal and distal to injury.
- Monitor the athlete for shock.

Box 9-3 Open Fracture Management

- Open fractures are a medical emergency. Activate EMS.
- Thoroughly irrigate soft tissue wounds and exposed bone, ideally with sterile saline solution, to remove debris.
- Cover the wound with a sterile dressing.
- With significant bleeding, apply careful, direct pressure to the sterile dressing to limit blood loss.
- Monitor the athlete for signs of shock while awaiting EMS arrival.

Box 9-4 Evaluating Neurovascular Status

- Bilateral sensation testing of skin distal to fracture site ("Does this feel the same on both sides?")
- Testing of motor function distal to fracture site (flexion and extension of wrist)
- Bilateral comparison of pulse distal to fracture site (see Chapter 2 for more information)
- Capillary refill test (see Chapter 2 for more information)

movement of the bone or joints both proximal and distal to an injured extremity. It is also of utmost importance that neurovascular status distal to an involved skeletal fracture be monitored frequently (Box 9-4).

Acute compartment syndrome may potentially arise subsequent to any skeletal fracture but is most often encountered in the forearm and lower leg. There is little area to accommodate edema in these anatomical locations. Abrupt increases in compartmental pressure as a result of excessive swelling cause diminished or absent pulses because of constricted blood vessels. The alteration of correct sensation may also be present as a consequence of nerve impingement. The defining clinical symptom of acute compartment syndrome is pain out of context to what is expected with contraction or lengthening of injured compartment musculature.[3,29] If inappropriately managed, this condition may prove limb threatening because the gradual onset of increased vascular pressure leads to an ischemic condition throughout the injured area.[3]

⭐ STAT Point 9-3. The defining clinical symptom of acute compartment syndrome includes pain out of context to what is expected with contraction or lengthening of injured compartment musculature.

On-site attempts at fracture realignment are occasionally used. The specific aims of fracture realignment are to relocate bony fragments for favorable healing; protect surrounding soft tissues at the injury site; and, most importantly, address associated neurovascular deficiencies.[3] Parameters to contemplate when attempting realignment of a skeletal fracture include an athletic trainer's competency with the technique, degree of displacement or angulation, acuity of injury, and accompanying neurovascular pathology. If distal pulses and sensation are intact, it is best to splint the angulated skeletal fracture in the position found. In the instance when pulses and sensation are absent, it is best to attempt realignment before splinting. Gentle traction

arterial pressure if necessary. Arterial pressure point techniques consist of locating an arterial pulse proximal to a fractured site and applying pressure to that specific pulse. This results in an occlusion of blood flow. (See Chapter 2 for more information.) The use of tourniquets for excessive blood loss is warranted only in extreme conditions because of the high incidence of complications.[29] Undetected occult fractures are usually responsible for excessive blood loss that is not readily identified and cannot be easily controlled. To reduce the potential for local infection, exposed bone must be thoroughly irrigated with sterile saline to remove contaminants and debris. This should be followed by the application of a sterile dressing.[3,29] Stability of both closed and open fractures may be best accomplished by limiting along the longitudinal axis of the bone while moving fractured ends into correct anatomical position will usually result in reestablishment of pulses and sensation and may lead to a reduction in pain. Increased pain or resistance to this procedure is reason to discontinue the realignment attempt. Administration of opioid analgesics by a physician or emergency medical services (EMS) greatly improves the injured athlete's tolerance to realignment techniques.

Splinting Techniques

The athletic trainer must be aware of splinting principles and techniques and the specific splints best used for immobilizing orthopedic injuries. From a practical standpoint it is economically difficult to possess every possible splinting device. It is best to acquire splinting supplies adequate for the majority of orthopedic injuries commonly encountered in sports. It should also be stressed that athletic trainers appropriately select emergency medical equipment that satisfactorily meets the inherent risks specific to sports. In the case of a traumatic emergency, athletic trainers should be reassured EMS would have access to additional splinting equipment for more extensive injuries. A well-composed emergency action plan should address these specific situations.

Once an injured extremity that is suspected of fracture has been properly evaluated, it should be splinted prior to transport from the field. This is especially true if the injured athlete is transported via cart or stretcher. Proper immobilization of the injury tends to diminish irritation and pain and consequently limits edema or effusion.[10,19] Furthermore, immobilization of skeletal fractures reduces the danger of magnified fragment displacement.[10,19,29] Accurate procedures for splinting an orthopedic injury must continually begin with an extensive visual inspection of the extremity. Lacerations, abrasions, and avulsions should be suitably cleansed and dressed with sterile supplies prior to application of a splint. It is also vital that an extremity be assessed for the sudden onset of acute compartment syndrome and neurovascular compromise before and after splinting.[3,10,19]

Five basic classes of splints are used in orthopedic sports medicine and emergency medical care. These include rigid, soft, formable, vacuum, and traction splints (Fig. 9-2). Rigid splints, which are constructed of stiff and sturdy materials, are most appropriately used for protecting and immobilizing misaligned skeletal fractures or gross joint instability. Soft splints use air pressure or bulky padding for immobilization and protection purposes of skeletal fractures and pathological joint instability. Varied forms of soft devices include pillow and air splints. A pillow splint is a comfortable piece of equipment commonly used with foot and ankle complex injuries that applies mild and steady pressure on the affected anatomy. A pillow splint is wrapped around the foot and ankle complex and then secured with either tape or triangular bandages.

Air splints are structured in a similar way to a fashioned cylinder and permit contouring specific to the injured anatomy. These particular devices rely on air pressure, which shapes and reinforces the splint to compress and immobilize an injured area. Air splints provide the advantage of supplemental compression that may be beneficial in limiting excessive hemorrhages. However, air splints must be regularly monitored and appropriately adjusted for alterations in temperature and atmospheric pressure that may cause changes in the rigidity of the splint once it has been applied. Moreover, caution should be advised when using a lower extremity air splint. These specific air splints typically cover the foot, which makes evaluating distal pulses and sensory perception problematic. Air splints are not to be used with humeral or femoral fractures because of their inability to adequately limit proximal joint **excursion.**

A formable splint is somewhat of a fusion device consisting of a semi-rigid shell and soft inner lining. The semi-rigid shell of formable splints is typically constructed of a pliable metal that permits manual contouring. This allows the splint to conform to the angulation of the injured anatomy for immobilization. The formable splint's soft inner lining is usually composed of foam and serves to support the injured area. Vacuum splints are constructed of fabric or vinyl material containing micro-Styrofoam beads

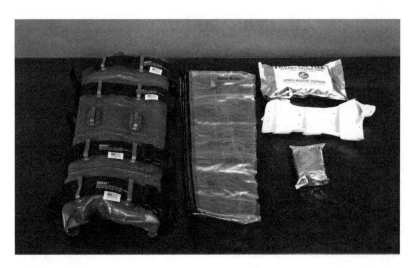

Figure 9-2. Assorted splinting materials and devices.

that are fixed and secured to the injured area by straps. A pump is used to draw air from the material to compress the Styrofoam beads together, thereby stiffening the splint. This allows the splint to conform to the affected anatomy, thereby increasing its versatility and adaptability for immobilizing an injured extremity.

Traction splints are often used to treat long-bone fractures, especially of the lower extremity. These splints exert a steady longitudinal pull on the axis of the affected anatomy to limit spasm of surrounding musculature. This potentially results in decreasing pain to facilitate realignment of fractured fragments. However, traction splints are used cautiously with upper extremity long-bone fractures because of the potential for susceptible pathology of respective neurovascular structures.[3,29] Traction splints are costly and require specialized instruction typically found in emergency medical technician curricula. As such, traction splints and their use should be left to EMS personnel.

Regardless of the specific splint selected, it is crucial to immobilize joints both proximal and distal to a fracture site to effectively manage the traumatic orthopedic injury. Splints should be adequately padded to protect the skin and soft tissues prior to their application.[10,19] This may be accomplished by the use of elastic stockinette or cotton Webril to envelop the injured extremity. Elastic wraps are typically used in splint application. Caution must be taken to avoid applying elastic wraps so tightly that circulation is hindered. In the case of skeletal fractures where edema or effusion is present, an extremity may substantially expand in girth. The fact that splints are not rigid cylinders is beneficial in that they may accommodate for such increases in anatomical area. This factor also assists with inhibiting detrimental circumferential pressures.[10,19] Furthermore, elastic wraps that are properly applied will secure the splint to an injured extremity and allow expansion of anatomical area because of swelling. The athletic trainer must consistently reassess neurovascular integrity prior to and following application of a splint. Vascular integrity of an injured extremity may also be evaluated via capillary refill time. Extended capillary refill time is indicative of potential vascular compromise.

Fractures of the Hand and Wrist

The most commonly fractured sites of the human skeletal system occur at the hand and wrist complex.[31] Attaining the necessary skills to properly manage these injuries is vital so that potentially debilitating conditions are prevented. When caring for injuries to the hand and wrist complex, preserving function opposed to form takes precedence.[15,50] Although all injuries to the hand and wrist deserve prompt examination and treatment, only open fractures and dislocations are considered true orthopedic traumatic emergencies. Conservative emergency medical care consists of splinting the injured hand and wrist complex in a position of function and immediately transporting the athlete to the nearest hospital.

Fractures of the Forearm

The most common type of distal radial fracture is the **Colles' fracture,** which is most often associated with falling on an outstretched arm with the wrist in extension.[15,31] The force associated with this mechanism of injury tends to displace fractured fragments dorsally. A Colles' fracture must be dealt with meticulously because severe morbidity may result from improper management. An additional traumatic distal radial fracture is known as the **Smith's fracture.**[15] This particular fracture is noted by volar displacement of distal fragments following injury. The mechanism of injury usually associated with a Smith's fracture is characterized by falling on an outstretched arm with the wrist in flexion. A Smith's fracture tends to be considerably unstable and requires urgent referral to an orthopedic specialist for consultation (Fig. 9-3). Suitable treatment for Colles' and Smith's fractures requires careful immobilization by application of a forearm splint in the position of presentation so as not to exacerbate angulation of fractured fragments.[10,19] Activation of EMS may be necessary to facilitate transport to the nearest hospital. While awaiting arrival of EMS, the athletic trainer must periodically monitor neurovascular function of the affected extremity. The athletic trainer should also be attentive for symptoms of acute compartment syndrome and shock.

Radial and ulnar shaft fractures are most often the result of a significant direct force. Radial shaft fractures are more prevalent at the middle and distal third because of the decreased cross-sectional area of the musculature. Management of displaced forearm fractures requires immobilizing the area, including the wrist and elbow joints, in the position found with a rigid splint. Immediate transport to

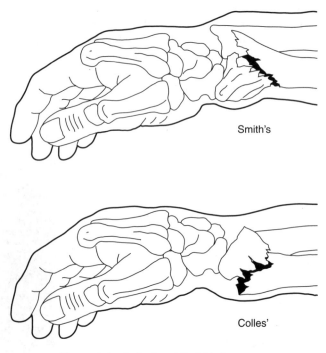

Figure 9-3. Colles' and Smith's fractures.

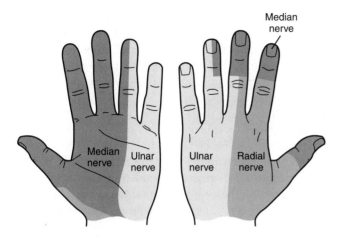

Figure 9-4. Sensory distributions throughout the hand.

the nearest emergency medical facility is also mandated for proper follow-up care.[29,54]

Management of forearm skeletal fractures must stress evaluation of the elbow and wrist joints for associated injury. Most important is assessing sensorimotor distribution of the radial, median, and ulnar nerves along the forearm and hand (Fig. 9-4). The athletic trainer must intermittently monitor neurovascular functions of the injured extremity and constantly screen for signs of acute compartment syndrome and shock while awaiting definitive care.

Fractures of the Elbow

Skeletal fractures of the elbow characteristically result from blunt trauma or falling on an outstretched arm. Although occult fractures of the elbow are uncommon, neurovascular pathology is of great concern when managing these injuries. Close attention should be paid to sensorimotor distribution of the median nerve because it is commonly injured with fractures to the distal humerus, regardless of displacement. Monitoring the brachial artery is also imperative because it is additionally vulnerable to injury. If the brachial artery sustains an injury that is not appropriately managed, **Volkman's ischemic contracture** may result.[25,54] Treatment for distal humeral fractures should include application of a comfortable compressive dressing and immobilization of the elbow with a rigid long-arm splint in the position of presentation.[10,19] If involvement of the humeral condyles is suspected, splinting should be more specific. If the lateral condyle is affected, splint the forearm in supination with the wrist in extension so as to alleviate tension on the wrist extensor musculature. If the medial condyle is fractured, the wrist should be splinted in pronation and flexion so as to ease tension on the wrist common flexor tendon. Properly controlling effusion and edema of the elbow complex is advantageous because a delayed onset of swelling can periodically result in neurovascular compromise. Urgent referral to an orthopedic specialist for advanced care is highly recommended. Significant complications such as misalignment

and decreased elbow joint range of motion are often probable if these fractures are not realigned correctly.

Special consideration should be given to the olecranon if suspected of fracture because adverse morbidity often ensues if managed poorly. Fracture of the olecranon is recognized as an intraarticular lesion and calls for intricate realignment to ensure favorable outcomes.[25,54] Displaced olecranon fractures routinely rupture the triceps aponeurosis and subject the ulnar nerve to compromise. As such, displaced fractures of the olecranon should be immobilized in the position of presentation with a rigid splint and warrant immediate activation of EMS for comprehensive care.[25,54] If these particular fractures prove to be nondisplaced, the affected forearm may be immobilized in a long-arm splint with the elbow joint flexed to 70 degrees and the wrist joint in neutral.[25,54] Complications that may arise from improper care include cubitus valgus or varus deformity, malunion, arthritis, and ulnar nerve palsy.

Fractures of the radial head and neck are commonly related to avulsion of the humeral lateral epicondyle or capitellar injury. It is important that these fractures be immobilized in a rigid long-arm splint and that the athlete immediately be transported to the nearest emergency medical facility for proper follow-up care.[10,19] Advanced diagnostics are usually required to assess potential displacement and degree of angulation prior to attempting realignment of the fracture. It is vital that athletic trainers assess integrity of the distal radioulnar joint subsequent to radial head and neck fractures. Violent mechanisms of injury to the radial head and neck may occasionally result in an **Essex-Lopresti fracture**.[54] This pathology manifests as rupture of the interosseous membrane and warrants immediate activation of EMS for comprehensive care. Substantial morbidity may result from negligible treatment of an Essex-Lopresti fracture.[25] In managing elbow skeletal fractures, it is of utmost importance that neurovascular processes be monitored intermittently with deficiencies or alterations accounted for. Moreover, athletic trainers must be alert for the potential onset of acute compartment syndrome secondary to skeletal fracture.

Fractures of the Humerus and Shoulder

Proximal humeral fractures typically occur in the athletic population as the result of trauma, most likely secondary to falling on an outstretched arm.[32] These fractures may also occur from a direct blow to the lateral aspect of the bone, although this is rare. On examining this specific pathology, athletic trainers may advise the injured athlete to hold the involved arm in an adducted position.[32] Symptoms usually include considerable pain, edema, and focal tenderness over the proximal humerus. The athletic trainer must thoroughly inspect the injured anatomy for any gross deformity that could place the brachial plexus, axillary nerve, and vascular structures in danger of compromise. Occasionally, a proximal humeral fracture can accompany a glenohumeral joint (GHJ) dislocation and most often occur from extreme forces imparted on the shoulder complex. Typically GHJ fracture-dislocations cause the anatomical area to be more susceptible to related rotator cuff lesions and brachial plexus and axillary neurovascular pathology.[5,32] Basic emergency medical care typically includes seating the athlete upright for elevation and placing the injured extremity in an appropriate arm sling and swathe.[5,32] The careful application of ice for pain and spasm control may be incorporated. In addition, prompt transport of the injured athlete to the nearest emergency medical facility is necessary for proper follow-up care. Potential complications resulting from inappropriate treatment include malunion healing, **myositis ossificans,** secondary GHJ stiffness, and arthritis. Adjunct complications for failure to recognize associated pathology to the greater and lesser tuberosities include nonunion healing of the respective osseous structures and tenosynovitis of rotator cuff musculotendinous tissues.[32] Special attention must be considered when caring for the skeletally immature athlete because **avascular necrosis** (AVN) may also result from inadequate management of these conditions.

Fractures to the humeral shaft are most often a consequence of either direct or indirect forces. A direct force to the humerus, such as a violent blow, frequently results in a transverse fracture of the bone. An indirect force, however, such as landing on an outstretched arm or the elbow, will likely result in a spiral fracture.[5] As a result of the large cross-sectional area of musculature spanning the humerus, realignment tends to be difficult. Assessment of neurovascular tissues subsequent to humeral shaft fractures, especially the radial nerve, is essential. Fractures to the middle and distal third of the humerus carry the potential for **radial palsy,** which is exemplified by wrist-drop or an inability to actively extend the wrist of the injured arm.[5] Hence, it cannot be overstressed that athletic trainers perform a complete examination of the shoulder and elbow joints to rule out occult injuries. The onset of neurovascular compromise necessitates immediate activation of EMS. Appropriate interventions for successfully managing humeral shaft fractures depends on the presence of displacement and the degree of angulation or accompanying neurovascular pathology. If displacement is not evident, the fracture may be immobilized with a rigid long-arm splint and the athlete must be transported to the nearest emergency medical facility for proper follow-up care.[5,10,19] However, if displacement is noted, the affected extremity should be immobilized with a rigid long-arm splint in the position of presentation and immediate activation of EMS for comprehensive care is warranted.[5] Failure to appropriately manage humeral shaft pathology may lead to nonunion or delayed union healing and radial nerve palsy.

Scapular Fractures

Fractures to the scapula are rare in athletics and require extreme forces.[49] Because of the violent nature of scapular fractures, suspicion of associated thoracic injuries must be assumed until definitely ruled out.[49] *(See Chapter 11 for more information.)* Proper immediate management of scapular fractures typically consists of immobilizing the injured extremity and activating EMS for comprehensive care.[5,49] Prompt activation of EMS is prudent because extreme forces eliciting scapular fracture may be associated with life-threatening thoracic injuries. The athletic trainer can best manage scapular fractures by having the injured athlete sit upright for elevation, immobilizing the affected extremity in a sling and swathe, and carefully applying ice for pain control.[5,49] Furthermore, athletic trainers must periodically monitor the injured athlete's vital signs while awaiting EMS to recognize the potential onset of life-threatening injures such as pneumothorax.

Clavicle

Clavicular fractures are frequent injuries encountered in sports. Fractures to the clavicle usually result from a direct force to the bone or are secondary to a traumatic force imparted onto the lateral aspect of the shoulder complex.[2] Because the clavicle is very superficial, fractures are usually obvious. However, its superficial orientation also warrants appreciation because improperly managed injuries are in potential danger of exacerbation into an open fracture.[1,2] Clavicular fractures may present with or without obvious anatomical deformity in addition to focal bone pain. Discomfort typically intensifies considerably with passive and active excursion of the shoulder complex, especially GHJ horizontal adduction. Moreover, fractures of the clavicle are usually classified by dividing the respective anatomy into thirds. Fractures to the intermediate and lateral thirds of the clavicle are most prevalent. Regardless of displacement, these fractures are best treated with a sling and swathe, careful application of ice for pain control, and urgent referral to an orthopedic specialist for consultation.[2] Traditionally, figure-eight bandages were indicated but they proved fairly cumbersome and yield a higher incidence of complications with less than optimal functional outcomes.[2]

The most severe yet least common type of clavicular fracture occurs at the medial third. This specific skeletal fracture carries significant potential for dire related injuries such as thoracic and neurovascular compromise (Fig. 9-5). Effective emergency medical care includes thoroughly monitoring the athlete's vital signs and placing the injured extremity in a sling and swathe. It cannot be understated that this identifiable pathology necessitates immediate activation of EMS for ruling out associated life-threatening injuries and ensuring comprehensive care. Acute complications are not typical, yet in certain circumstances pneumothorax or hemothorax may result and lesions to the brachial plexus or subclavian vasculature are possible.[1] As such, athletic trainers must perform a complete adjunct examination of pulmonary and neurovascular functions during routine management of clavicular fractures.

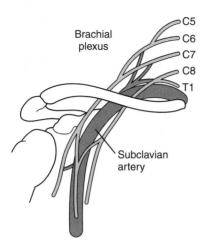

Figure 9-5. Neurovascular structures posterior to the clavicle.

Fractures of the Thorax

Sternum

Sternal fractures result from high-energy trauma in contact sports and usually from a blunt force directed to the anterior thorax. Extreme trunk hyperflexion injuries may also generate fractures of the sternum, although such injuries are rare.[23] Physical examination of sternal injuries generally elicits focal pain at the site of contact. Furthermore, tenderness and occasional crepitus may be present with palpation of the fractured bone. A moderate number of these specific injuries will also present with difficulty breathing, which may indicate significant cardiopulmonary contusion.[38] Palpitations may be noted secondary to dysrhythmia, which is an additional sign of cardiac pathology.[38] Emergency medical care of sternal fractures involves having the athlete assume a comfortable position to facilitate respiration and periodic evaluation of vital signs. Appropriate management also consists of monitoring for potential associated life-threatening pathology such as pneumothorax, hemothorax, cardiopulmonary contusion, and neurovascular compromise.[39] The immediate activation of EMS is mandated for comprehensive care of sternal fractures.[23,38] Splinting or supportive prophylactic materials affixed to the sternum are often contraindicated because it may increase respiratory restriction and exacerbate an underlying pulmonary injury.

Fractures of the Lower Extremity

Pelvis

Pelvic fractures, although a rare circumstance in athletics, represent a serious emergency medical situation. The disruption of pelvic integrity necessitates a substantial degree of force. As such, pelvic fractures are most often the result of violent mechanisms of injury. These specific injuries typically result from a fall from a significant height in extreme sports or vehicular accidents in motor sports. Because of the considerable forces and mechanisms involved with pelvic fractures, associated injuries to internal organs and extensive vascular structure systems are common.[21,45] Symptoms specific to pelvic fractures include extreme pain and tenderness throughout the injured area and hematuria indicating internal hemorrhage.[21,45] Other clinical indications include **Destot sign,** indicated by formation of a hematoma above the inguinal region. **Roux sign** indicates bilateral distance discrepancies between the greater trochanter and anterior superior iliac spines, signifying an acetabular fracture. Extensive neurovascular deficiencies throughout the lower extremities may also be noted subsequent to pelvic pathology.

The most important role of the on-site athletic trainer in managing pelvic fractures includes immediate activation of EMS for immediate transport to the nearest emergency medical facility.[21,45] A thorough monitoring of the injured athlete's vital signs must also be routinely conducted while awaiting definitive care. The athletic trainer should ensure that excessive pelvic girdle movement is avoided to limit pain and internal bleeding. Complications specific to inappropriate management of pelvic fractures and related injuries account for an elevated incidence of intrapelvic compartment syndrome, digestive and reproductive systems dysfunctions, and internal infections subsequent to disruption of urinary and bowel structures.

Femur

The femur is known to be the largest and strongest bone in the body. This bone also possesses a rich vascular supply and is surrounded by a dense cross-sectional area of musculature. As a result of the femur's anatomical composition and orientation, an extremely significant force is required to disrupt its integrity. In the event of a fracture, the musculature surrounding the femur will usually contract, causing additional displacement of the fractured ends. Of even greater concern is the extreme amount of blood loss, which is expected because of the bone's extensive vascular supply. Three classes of femoral shaft fractures are typically described: Type I (spiral or transverse, which represents the most common); Type II (comminuted); and Type III (open).[47] Complications associated with femoral fractures are common.

On examination of the injury site, athletic trainers will commonly note obvious deformity and significant pain. Considerable focal tenderness and crepitus typically accompany palpation of the injured bone. The quadriceps musculature may exhibit significant swelling as the result of a hematoma. A neurovascular examination of the lower leg should be performed and repeated frequently. Because of extreme forces required for fracturing the femur, accompanying injuries must be ruled out. Tachycardia and hypotension may result from extensive blood loss and are indicative of hypovolemic shock.[47] Although concern for lesions to nervous tissues is inherent, these injuries are rare because of the dense cross-sectional area of musculature shielding nerves.[6]

Moreover, adequately assessing neurological function is often compromised as a result of considerable pain subsequent to femoral fractures.[6,29] While awaiting the arrival of EMS, the athletic trainer should immobilize the affected extremity in the position of presentation with a rigid splint. An open fracture should be irrigated, ideally with sterile saline solution, to cleanse the bone and soft tissues of contaminants and debris.[3,29] This must be followed with the application of a sterile dressing to shield the wound.[3,29] Successful realignment of femoral fractures often requires intravenous opioid analgesic administration for pain control. Femoral fractures are generally effectively stabilized with implementation of a traction splint by EMS personnel (Fig. 9-6).[6,47]

Patella

Fractures to the patella may be the result of both indirect and direct mechanisms of injury. Indirect trauma is most prevalent with patellar fractures and occurs as the result of a violent quadriceps contraction.[48] This abrupt contraction may cause a displaced transverse fracture to the patella and render the knee joint void of the quadriceps extensor mechanism. As a result the athlete will be unable to actively extend the knee joint or perform a straight leg raise against gravity. Direct trauma is uncommon but results in a comminuted fracture and should raise suspicion for associated tibiofemoral injuries.[48] Fractures of the patella usually elicit notable pain, ecchymosis, and edema or effusion.[6] Closed patellar fractures should be splinted with a knee joint immobilizer and the athlete should be referred to an orthopedic surgeon. Careful application of ice may be effective for pain relief. Open patellar fractures should be splinted with a knee joint immobilizer after the wound is appropriately cleaned and dressed for transport to a hospital by EMS.

Tibia and Fibula

The tibia is the largest bone in the lower leg and accepts the majority of weight-bearing forces compared to the fibula during correct physiological gait. The fibula serves primarily as a point of attachment for tendons and ligaments. Because of the dense cortex of the tibia, a large force is typically necessary to yield a fracture.[17] However, the tibia remains the most frequently fractured long bone in the human skeletal system and is often associated with open fractures.[3]

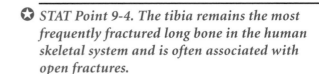

✪ *STAT Point 9-4. The tibia remains the most frequently fractured long bone in the human skeletal system and is often associated with open fractures.*

The most common mechanism of injury for tibial and fibular fractures is direct trauma and indirect torsional forces. Substantial direct force to the tibia often produces a transverse or comminuted displaced open fracture with associated fibular fracture. Indirect torsional mechanisms of injury may result in spiral or oblique fractures and are less likely to yield displaced fragments or coupled soft tissue pathology. As a result of the abundant muscular and vascular tissues in the lower leg, complications secondary to trauma or inadequate management are possible. The tibia is closely joined to the fibula by a sturdy interosseous membrane and, with the close proximity of the bones, a displaced fracture of either one tends to yield fracture in the other (Fig. 9-7).

Tibial and fibular fractures often present with extreme pain and edema of the lower leg and an obvious anatomical deformity. Although vascular tissues are not commonly injured in these circumstances, periodic assessment of dorsal pedal and posterior tibial pulses and capillary refill are necessary to recognize the onset of acute compartment syndrome.[3,29,48] This includes noting any symptoms of exaggerated pain, pallor, paresthesia, or paralysis. When caring for closed fractures, it is best to immobilize the lower leg in the position found with a rigid or vacuum splint and immediately activate EMS for transport to a hospital. Remember that open fractures pose an urgent emergency situation and must be carefully managed as previously noted. It is also of utmost importance that neurovascular status distal to the involved fracture be monitored closely. The athletic trainer must monitor the injured athlete for developing signs of shock while awaiting arrival of EMS.

Fractures of the Foot and Ankle

Foot

Although foot fractures commonly occur in sports, they are rarely severe enough to be considered a true medical emergency. Conservative management usually consists of

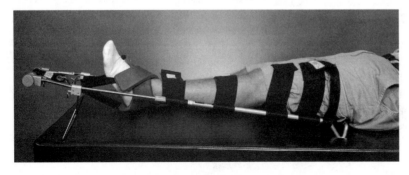

Figure 9-6. Immobilized femur in a traction splint.

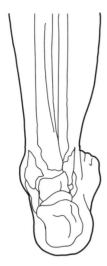

Figure 9-7. A displaced tibial–fibular fracture.

appropriately splinting the injured area and advising the use of crutches until definitive diagnosis. One exception is the **Lisfranc fracture.** Although rarely encountered in sports, Lisfranc fractures are serious orthopedic traumatic emergencies.[11] This injury usually is the result of substantial torsional stress, and physical examination reveals significant swelling and pain at the tarsometatarsal joint. Point tenderness is also prominent at the base of the third metatarsal. Displaced Lisfranc fractures are clinically evident, thereby facilitating definitive diagnosis. However, this pathology is typically misdiagnosed as minimally or nondisplaced fractures on clinical examination.[11] This unique fracture is sometimes deemed catastrophic because of the high incidence of complications and warrants immediate transportation of the injured athlete to the nearest emergency medical facility because surgical intervention is typically required. The role of athletic trainers in correctly managing this fracture should include immobilizing the foot in a posterior ankle splint or walking boot and advising the use of crutches for nonweight-bearing ambulation.[53,55] Failure to promptly recognize this significant injury may delay adequate care and yield unsuccessful outcomes. Common complications secondary to improper management of Lisfranc fractures include post-traumatic arthritis and reflex sympathetic dystrophy.

Ankle

The ankle is the most commonly injured joint in the human skeletal system.[11,14,56] Ankle fractures typically refer to pathology of the distal tibia and fibula and the talus and calcaneus. The most common mechanism of injury is hyperinversion of the joint. Although the ankle joint is less susceptible to hypereversion mechanisms of injury, pathology subsequent to this specific mode tends to produce significant damage. Ankle injuries frequently result in loss of playing time throughout sports. However, rarely do these fractures rise to the level of a true medical emergency unless an

open fracture occurs. The **Ottawa rules** are a useful guide to athletic trainers for quickly establishing the potential severity of ankle pathology (Box 9-5).[51] Any athlete presenting with significant posterior ankle pain or the failure to bear body weight should be immediately removed from athletic activity and referred to a physician.[51]

When assessing a potential ankle fracture, the inability to bear weight on the affected extremity should raise suspicion of significant ankle injury. Careful inspection for any open wounds is of utmost importance. Unrecognized open fractures are a risk for serious infection. Common findings specific to ankle fractures typically include obvious deformity, edema or effusion, ecchymosis, and point tenderness along the injured bone. Principal management of ankle fractures is dependent on multiple factors, with the preservation of anatomical integrity and correct physiological joint function being critically important in preserving later gait and weight-bearing function. As such, immediate activation of EMS or transport of the athlete to the nearest emergency medical facility is mandated with severe cases of injury for comprehensive care. Furthermore, when caring for ankle fractures, it is extremely important that the athletic trainer periodically monitor neurovascular functions of the foot and ankle. Immobilization of the ankle joint in the position of presentation with a posterior ankle splint, sugar tong/short-leg stirrup splint, or walking boot will assist in pain control and limit displacement of fragments, thereby sustaining soft tissue integrity.[10,19,55] The use of crutches may also be advised for nonweight-bearing ambulation to further protect the affected area.

Fundamentals of Joint Dislocations

Dislocations of the shoulder, elbow, hip, knee, ankle, and sternoclavicular joints constitute traumatic orthopedic emergencies as a result of the potential for neurovascular compromise and resultant disability if not treated immediately.[7] Definitive treatment for dislocated joints comprises reducing the injury to correct anatomical position. Whether this occurs on-site or in a hospital depends on the competency of the athletic trainer. A properly trained athletic trainer may attempt joint reduction with prior approval of the team physician; this approval should be written and should clearly refer to specific joints and types of dislocations. This is especially indicated if the arrival of EMS or transport to a hospital will be prolonged. Early reduction following joint dislocation is less difficult than prolonged reduction. This is because of muscle spasms and guarding from pain, which will increase over time and hinder such efforts.[7] Reduction attempts should be performed only after a thorough examination of the joint. Furthermore, neurovascular status must be monitored before, during, and after any attempts. As a general rule, most EMS providers are not specifically trained nor permitted to reduce joint dislocations. Significant resistance or greatly increased pain are reasons to abort reduction attempts and may indicate an associated fracture. Dislocations that are not reduced should be splinted in the position found and the athlete should be transported to a hospital immediately. If reduction is successful, distal neurovascular function should be rechecked, followed by careful application of ice and splinting the area in a position of function. The athlete should be seen as soon as possible by an orthopedic surgeon for further evaluation of joint function.

In most cases only dislocations of the patella, shoulder, fingers, or toes should be reduced on the field if required immediately. Reductions of the elbow, hip, or knee joints are regarded as difficult and should only be attempted by an appropriate medical specialist. This difficulty is attributed to challenging reduction techniques, the high likelihood of concomitant fractures, and severe complications from incompetent attempts. The athletic trainer covering sports without a physician present should obtain or develop written clinical standards and field protocols pertaining to the management of joint dislocations. In any event, all dislocations, whether reduced in the field or not, must be evaluated by an orthopedic surgeon as soon as possible.

Dislocations of the Hand

Dislocations at the hand, especially of the digits, are common in sports activities.[26,35] Mechanisms of injury may present as either significant or marginal trauma and usually consist of axial loading, compression, hyperextension, and valgus or varus forces on the respective joint.[22] Although these injuries are painful and frequently grotesque, they seldom arise to the level of an emergency unless open. Proper

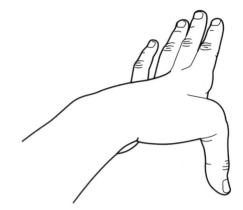

Figure 9-8. Dislocated thumb.

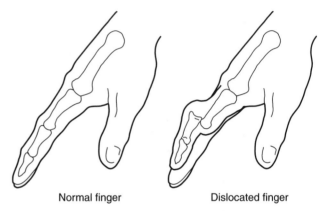

Normal finger   Dislocated finger

Figure 9-9. Dislocated finger (proximal interphalangeal joint).

treatment of joint dislocations to the hand is mandated because improper care may result in long-term disability and poor anatomical function. This is especially true for dislocations of the thumb (Fig. 9-8). As such, reduction attempts of thumb dislocations should be limited to a hospital setting. Reduction of common finger dislocations requires firm traction along the longitudinal axis of the joint and gentle movement so as to return the joint to normal anatomical alignment (Fig. 9-9). If the reduction is successful, treatment consists of applying ice and splinting in a position of function such as buddy taping. If reduction is unsuccessful or is not attempted, then treatment is to splint in the position found and immediately transport to a hospital. Only rarely should EMS be used for transporting an injured athlete with a dislocation to the hand.

Dislocations of the Elbow

The elbow is characteristically a stable joint requiring a significant force to disrupt its integrity and result in dislocation. As such, a fair number of dislocations are often accompanied by concomitant fractures.[39] The elbow joint is susceptible to anterior and posterior dislocation, with the latter being more prevalent.[12] With anterior dislocations, a significant force is

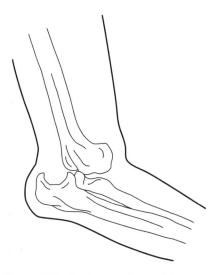

Figure 9-10. Posterior elbow dislocation.

typically directed to the posterior aspect of a flexed elbow. This mechanism of injury results in the olecranon displacing anteriorly respective to the humerus. In the more common posterior dislocation, the mechanism of injury is often described as a fall on an outstretched arm. This condition will usually present in an obvious deformity with an exaggerated protrusion of the olecranon posteriorly (Fig. 9-10).[8] Clinical symptoms for both dislocations include intense pain focal to the elbow joint and a rapid onset of effusion.[12,39] Emergency medical care should consist of immobilizing the anatomy in the position of presentation with a rigid, air, or vacuum splint.[12] Because of the complexity of the elbow joint, a high incidence of neurovascular compromise and associated fractures typically accompany such dislocations. Therefore, it is highly suggested only competent orthopedic specialists perform specific on-site reductions. Therefore, elbow joint dislocations require the immediate activation of EMS for comprehensive care and transport to the nearest medical facility. While awaiting EMS, the athletic trainer must periodically monitor neurovascular status. Complications resulting from inadequate management include brachial artery occlusion, medial or ulnar nerve pathology, and myositis ossificans and arthritis. The athletic trainer must also remain cognizant of the possibility of spontaneous reduction of the dislocation and remain vigilant for warning signs of any of the previously mentioned complications. If a spontaneous reduction of a dislocation is suspected, the athletic trainer should evaluate stability of the elbow complex and appropriately splint the area. The injured athlete must also be immediately transported to the nearest emergency medical facility for proper follow-up care.[8]

Dislocations of the Shoulder

Of large articulations throughout the human skeletal system, the GHJ is one most predisposed to dislocate during athletic activities.[8] The majority of GHJ dislocations are

described as anterior and posterior.[37] Inferior dislocations are typically associated with concomitant fracture and significant neurovascular compromise, although such injuries are rare.[37] Glenohumeral joint dislocations are widespread in contact or collision sports participation and are often the result of direct trauma. The mechanism of injury most often eliciting an anterior dislocation is that of a direct extreme external rotation and abduction force applied to the GHJ. Posterior dislocations of the GHJ occur as the result of a significant direct force that drives the humeral head posteriorly, thereby disrupting its integrity with the glenoid. Athletes sustaining GHJ dislocations often present with a significant amount of pain and tendency to cradle the injured extremity.[8] There is also an unwillingness and inability to generate range of motion within the affected shoulder complex. Assessing a GHJ dislocation is best accomplished through visual inspection of the involved anatomy for obvious deformity. This usually consists of an exaggerated protrusion of the humeral head and hollow area inferior to the acromion.[8,37]

Emergency medical care of GHJ dislocations should begin with a thorough examination to rule out associated neurovascular compromise and potentially related fractures. Significant spasm of surrounding musculature is usually quickly noted subsequent to GHJ dislocations. This protective guarding mechanism can pose a considerable challenge in reducing the joint dislocation. Prompt competent joint reduction on the field of play typically necessitates less force. Furthermore, early reduction can provide considerable relief from pain in addition to diminishing the potential for **iatrogenic** pathology.[27,36,37] Although ideally radiographic images of the injured joint should be obtained prior to and following reduction to rule out related fractures, the benefits of early reduction usually outweigh the involved risks.[27,36,37] This is especially evident in those individuals suffering from chronic GHJ instability and recurrent dislocations. Within this particular population concomitant fractures rarely present.[37]

Three commonly used modes of reduction include the **self-reduction technique,** the **gravity (modified Stimson's) method,** and **traction/external rotation procedure.** Self-reduction calls for the athlete with a GHJ dislocation to interlock his or her fingers and grasp the flexed knee of the unaffected side. The athlete then gradually leans backward, inducing slight traction to the GHJ, which ideally yields relocation.[37]

The gravity (modified Stimson's) method requires the athlete to lay prone with the injured extremity draped over an examination table or similar surface. The athletic trainer then grasps the wrist of the affected extremity and applies a minimal amount of gravity-assisted traction. The gravity-assisted traction aims to gradually stretch the surrounding musculature in spasm, thereby facilitating relocation of the GHJ (Fig. 9-11).[27,37]

The traction/external rotation procedure begins with the injured athlete in a supine position followed by the athletic trainer inducing mild and continual traction along the humeral axis of the affected extremity. In many cases, this will

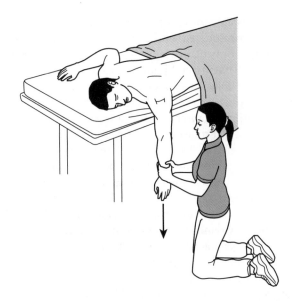

Figure 9-11. Gravity (modified Stimson's) method.

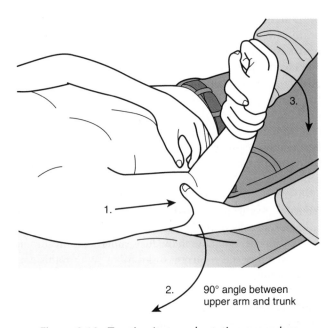

3.

1.

2.   90° angle between
upper arm and trunk

Figure 9-12. Traction/external rotation procedure.

significantly decrease pain. The athletic trainer then slowly and passively guides the GHJ to approximately 90 degrees of abduction while maintaining the mild traction. Once this has been accomplished the GHJ should be gradually externally rotated to correct physiological terminal range. This position is held steadily to relieve muscle spasm. Once the protective muscle spasm has been decreased, the GHJ dislocation should reduce spontaneously and be felt by both the injured athlete and athletic trainer (Fig. 9-12).[36] If reduction in this position proves unsuccessful, the clinician may attempt to gradually increase GHJ abduction to 120 degrees while steadily maintaining traction and GHJ external rotation. The athletic trainer must remain cognizant that aggressive traction or countertraction is not used in this joint reduction mode.[36] Following relocation of the articulation, the GHJ is

returned to 0 degrees of abduction and internally rotated until the hand comes into contact with the torso, all while maintaining steady traction.

It is imperative the athletic trainer periodically reassess neurovascular functions following reduction. An arm sling should be used for comfort, with careful application of ice for pain control.[8,37] Referral to an orthopedic specialist for urgent consultation is highly recommended following GHJ dislocations. If a GHJ dislocation cannot be reduced easily, it must be appropriately splinted in a position of comfort and the injured athlete must be transported to a hospital by EMS.

Dislocations of the Thorax

The sternoclavicular joint (SCJ) has a dense network of ligamentous and capsular tissues that maintain the joint and make dislocations rare. Therefore, an extreme force is required to compromise integrity of the SCJ. Anterior dislocations of the SCJ are more prevalent and usually are associated with an indirect mechanism of injury.[13] This includes a blow to the anterior aspect of the shoulder complex transmitting force to the SCJ, which results in its disruption. Conversely, direct forceful contact to the superior portion of the sternum or medial clavicle often results in posterior dislocations of the SCJ.[13] Significant morbidity is typically not associated with anterior SCJ dislocations. However, complications with regard to posterior SCJ dislocations are prevalent. These include pneumothorax, lesions to the superior vena cava and trachea, and occlusion of the subclavian vasculature.[13] Potential complications subsequent to posterior SCJ dislocations are severe and, if not properly managed in a swift manner, may result in death. Athletes sustaining SCJ dislocations usually complain of chest and shoulder pain exacerbated by excursion of the shoulder complex or assumption of a supine position. Perceived pain is usually more intense with posterior SCJ dislocations.[30] Physical observation may also reveal the athlete tending to lean the head toward the injured anatomy and cradling the affected arm in GHJ adduction.[30] Edema and focal tenderness about the injured joint is also present. Careful inspection should be given with posterior SCJ dislocations. In this instance, edema or effusion may potentially obscure deformities and yield a false impression of the injury.[13] Other symptoms that may be indicative of additional pathology include dyspnea, **dysphagia,** and paresthesia.[13,30] Appropriate management should consist of monitoring vital signs and immediate activation of EMS for transport to a hospital. For comfort the injured athlete may remain seated upright with the affected arm placed in a sling while awaiting arrival of EMS for comprehensive care (Fig. 9-13).

✪ *STAT Point 9-5. Potential complications subsequent to posterior SCJ dislocations are severe and, if not properly managed in a swift manner, may result in death.*

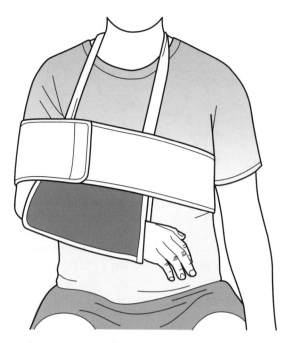

Figure 9-13. Shoulder sling.

Dislocations of the Hip

Dislocations of the hip joint represent a traumatic orthopedic emergency that calls for swift and appropriate management. This includes immediate activation of EMS for rapid treatment and transport. The common mechanism of injury resulting in hip joint dislocations is violent direct trauma.[58] Hip joint dislocations are classified in terms of their anatomical orientation and are described as anterior, posterior, or central (Box 9-6).[58] Less common anterior hip joint dislocations most often result from a substantial force imparted on an abducted leg, which levers the femoral head anteriorly from the acetabulum. A second mechanism of injury triggering anterior dislocation of the hip may occur subsequent to a forceful direct blow to the posterior aspect of the joint. This compromises the joint's anterior ligamentous structures and results in protrusion of the femoral head from the acetabulum. The more prevalent posterior dislocations usually result

from a significant force transmitted along the femoral shaft while both knee and hip joints are in a flexed position. The final type of hip joint dislocation, termed central, is best labeled a fracture-dislocation.[45] The central hip dislocation typically ensues following application of a significant direct force to the lateral aspect of the joint. This mechanism of injury results in the femoral head being driven medially into the acetabulum resulting in concomitant fractures.

Typical biomechanical presentation of the injured lower extremity subsequent to respective hip joint dislocations may be obvious.[58] On visual inspection of the injured athlete who has suffered an anterior hip dislocation, the lower extremity tends to be abducted and externally rotated. Conversely, following posterior hip joint dislocations the injured lower extremity may present in a position of adduction and internal rotation. As a result of complexity of central hip joint dislocations, the affected lower extremity may demonstrate a subtle shortening, depending on the degree of penetration of the femoral head into the acetabulum.

Common complaints unique to anterior dislocations consist of considerable pain throughout the hip and inability to generate any joint excursion. Symptoms of **paresis** may further indicate associated pathology to the femoral nerve. Pallor and diminished distal pulses should raise suspicion of femoral artery compromise. A sign specific to posterior hip dislocations is notable pain throughout the joint, which at times may be focalized to the gluteal region. With posterior displacement of bony fragments, potential compromise of the sciatic nerve may result. This elicits referred pain throughout the posterior aspect of the affected leg. Injury to vascular structures is rare subsequent to posterior hip joint dislocations, yet this should not deter the athletic trainer from conducting a thorough assessment for such functions of the injured lower extremity.[58]

The incidence of mortality associated with catastrophic hip joint dislocations is most often the result of accompanying pelvic or thoracic pathology.[21,58] Hence, it is mandatory for thorough assessments of such related injuries when managing traumatic hip joint dislocations. As a result of the intricate nature of hip joint dislocations, attempts at on-site reduction by those other than an orthopedic specialist are discouraged. With the increased incidence of associated pathology the athletic trainer should monitor for such injuries, periodically assess vital signs, and immobilize the hip in the position found while awaiting EMS arrival. Complications of hip joint dislocations include osteoarthritis, femoral neurovascular compromise specific to anterior dislocation, chronic hip joint instability, AVN of the femoral head, and sciatic nerve pathology subsequent to posterior dislocation (Box 9-7). The probability of AVN is significantly increased with delayed reduction or repeated failed attempts at relocating the hip joint dislocation.

Box 9-6 Comparison of Hip Dislocations

- *Anterior hip dislocation:* Lower extremity abducted and externally rotated

- *Posterior hip dislocation:* Lower extremity adducted and internally rotated

- *Central hip dislocation:* Lower extremity may demonstrate a subtle shortening depending on the degree of penetration of the femoral head into the acetabulum

---

⭐ *STAT Point 9-6. The probability of AVN is significantly increased with delayed reduction or repeated failed attempts at relocating the hip joint dislocation.*

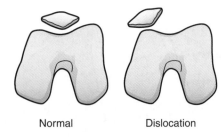

Figure 9-14. Patellar dislocation

Box 9-7   Complications of Hip Joint Dislocations

- Osteoarthritis
- Femoral neurovascular compromise specific to anterior dislocation
- Chronic hip joint instability
- Avascular necrosis of the femoral head
- Sciatic nerve pathology subsequent to posterior dislocation

Dislocations of the Knee

Tibiofemoral Joint

Dislocations of the tibiofemoral joint are rarely encountered in orthopedic sports medicine.[59] This dislocation is described as complete displacement of the tibia from the femur with rupture of three or more articulating ligaments. The perplexing issue involving these dislocations is that a majority of cases often reduce spontaneously before initial emergency medical care is rendered.[18,59] The etiology of knee dislocations is associated with an extreme violent force to the joint, which usually ruptures both cruciate ligaments and at least one collateral ligament. In rare instances only a single cruciate ligament is completely ruptured. The classification system of knee joint dislocations is based on orientation of tibial displacement relative to the femur.[18,57,59] More specifically, these dislocations are described as anterior, posterior, medial, lateral, and rotational. Dislocations termed rotational can be categorized by orientation of the displaced tibial plateau, with the occurrence of posterolateral being most common. Finally, knee joint dislocations can also be expressed as open or closed and either reducible or irreducible.

Knee joint dislocations constitute a traumatic orthopedic emergency and require immediate activation of EMS. Management of knee dislocations requires frequent monitoring of distal pulses and sensory distribution. The high prevalence of associated neurovascular pathology is of utmost concern regarding knee joint dislocations. Particular interest is specific to the popliteal artery and peroneal nerve.[57] Both of these respective vascular and nervous tissues are subject to significant traction or entrapment subsequent to knee joint dislocation. Therefore, it is stressed that athletic trainers be observant for signs of cyanosis and escalating hematoma because these symptoms may be indicative of vascular compromise. Knee joint dislocations are best immobilized in the position found with a rigid splint. The athletic trainer must frequently monitor neurovascular status while awaiting arrival of EMS.[57] If the athletic trainer were to encounter a knee joint dislocation suspected of spontaneous reduction, the involved lower extremity should be stabilized in a knee joint immobilizer set to 30 degrees of flexion. The injured athlete must then be urgently transported to the nearest emergency medical facility for follow-up care.[18,59]

Patellofemoral Joint

Dislocations of the patella most often occur when a partially flexed knee is exposed to simultaneous valgus and extensor forces. As a result, the patella typically dislocates laterally in relation to the knee complex (Fig. 9-14). Associated injury to adjacent neurovascular structures is rare. Isolated reductions of patellar dislocations are not as intricate as the relocation techniques of other joint dislocations. Examination of the knee will display obvious deformity, swelling, and consequent pain. The injured athlete will be unable to ambulate or actively extend the knee from a flexed position.

To successfully reduce a dislocated patella the athletic trainer begins by passively flexing the hip to relieve quadriceps tension. The athletic trainer then fully extends the knee gently while applying firm pressure directed medially to the lateral border of the patella (Fig. 9-15). Successful reduction results in immediate pain relief and loss of obvious anatomical deformity. Treatment of patellar dislocations includes immobilization of the knee joint in full extension with a brace, application of ice, and referral to an orthopedic specialist. If reduction attempts prove unsuccessful, the knee joint should be immobilized in the position found and the injured athlete should be transported to a hospital.

Dislocations of the Ankle

Dislocations of the ankle are a result of substantial forces imparted to the joint, which disrupts the integrity of the articulating structures and often results in associated fractures.[33] As with any joint dislocation, neurovascular injury is of great concern. This is especially true with regard to preservation of the talus, which lacks substantial blood supply. Four types of joint dislocations are generally noted at the ankle and include posterior, anterior, lateral, and superior.[20,33,44] Posterior dislocations represent the most prevalent type encountered and are subsequent to a force that displaces the talus posteriorly relative to the tibia.[20,33] As a result of the greater cross-sectional area of the anterior talus, the

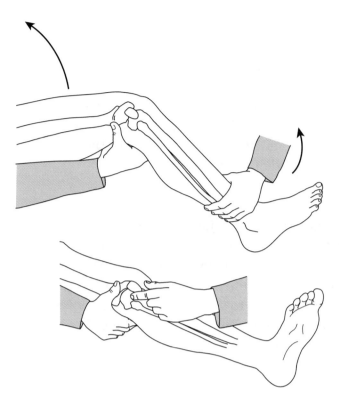

Figure 9-15. Proper hand placement for reducing a dislocated patella.

posterior displacement of this bone may potentially disrupt the tibiofibular syndesmosis and consequently yield fractures.[44] Anterior dislocations are commonly the product of an anteriorly directed force on the posterior aspect of the ankle while the foot is suspended in the open kinetic chain. This dislocation may also result from a significant

posteriorly directed force imparted to the anterior aspect of the tibia, as the foot remains fixed in the closed kinetic chain. Lateral dislocations are associated with hyperinversion, hypereversion, or excessive rotatory excursion of the ankle joint and are typically accompanied by malleolar and distal fibular fractures. Superior joint dislocations are most often the product of the talus displacing superiorly within the ankle mortise and usually are encountered subsequent to violent falls from a considerable height.

Physical examination of the ankle joint following dislocation often reveals obvious anatomical deformity, significant effusion, and considerable pain. These specific conditions warrant immediate activation of EMS because of complexities involved for reducing the respective joint dislocations.[20] While awaiting definitive care the athletic trainer must monitor the athlete's neurovascular status frequently. Furthermore, the ankle must be appropriately splinted in the position found.[20] The high potential for associated fractures precludes reduction attempts on the field. Early reduction at a hospital diminishes the likelihood for associated AVN or neurovascular compromise.

The athletic trainer assumes the responsibilities of medical emergency management, triage, and judgment concerning return to play during sporting events. As such, athletic trainers must be properly prepared to recognize traumatic life- and limb-threatening situations. As allied health professionals, athletic trainers should be competent in providing preliminary emergency medical care of such conditions and regulating appropriate referral when necessary. All athletic trainers should be cognizant of clinical standards and field protocols pertaining to the correct management of orthopedic trauma. This helps ensure that optimal successful outcomes are highly likely when rendering emergency medical care of orthopedic sports injuries.

EMERGENCY ACTION

Prompt emergency medical care of the suspected humeral shaft fracture would consist of temporarily stabilizing the affected anatomy in the position found and assessing neurovascular status, especially of the radial nerve. The athletic trainer must be cognizant that fractures to the middle and distal third of the humerus carry the potential for radial palsy. This is exemplified by wrist-drop or an inability to actively extend the wrist of the involved arm. A complete examination of the shoulder, elbow, and wrist joints must be performed to rule out occult injuries. The onset of neurovascular compromise as evidenced by the inability of the athlete to actively extend the wrist of the injured extremity necessitates immediate activation of EMS for transport. The involved arm should be immobilized in the position found with a rigid long-arm splint for transport off the field of play and to the nearest emergency medical facility. The athletic trainer must also periodically monitor for symptoms indicative of acute compartment syndrome while awaiting arrival of EMS.

CHAPTER HIGHLIGHTS

- Clinical symptoms of fractures generally involve significant focal bone pain, osseous anatomical deformity, edema, and ecchymosis.

- The most commonly fractured sites of the human skeletal system occur at the hand and wrist complex.

- Attaining the necessary skills to properly manage these fractures is vital to prevent potentially debilitating conditions.

- The joints proximal and distal to a potential fracture must be assessed for associated injuries.

- Stability of a fracture may be accomplished by limiting excursion of the bone or joints both proximal and distal to the affected area.

- It is of utmost importance that neurovascular status distal to an involved fracture be monitored frequently with deficiencies or alterations accounted for.

- Open fractures tend to increase the incidence for infection and are considered true traumatic orthopedic emergencies. Therefore, any bleeding noted in the vicinity of a fracture should be considered open and managed as such.

- Significant vascular compromise that leads to profuse bleeding or absent pulses jeopardizes not only the integrity of the associated extremity but also may create a life-threatening scenario. As such, bleeding must be controlled with direct pressure and exposed bone should be irrigated and dressed with sterile materials to reduce the potential for local infection.

- It is extremely important that athletic trainers monitor for the onset of acute compartment syndrome associated with traumatic fractures. If this condition is not appropriately managed, it can prove limb-threatening secondary to ischemia.

- Five basic classes of splints are used in orthopedic sports medicine and emergency medical care. These include rigid, soft, formable, vacuum, and traction splints.

- The athletic trainer must remember to reassess neurovascular integrity immediately and periodically following the application of a splint.

- Gross joint instability resulting from dislocation constitutes a traumatic orthopedic emergency.
- Standard emergency medical care principles state that joint dislocations are to be immobilized in the position found and the that athlete must be referred to the nearest hospital for comprehensive care.
- To decrease pain and prevent further injury to the joint or surrounding anatomical structures, practical attempts at prompt reduction on the field of play can be attempted by the athletic trainer. The dislocations in this context are the shoulder, fingers, and patella.
- Reductions of the elbow, hip, and knee joints are regarded as difficult and not recommended for the athletic trainer. This is because of the challenging reduction procedures, high likelihood of associated fractures, and severe complications from inadequate attempts.

Chapter Questions

1. Based on the orientation of fragments, skeletal fractures may be described as all but the following:
   A. Transverse
   B. Oblique
   C. Comminuted
   D. Central

2. Knee joint dislocations are described as anterior, posterior, medial, lateral, and _____:
   A. Central
   B. Rotational
   C. Superior
   D. Complicated

3. Dislocations of all but what joint highly result in neurovascular compromise?
   A. Sternoclavicular
   B. Knee
   C. Elbow
   D. Shoulder

4. Potential complications resulting from SCJ dislocations do not result in lesions to the _____:
   A. Superior vena cava
   B. Subclavian vasculature
   C. Scapular circumflex artery
   D. Trachea

5. What splints must be regularly monitored and adjusted for changes in temperature as well as atmospheric pressure?
   A. Air
   B. Pillow
   C. Rigid
   D. Formable

6. Which of the following is not a type of femoral fracture?
   A. Type I: spiral or transverse
   B. Type II: comminuted
   C. Type III: open
   D. Type IV: superior

7. Traction splints are often used to immobilize long-bone fractures, especially of the _____:
   A. Humerus
   B. Fibula
   C. Femur
   D. Radius

8. What is the most frequently fractured long-bone in the human skeletal system?
   A. Humerus
   B. Fibula
   C. Femur
   D. Tibia

9. The most commonly fractured sites of the human skeletal system occur where?

A. Hand and wrist

B. Shoulder

C. Lower leg

D. Foot and ankle

10. Which of the following joints is most predisposed to dislocate during athletic activities?

A. Hip

B. Elbow

C. Shoulder

D. Ankle

■ *Case Study 1*

During a soccer match an athlete experiences a violent slide tackle to the fibula. Following examination of this traumatic orthopedic injury, the athlete is suspected to have sustained a closed nondisplaced fibular fracture. After providing appropriate treatment, the sports medicine staff decide to transport the injured athlete off the field of play. However, shortly following the initial mechanism of injury the athlete begins to report increasing discomfort throughout the affected area. This continues until the athlete complains of escalating pain significantly out of context to what is expected with such a fracture.

Case Study 1 Questions

1. What is the potential prognosis for this case?

2. What would be the appropriate emergency medical care?

3. What is the role of the athletic trainer in managing this situation?

■ *Case Study 2*

A basketball player falls forcefully on an outstretched arm after being knocked off balance while going for a rebound. The athletic trainer providing event coverage is summoned to the court, where it appears the athlete has suffered an elbow dislocation. After noting orientation of the olecranon, the athletic trainer's impression is that the elbow joint has dislocated posteriorly. Clinical symptoms include a rapid onset of effusion, and the injured athlete conveys that he is in a substantial amount of pain. After the athletic trainer has adequately examined the orthopedic injury, a member of the support staff immediately activates EMS. The athletic trainer effectively splints the involved extremity and advises the injured athlete to remain in the position of presentation until arrival of EMS.

Case Study 2 Questions

1. Are there additional responsibilities of the athletic trainer in managing this trauma?

2. Why should the athletic trainer defer reducing this specific joint dislocation?

3. What complications can arise from inadequate emergency medical care?

References

1. Allman FL Jr. Fractures and ligamentous injuries of the clavicle and its articulation. J Bone J Surg Am. 1967;49: 774–784.

2. Andersen K, Jensen PO, Lauritzen J. Treatment of clavicular fractures. Figure-of-eight bandage versus a simple sling. Acta Orthop Scand. 1987;58:71–74.

3. Axe MJ. Limb-threatening injuries in sport. Clin Sports Med. 1989;8:101–109.

4. Benson LS, Bailie DS. Proximal interphalangeal joint injuries of the hand. Part II: Treatment and complications. Am J Orthop. 1996 Aug;25(8):527–530.

5. Blake R, Hoffman J. Emergency department evaluation and treatment of the shoulder and humerus. Emerg Med Clin North Am. 1999;17:859–876.

6. Bruns W, Maffuli N. Pediatric and adolescent sports injuries. Lower limb injuries in children in sports. Clin Sports Med. 2000;19(4):637–662.

7. Burgess AR, Poka A. Musculoskeletal trauma. Emerg Med Clin North Am. 1984;2:871–882.

8. Burra G, Andrews JR. Acute shoulder and elbow dislocations in the athlete. Orthop Clin North Am. 2002;33: 479–495.

9. Burt CW, Overpeck MD. Emergency visits for sports-related injuries. Ann Emerg Med. 2001 Mar;37: 301–308.

10. Chudnofsky CR. Splinting techniques. In: Roberts J, Hedges J. Clinical procedures in emergency medicine, 3rd ed. Philadelphia: WB Saunders; 1998:852–873.

11. Clanton TO, Porter DA. Primary care of foot and ankle injuries in the athlete. Clin Sports Med. 1997;16:435–466.

12. Cohen MS, Hastings H. Acute elbow dislocation: Evaluation and management. J Am Acad Orthop Surg. 1998 Jan-Feb;6(1):15–23.

13. Cope R. Dislocations of the sternoclavicular joint. Skeletal Radiol. 1993;22(4)233–238.

14. Daffner RH. Ankle trauma. Radiol Clin North Am. 1990 Mar;28(2):395–421.

15. Daniels JM II, Zook EG, Lynch JM. Hand and wrist injuries: Part II. Emergent evaluation. Am Fam Physician. 2004;69:1949–1956.

16. Easter A. Management of patients with multiple rib fractures. Am J Crit Care. 2001 Sept;10(5):320–327.

17. Edwards PH, Grana WA. Physeal fractures about the knee. J Am Acad Orthop Surg. 1995;3:63–69.

18. Frassica FJ, Stim FH, Staeheli JW, et al. Dislocation of the knee. Clin Orthop. 1991 Feb;(263):200–205.

19. Geiderman JM. Orthopedic injuries: Management principles. In: Rosen P, Harkin R, Danzl D, eds. Emergency medicine: Concepts and clinical practice, 4th ed. St Louis: Mosby-Year Book; 1998:602–624.

20. Graeme KA, Jackimczyk KC. The extremities and spine. Emerg Med Clin North Am. 1997 May;15(2):365–379.

21. Harrington KD. Orthopedic management of extremity and pelvic lesions. Clin Orthop. 1995 Mar;(312):136–137.

22. Hossfeld G, Uehara D. The hand in emergency medicine. Emerg Med Clin North Am. 1993;11:781–796.

23. Johnson I, Branfoot T. Sternal fracture—A modern review. Arch Emerg Med. 1993 Mar;10(1):24–28.

24. Kay RM, Matthys GA. Pediatric ankle fractures: Evaluation and treatment. J Am Acad Orthop Surg. 2001;9:268–278.

25. Kuntz DG Jr, Baratz ME. Fractures of the elbow. Orthop Clin North Am. 1999;30:1–37.

26. Lee SJ, Montgomery K. Athletic hand injuries. Orthop Clin North Am. 2002;33:547–554.

27. Lippert FG. A modification of the gravity method of reducing anterior shoulder dislocations. Clin Orthop. 1982;259–260.

28. Mann DC. Distribution of physeal and nonphyseal fractures of long bones in children aged 0–16 years. J Ped Orthop. 1990;10:713–716.

29. Marder RA, Chapman MW. Principles of management of fractures in sports. Clin Sports Med. 1990;9:1–11.

30. Marker LB, Klareskov B. Posterior sternoclavicular dislocation: An American football injury. Br J Sports Med. 1996 Mar;30(1):71–72.

31. Mastey RD, Weiss AP, Akelman E. Primary care of hand and wrist athletic injuries. Clin Sports Med. 1997;16: 705–724.

32. Misra A, Kapur R, Maffulli N. Complex proximal humeral fracture in adults—A systematic review of management. Injury. 2001;32:363–372.

33. Moehring HD, Tan RT, Marder RA, et al. Ankle dislocation. J Orthop Trauma. 1994;8(2):167–172.

34. Nunley JA. Fractures of the base of the fifth metatarsal. Orthop Clin. 2001;32:171–180.

35. Palmer RE. Joint injuries of the hand in athletes. Clin Sports Med. 1998;17:513–531.

36. Plummer D, Clinton J. The external rotation method for reduction of acute anterior shoulder dislocations. Emerg Med Clin North Am. 1989;7:165–175.

37. Quillen DM, Wuchner M, Hatch RL. Acute shoulder injuries. Am Fam Physician. 2004 Nov;70(10): 1947–1954.

38. Rashid MA, Ortenwall P, Wilkstrom T. Cardiovascular injuries associated with sternal fractures. Eur J Surg. 2001 Apr;167(4):243–248.

39. Ratting AC. Elbow, forearm and wrist injuries in the athlete. Sports Med. 1998 Feb;25(2):115–130.

40. Rosenburg GA, Sferra JJ. Treatment strategies for acute fractures and nonunions of the proximal fifth metatarsal. J Am Acad Orthop Surg. 2000;8:332–338.

41. Rossi F, Dragoni S. Acute avulsion fractures of the pelvis in adolescent competitive athletes. Skeletal Radiol. 2001;30:127–131.

42. Sailer S, Lewis S. Rehabilitation and splinting of common upper extremity injuries in athletes. Clin Sports Med. 1995;14:411–446.

43. Salter RB, Harris WR. Injuries involving the epiphyseal plate. J Bone Joint Surg Am. 1963;45A:587–622.

44. Schuberth JM. Diagnosis of ankle injuries: The essentials. J Foot Ankle Surg. 1994;33(2)214.

45. Smith JM. Pelvic fractures. West J Med. 1998 Feb; 168(2):124–125.

46. Stanish WD. Lower leg, foot, and ankle injuries in young athletes. Clin Sports Med. 1995;14:651–668.

47. Starr AJ, Hunt JL, Reinert CM. Treatment of femur fractures with associated vascular injury. J Trauma. 1996 Jan;40(1):17–21.

48. Steele PM, et al. Management of acute fractures around the knee, ankle and foot. Clin Fam Pract. 2000;2(3):661.

49. Stephens NG, Morgan AS, Corvo P, et al. Significance of scapular fracture in the blunt-trauma patient. Ann Emerg Med. 1995 Oct;26(4):439–442.

50. Stewart C, Winograd S. Hand injuries: A step by step approach for clinical evaluation and definitive management. Emerg Med Rep. 1997;18:223–234.

51. Stiell IG, McKnight RD, Greenberg GH. Implementation of the Ottawa ankle rules. JAMA. 1994:271(11):827–832.

52. Valkosky GJ, Pachuda NM, Brown W. Midfoot fractures. Clin Podiatr Med Surg. 1995 Oct;12(4):773–389.

53. Vouri JP, Aro HT. Lisfranc joint injuries: Trauma mechanisms and associated injuries. J Trauma. 1993 Jul;35(1):40–45.

54. Watson JT. Fractures of the forearm and elbow. Clin Sports Med. 1990;9:59–83.

55. Wedmore IS, Charette J. Emergency department evaluation and treatment of ankle and foot injuries. Emerg Med Clin North Am. 2000 Feb;18(1):85–113.

56. Wexler RK. The injured ankle. Am Fam Physician. 1998 Feb 1;57(3):474–480.

57. Yeh WL, Tu YK, Hsu RW. Knee dislocation: treatment of high-velocity knee dislocation. J Trauma. 1999 Apr;46(4):693–701.

58. Yound EC, Cornwall R. Initial treatment of traumatic hip dislocations in the adult. Clin Orthop. 2000 Aug;(377):24–31.

59. Zoys GN. Knee dislocations. Orthop. 2001 Mar;24(3):294–299.

Suggested Readings

1. Orthopaedic Trauma Association: www.ota.org

2. American Orthopaedic Association: www.aoassn.org

3. American Trauma Society: www.amtrauma.org

4. Orthopaedic Research Society: www.ors.org

5. United States Bone and Joint Decade: www.usbjd.org

6. Trauma Care of America: www.traumacare.com

7. International Society for Fracture Repair: www.fractures.com

Chapter 10

Abdominal Emergencies

David Stone, MD, and Scott Wissink, MD

KEY TERMS

Abdomen	Hilum	Pancreas
Abdominal splinting	Kehr's sign	Pancreatitis
Ballone sign	Kidney	Parenchymal injury
Contrast material	Laparotomy	Peritonitis
Cullen's sign	Liver	Spleen
Ectopic pregnancy	Nephrectomy	Thrombosis
Epigastrium	Omental infarction	Turner's sign

 EMERGENCY SITUATION

At practice, a football player attempts to recover a fumble and dives on a loose ball. Two other players fall on top of him as he lands on the ball. He has the wind knocked out of him and he must be helped off the field. He complains of mild abdominal pain, which is localized to the periumbilical area. His blood pressure is 138/72, and his pulse is 96. His abdominal examination demonstrates localized abdominal discomfort on palpation with no rebound tenderness. He has discomfort when contracting his abdominal muscles. He is given an ice bag for the abdomen, and his examination is repeated 15 minutes later. At that time, his blood pressure is 110/68, his pulse is 64, and he has only minimal abdominal tenderness. He expresses a desire to return to practice. As the athletic trainer, what actions should you take?

Sports-related abdominal emergencies are uncommon. In a 30-year period, Bergovist et al.[1] were able to document only 136 abdominal injuries requiring hospitalization in a Swedish county. The dominant age group was 10 to 20 years old, and soccer was the most commonly involved sport, accounting for almost half the injuries. The most common diagnosis was an abdominal wall contusion, accounting for 60 of the 136 injuries studied. The **kidney** was the most commonly injured organ and was four times more frequently injured than the **spleen,** the next most commonly injured organ. The authors noted that the abdominal symptoms on admission to the hospital were usually not dramatic, with only eight patients demonstrating signs of clinical **peritonitis.** Four of the patients were diagnosed with delayed splenic rupture.

In a search of the National Pediatric Trauma Registry, Wan et al.[2] found that sports were responsible for only 6.64% of the cases reported to the trauma centers in the study and comprised only 0.56% of the injuries. Of the injuries, 84% occurred in children between the ages of 12 and 18 years. American football was the most frequently involved sport, with baseball and basketball the next most common. The spleen was the most frequently injured organ across all age groups, with 96 cases, and the kidney was second with 42 cases. Ryan[3] noted that the relative infrequency of abdominal injuries put them at risk to go undiagnosed because they are internal and concealed.

✪ *STAT Point 10-1. The relative infrequency of abdominal injuries puts them at risk to go undiagnosed because they are internal and concealed.*

Initial Evaluation

It is important for the athletic trainer and physician to remember that the infrequent nature of abdominal injuries is a pitfall in their management. Differentiating benign injuries from injuries that require transfer to a hospital is often challenging, and the difference may not be obvious on the initial examination. Repeated monitoring of vital signs and abdominal examinations are imperative regardless of the severity of the trauma involved and should be done at intervals until the athlete has either clearly improved or clearly requires transport for imaging studies and blood work. It should also be remembered that in the general population unrecognized abdominal injury is a frequent cause of preventable death[3] and can be masked by head injury, orthopedic injury, medications, or ergogenic aids.[4] Physical examination has been found to be accurate in only 65% of cases of blunt abdominal trauma,[5] and up to one third of patients who initially have a benign abdominal examination will require emergency **laparotomy.**[6] The failure of the physical examination alone to adequately determine the presence of a true abdominal emergency makes further studies almost routine in the evaluation of abdominal trauma. Generally, the team physician will determine if tests can be obtained in

an outpatient setting or if referral to the hospital emergency department is required, but the athletic trainer should be able to evaluate the athlete and make the decision if no physician is available. The evaluation itself consists of two parts: the history and the physical examination.

✪ *STAT Point 10-2. Repeated monitoring of vital signs as well as the abdominal examination is imperative regardless of the severity of the trauma involved, and should be repeated at intervals until the athlete has either clearly improved, or clearly requires transport.*

✪ *STAT Point 10-3. In the general population unrecognized abdominal injury is a frequent cause of preventable death,[3] and can be masked by head injury, orthopedic injury, medications, or ergogenic aids.[4]*

History

A good history is important in determining which abdominal organs are at risk of injury and the severity of the injury (Box 10-1). If the episode was not observed, asking coaches, teammates, and other personnel at the event to describe what happened is critical. The location of the trauma, velocity of impact, and the presence of pads or other protective devices are all important in assessing the severity of the injury and organs at risk. Deceleration injuries are associated with injury to the **liver,** spleen, kidney, or abdominal viscera because these organs continue moving while the body stops.[7] A direct blow to a specific area can result in rib fracture and injury to the abdominal organs behind it. Once the mechanism of injury has been obtained, a description of the pain and its location should be obtained. The history should include the location of the pain and whether it is diffuse or localized; whether the onset was immediate or slowly progressive; and its relationship to coughing, laughing, and

---

Box 10-1   History Summary

- Mechanism of injury?
- Location of pain?
  - Diffuse? Local?
  - Fast or slow onset?
- Any referred pain?
- Prior history of abdominal injury or surgery?
- Allergies?

movement. If activities such as coughing, laughing, or general movement increase the pain, peritonitis could be the involved. Localized pain is often considered evidence of abdominal wall contusion, whereas diffuse pain is associated with intraperitoneal irritation.[7] Radiation of pain to the shoulder (**Kehr's sign**) is associated with abdominal bleeding that irritates the diaphragm. Loss of appetite in athletes is considered by some authors to be an important sign.[8] The history of prior abdominal trauma, prior abdominal surgery, use of medications and ergogenic aids, and any prior medical conditions provides information that also may increase concern and make transport more likely. Finally, allergies to medications and to the **contrast material** used in some imaging studies should be reviewed.

Physical Examination

Physical examination should begin with evaluation of the airway, breathing, and circulation (ABCs). Blood pressure, pulse, and respiratory rate should be obtained to provide baseline data; serial measurements are important to monitor for evidence of circulatory collapse and shock. If evidence of circulatory collapse is present, immediate transfer should be arranged.

The abdominal examination begins with inspection. A brief evaluation for asymmetry, distension, **abdominal splinting,** and prior surgical scars should be undertaken. Ecchymosis in the periumbilical area (**Cullen's sign**) or in the flanks (**Turner's sign**) is usually not seen acutely and may not be present for several hours after acute abdominal trauma. Abrasions may be present and provide clues to location of trauma. The contour of the **abdomen** should be observed. Auscultation for bowel sounds is not often important in the acute setting because electrolyte imbalances or hydration status may alter bowel sounds. When pain is severe posteriorly, a back examination is warranted to look for posterior rib fractures, and, at that time, a quick neck evaluation may need to be performed to rule out cervical spine injury. The presence of a rib fracture is associated with a splenic injury in 20% of cases if it is on the left and in 10% of hepatic injuries if it is on the right side in the lower six ribs.[9,10] In specific cases, palpation of the iliac crest and pelvis to look for pelvic fractures may also be considered. Superficial palpation followed by deep palpation should be performed to evaluate for guarding, peritoneal rebound, and tenderness (Box 10-2). Some professionals do not believe deep palpation is effective and think it should be avoided.[8] In rare cases, examination by a physician of the external genitalia and rectum will need to be performed, predominantly in cases of pelvic trauma.[11] When performing a physical examination, the examiner should be able to evaluate all abdominal quadrants and to assess their contents (Box 10-3).

> ✪ *STAT Point 10-4. The presence of a rib fracture is associated with a splenic injury in 20% of cases if it is on the left, and in 10% of hepatic injuries if it is on the right side in the lower six ribs.*

Box 10-2 Rebound Tenderness

Palpate gently but firmly and deeply and then quickly release pressure. If there is increased pain during or after the release, the patient has rebound tenderness, indicative of peritoneal inflammation (peritonitis). This is a serious condition, warranting immediate referral to a physician.

Box 10-3 Physical Examination Summary

- ■ **ABCs**
- ■ **Vital signs**
  - • **Blood pressure**
  - • **Pulse rate**
  - • **Respiration rate**
- ■ **Visual inspection**
- ■ **Palpation**
  - • **Superficial**
  - • **Deep**

Specific Injuries

Abdominal Wall Contusion

As noted by Bergqvist,[1] the most common traumatic injury in sports is an abdominal wall contusion. Contusions in the region of the **epigastrium** may result in transient dyspnea ("getting the wind knocked out").[7] This injury can usually be treated with a period of rest. The athlete can return to play when symptoms subside, often in a matter of several minutes. However, it is possible for a player to suffer a direct blow to the abdomen and recover adequately to return to play only to have symptoms later in the game or afterward and ultimately be diagnosed with a hollow organ injury[12] or injury to a solid organ.[13] The easy misdiagnosis of a severe abdominal injury requiring surgery with slow or unusual presentations has been documented in other case reports.[14,15] However, a blow to the abdomen can also cause a hematoma in the rectus abdominus, which can mimic an acute abdominal internal injury. These athletes will usually complain of sudden abdominal pain with rapid swelling but will improve by being placed in postures that relax the abdominal wall musculature, usually a forward flexed position. Active contraction of the abdominal muscles will worsen symptoms. Swelling of the abdominal wall and abdominal mass below the umbilicus may be present.[7] If the diagnosis of abdominal wall contusion is made, initial icing to reduce bleeding and metabolic requirements of injured tissues is usually recommended. Padding for protection or a flak jacket if available may further reduce risk of reinjury if the athlete decides to return to play. Continued observation for intraabdominal injury is a necessity.

✪ *STAT Point 10-5. It is possible for a player to suffer a direct blow to the abdomen, recover adequately to return to play only to have symptoms later in the game or afterwards and ultimately be diagnosed with a hollow viscus injury[12] or injury to a solid organ.*

Splenic Injuries

Injuries to the spleen are most often caused by direct trauma to the left lower chest wall or left upper abdominal quadrant (Fig. 10-1).[8] The initial presentation may include fainting, dizziness, and weakness from blood loss[17] but often is confined to left upper quadrant tenderness with or without left shoulder pain (Kehr's sign).[18] A left upper quadrant mass, abdominal distension, and abdominal rigidity are also frequent physical examination findings.[17] **Ballone sign**—fixed dullness in the left flank and shifting position dullness in the right flank—has been described as an infrequent finding.[19] The capsule of the spleen can contain bleeding, and physical examination findings are occasionally delayed in their presentation. Delayed rupture of the spleen is an uncommon complication of splenic injury[20] but an important concern in management.

✪ *STAT Point 10-6. The capsule of the spleen can contain bleeding and physical examination findings are occasionally delayed in their presentation.*

Plain x-rays may demonstrate an enlarged spleen if a subcapsular hematoma with an intact capsule is present. An enlarged spleen may also displace the stomach anteromedially and the left kidney, left transverse colon, and splenic flexure inferiorly. On x-ray, haziness of the abdomen, bulging flanks, and displacement of small bowel loops are associated with signs of free peritoneal fluid, such as blood.[17]

Use of ultrasound to diagnose splenic injuries is common, and sensitivity in diagnosing splenic injuries is greater than for other abdominal organs.[21] However, the appearance of the spleen on sonograms can vary widely. Siniluoto et al.[22] demonstrated that repeat ultrasound evaluation will ultimately pick up splenic injuries if the examination is followed for 1 to 3 days. Many trauma centers use ultrasound as a screening test because it can be performed rapidly, and a focused examination can be performed as a low-cost method for triaging patients with blunt abdominal trauma.[23] Some authors use ultrasound to follow patients because of its low cost and lack of ionizing radiation.[23] The "gold standard" test to evaluate an injury to the spleen is computed tomography (CT) scanning.[23] Findings on CT scan include capsular disruptions, subcapsular and intrasplenic hematomas, single and multiple fractures, and shattered and fragmented spleens.[23] Sensitivity and specificity of CT scan in the diagnosis of splenic injury are generally in the range of 96%.[24]

Box 10-4 provides Buntain's classification of splenic injury, which has been shown to correlate with the time

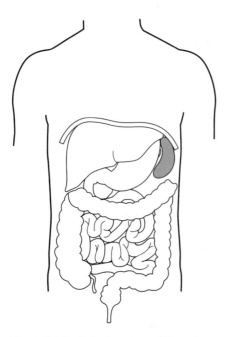

Figure 10-1. Anterior view of the spleen.

Box 10-4 Buntain's Classification of Splenic Injury

- ■ **Grade I:** Localized capsular disruption or subcapsular hematoma without significant parenchymal injury

- ■ **Grade II:** Single or multiple capsular and parenchymal disruptions that do not extend into **hilum** or involve major vessels

- ■ **Grade III:** Deep fractures, single or multiple, extending into the hilum and involving major blood vessels

- ■ **Grade IV:** Completely shattered or fragmented spleen or separated from its normal blood supply at the pedicle

required for radiologic healing and return to activity. The American Association for the Surgery of Trauma (AAST) classification has been shown to correlate with an increased risk for operative management.[25] The majority of injuries to the spleen can be treated nonoperatively, with more than half of the higher-grade injuries managed nonoperatively. However, patients who do not stabilize with minimal resuscitation, those with recurrent hemodynamic instability, and those with the presence of pooling or "blush" in the spleen on the initial CT scan with intravenous contrast all predict the failure of nonoperative management.[25]

On the field, the athletic trainer should obtain baseline vital signs, perform an abdominal examination, reassess vital signs for evidence of vascular instability, and decide if triage to the emergency room is required. If vital signs appear stable and abdominal pain does not increase with cough, sneeze, or rapid movements (all seen with peritoneal irritation), observation is a reasonable option. If there is any evidence of vascular instability, transport should be considered. Placement of an IV for fluid challenge if a question of vascular instability is present should be considered only when transportation to a hospital cannot be easily accomplished.

Liver Injuries

Liver injuries are uncommon in sports. Bergovist[1] noted only 6 injuries to the liver of the 136 patients documented. Wan[2] reported only 13 injuries to the liver in the 10-year period of his study. The usual mechanism of injury is either a direct blow to the right upper quadrant of the abdomen or a deceleration type of injury that lacerates the relatively thin capsule of the liver (Fig. 10-2). The initial complaint is usually right upper quadrant tenderness, but right lower quadrant complaints are occasionally described.[26] Like the spleen,

the physical examination for liver injuries begins with the ABCs followed by blood pressure, pulse rate, and respirations. In cases of blunt abdominal trauma, associated injuries to other abdominal structures are seen 4% to 15% of the time.[27] As with the spleen, on-field decisions about transport are based on an evolving physical examination and hemodynamic stability. Diagnostic testing is used to define the extent of injury and permit continued nonoperative management. CT scan is regarded as the best test to evaluate liver injuries and for the presence of blood in the abdomen.[28] Use of alanine aminotransferase (ALT) and aspartate aminotransferase (AST) has been shown to correlate with the presence of abdominal injury in both adults[29] and children[30] and can be used as screening laboratory tests in patients who are hemodynamically stable. These enzymes are elevated in cases without a radiologically definable liver injury. The American Association for the Surgery of Trauma Organ Injury Scale Classification of liver injuries[31] is provided in Table 10-1.

Renal Injuries

As noted, renal trauma is one of the most common abdominal emergencies in sports (Fig. 10-3). As with other abdominal injuries, signs of renal trauma may not be present immediately after the injury. The most common presenting symptom is flank pain, and hematuria is the most frequent finding on examination.[32] The vast majority of these injuries are mild,[2] but the need for **nephrectomy** can be as high as 10% to 12%,[2,33] and another 10% will have injuries severe enough to require surgery.[34] Unfortunately, hematuria associated with athletic activity is well recognized and in rare cases can be difficult to distinguish acutely from renal trauma. Boone et al.[35] found that 16% of football players had gross hematuria and that hematuria peaked during games. In general, sports hematuria resolves with rest. Cases of suspected renal trauma should be treated in the same way as other abdominal injuries with repeated evaluations of vital signs and abdominal examinations for evolving evidence of significant injury. CT scan remains the test of choice for renal injuries. In confusing cases with a history of trauma and sports hematuria, repeated urinalysis with and without activity can be used to distinguish sports hematuria from abdominal trauma with acute renal injury.[36] Renal vein **thrombosis** following martial arts trauma is a rare entity and presents with flank pain and microscopic hematuria.[37] CT scan is diagnostic.

Intestinal Injuries

Injury to the duodenum and jejunum rarely is reported with abdominal trauma in sports. Duodenal injury is most commonly associated with a direct blow to the epigastric area and often is found in conjunction with an injury to the **pancreas** (Fig. 10-4).[38] Signs and symptoms are notoriously subtle, and a CT scan with contrast is considered the best test to evaluate for this injury. A high degree of suspicion is important in

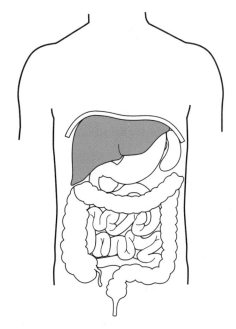

Figure 10-2. Anterior view of the liver.

Table 10-1   American Association for the Surgery of Trauma Organ Injury Scale: Liver

Grade	Description of Injury
I	*Hematoma:* Subcapsular, nonexpanding, less than 10% of surface area *Laceration:* Capsular tear, nonbleeding, less than 1 cm parenchymal depth
II	*Hematoma:* Subcapsular, nonexpanding, 10%–50% of surface or intraparenchymal, nonexpanding, less than 2 cm in diameter *Laceration:* Capsular tear, active bleeding 1–3 cm parenchymal depth, less than 10 cm in length
III	*Hematoma:* Subcapsular, greater than 50% surface area or expanding; ruptured subcapsular hematoma with active bleeding; intraparenchymal hematoma greater than 2 cm or expanding *Laceration:* Greater than 3 cm parenchymal depth
IV	*Hematoma:* Ruptured intraparenchymal hematoma with active bleeding *Laceration:* Parenchymal disruption involving 25%–50% of hepatic lobe
V	*Hematoma:* Parenchymal disruption involving more than 50% of hepatic lobe *Vascular:* Juxtahepatic venous injuries (i.e., retrohepatic vena cava/major hepatic veins)
VI	*Vascular:* Hepatic avulsion

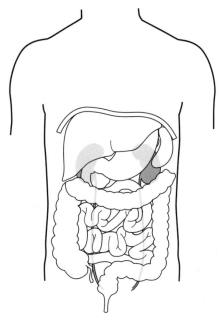

Figure 10-3. Anterior view of the kidneys.

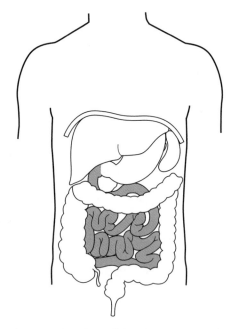

Figure 10-4. Anterior view of the duodenum and jejunum.

these cases because a delay in diagnosis and surgical intervention has been shown to increase mortality.[39]

Jejunal injuries are also extremely rare and have variable presentations.[40,41] In some cases athletes have returned to play, only to have symptoms after play and ultimately require surgery. Although CT scan with contrast is the test of choice, it may initially be negative. The athletic trainer covering practices and games without a physician should continue to evaluate the athlete with suspicion of these injuries throughout the competition or practice and after the game.

Pancreatic Injuries

Pancreas injuries are extremely rare and often difficult to diagnose (Fig. 10-5).[42] Onset is often gradual with slow progression of symptoms. Laboratory testing of serum amylase levels can be diagnostic, but the levels are often slow to rise. CT scan is the initial imaging study of choice and can show lacerations of the pancreas but may not diagnose injuries to the pancreatic duct, which often require endoscopic retrograde cholangeography (ERCP). Athletic

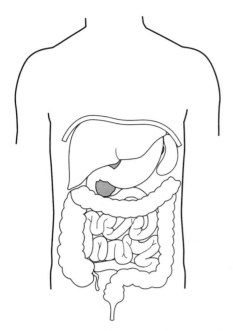

Figure 10-5. Anterior view of the pancreas.

trainers should approach suspected pancreatic injury in the same way they approach all abdominal injuries—with a high degree of suspicion until the injury is shown to be benign.

Nontraumatic Abdominal Injuries

Abdominal complaints are common in many sports.[43,44] Gastrointestinal symptoms are classically mild and consist of cramping, bloating and watery stools, and (rarely) bloody stools and are often associated with a change in mileage or intensity in runners.[45] However, rarely, severe abdominal conditions occur without trauma that requires rapid recognition and management. Marathon **pancreatitis** is a rare condition that presents with abdominal pain during a race and becomes progressively more painful on completion of the race. The etiology is unknown, although some authors postulate dehydration and others suggest ischemia. It appears to be more common in females and mostly in younger runners. CT scan demonstrates edema of the pancreas, and blood tests document injury to the pancreas. Treatment is supportive, but **omental infarction** was noted with one case, and laparotomy was performed.[46] Rupture of adhesions of the omentum from prior surgery has also been described with running,[47] resulting in massive intraabdominal bleeding requiring laparoscopy. Pubic symphysis staphylococcal infection after marathon running has also been described with patients presenting with pelvic, abdominal, and hip pain accompanied by fever and pubic symphysis pain. Ultrasound and CT scan were normal, but magnetic resonance imaging (MRI) of the pubic symphysis clearly demonstrated the infection.[48] Infectious pubic symphysitis must be distinguished from mechanical pubic symphysitis, and a history of infectious symptoms such as chills, sweats, and fever should be a required part of the history of all patients with pubic symphysitis.

Appendicitis

The diagnosis of appendicitis and its initial management are typically based on clinical more than radiologic or laboratory findings (Fig. 10-6). Unfortunately, appendicitis often presents with atypical symptoms, and diagnosis is often in doubt.[49] A thorough history and physical examination should be stressed in the early diagnosis of appendicitis, with the use of laboratory and imaging studies used to support the clinical impression. Right lower quadrant tenderness, abdominal rigidity, guarding, rebound tenderness, pain aggravated by coughing or movement, and duration of pain are the classic findings on examination and are the most common findings predicting appendicitis.[50] Symptoms of loss of appetite, nausea, and a low-grade fever are often present at the onset, although they are passed over until progression of the clinical picture occurs. Pain that begins in the periumbilical area and then shifts to the right lower quadrant of the abdomen is also highly predictive. The combination of clinical findings with the use of laboratory tests has been shown to increase the diagnostic accuracy of appendicitis when two or more descriptors of inflammation are increased.[51] The athletic trainer, who is faced with progressive abdominal complaints and suspects appendicitis, should perform a good history and physical examination and, if possible, arrange for a complete blood count, urinalysis, amylase, liver function studies, erythrocyte sedimentation rate, C-reactive protein, and

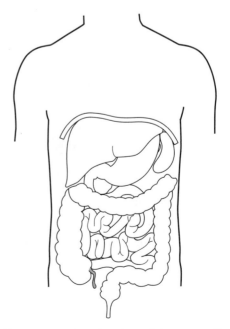

Figure 10-6. Anterior view of the appendix.

potentially a CT scan. Although CT scans are generally considered an excellent diagnostic test for appendicitis,[52,53] in some studies, there is a high false-negative rate and low sensitivity.[54] The most crucial issue in the management of appendicitis concerns transfer to a hospital and, ultimately, whether the patient needs surgery. Spontaneous resolution of appendicitis is common,[55] but the athletic trainer and team physician should err on the side of evaluating the abdominal pain, especially in situations in which air travel or a long bus trip is involved and the diagnosis of appendicitis would change travel plans. The athletic trainer should also be cautious about leaving an athlete with possible appendicitis in a situation where there is no one to observe the athlete because rapid deterioration is possible.

✪ *STAT Point 10-7. Pain which begins in the peri-umbilical area and then shifts to the right lower quadrant of the abdomen is highly predictive of appendicitis.*

Ectopic Pregnancy

Ectopic pregnancy is the implantation of a fertilized ovum outside of the endometrial cavity (Fig. 10-7). It is a major cause of morbidity and mortality in women and, if undiagnosed,

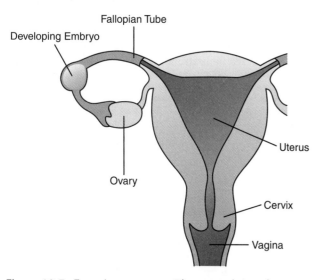

Figure 10-7. Ectopic pregnancy. The normal site of ovum implantation is in the uterus. An ectopic pregnancy almost always involves implantation of the ovum in a fallopian tube, although other sites are possible. If the pregnancy continues and the fallopian tube ruptures, there may be life-threatening intraabdominal bleeding.

can result in rupture of the fallopian tube, massive hemorrhage, and death. Major risk factors include prior damage to the fallopian tube from pelvic inflammatory disease, prior ectopic pregnancy, and prior tubal surgery. Cigarette smoking, increasing age, and more than one lifetime sexual partner have been weakly linked to an increased risk. The condition typically presents with abdominal or pelvic pain, but presentation can be extremely variable, and there is often a delay in reporting symptoms.[56]

✪ *STAT Point 10-8. Ectopic pregnancy is a major cause of morbidity and mortality in women, and if undiagnosed, can result in rupture of the fallopian tube, massive hemorrhage and death.*

Evaluation should begin with vital signs looking for evidence of hypotension, elevated pulse rate, and abdominal rigidity and guarding; however, physical examination findings are often subtle and the athletic trainer should arrange a pelvic examination by an experienced clinician or arrange for screening using transvaginal ultrasound.[57]

The diagnosis of ectopic pregnancy can be enhanced by the use of "discriminatory cutoff." Determining the age of a pregnancy by history can be difficult, and beta-human chorionic gonadatropin (β-hCG) is often used as a marker of gestational age. When β-hCG reaches a specific level, usually 1500 to 2500, an intrauterine pregnancy should be visualized. The absence of an intrauterine pregnancy implies an abnormal location and increases concern for an ectopic pregnancy.[58] When levels are below the discriminatory cutoff, serial measurements can be made and the athlete can be observed,[59] but when levels are above the cutoff and no intrauterine pregnancy is seen on ultrasound, surgery is recommended.[59]

The suspected presence of an ectopic pregnancy should be addressed acutely by referral to a competent obstetrician. Evidence of hypotension and circulatory collapse should be addressed by placement of an intravenous catheter and volume expansion.

Even for a physician, injuries to the abdomen can be difficult to accurately evaluate in the field without access to imaging and laboratory studies. Nevertheless, athletic trainers must be competent in assessing these types of injuries. If missed, some types of injuries can be fatal. Fortunately, injuries to the abdomen are relatively uncommon. The kidney is the most frequently injured organ, followed by the spleen. Injuries to the liver, pancreas, and intestines are rare. A good history and physical examination, although usually not conclusive in abdominal injuries, are management tools for athletic trainers.

EMERGENCY ACTION

Because the athlete's condition has improved, you decide to functionally test the athlete by having him perform running, cutting, and stance and start movements. He does so with minimal discomfort. You discuss your findings with your team physician and conclude that this is most likely an abdominal wall contusion. You explain to the athlete what to be aware of and allow the athlete to return to play.

CHAPTER HIGHLIGHTS

- The spleen is the most frequently injured organ across all age groups; the kidney is second.

- Physical examination has been found to be accurate in only 65% of cases of blunt abdominal trauma, and up to one third of patients who initially have a benign abdominal examination will require emergency laparotomy.

- Generally, the team physician will determine if tests can be obtained in an outpatient setting or if referral to the hospital emergency department is required, but the athletic trainer should be able to evaluate the athlete and make the decision if no physician is available.

- The initial presentation of a splenic injury may include fainting, dizziness, and weakness from blood loss but often is confined to left upper quadrant tenderness with or without left shoulder pain (Kehr's sign).

- The "gold standard" test to evaluate an injury to the spleen is a CT scan.

- The majority of injuries to the spleen can be treated nonoperatively, with more than half of the higher-grade injuries managed nonoperatively.

- If vital signs appear stable and abdominal pain does not increase with cough, sneeze, or rapid movements (all seen with peritoneal irritation), observation is a reasonable option for suspected splenic injuries.

- With liver injuries, the initial complaint is usually right upper quadrant tenderness, but right lower quadrant complaints are occasionally described.

- CT scan is regarded as the best test to evaluate for liver injuries.

- The most common presenting symptom for kidney injury is flank pain, and hematuria is the most frequent finding on examination.

- Cases of suspected renal trauma should be treated in the same way as other abdominal injuries, with repeated evaluations of vital signs and abdominal examinations for evolving evidence of significant injury.

- Duodenal injury is most commonly associated with a direct blow to the epigastric area and often is found in conjunction with an injury to the pancreas.

- Athletic trainers should approach suspected pancreatic injury in the same way they approach all abdominal injuries—with a high degree of suspicion until the injury is shown to be benign.

- Infectious pubic symphysitis must be distinguished from mechanical pubic symphysitis, and a history of infectious symptoms such as chills, sweats, and fever should be a required part of the history of all patients with pubic symphysis.

- The suspected presence of an ectopic pregnancy should be addressed acutely by referral to a competent obstetrician.

Chapter Questions

1. The most commonly injured organ in the abdomen is the _____:
   A. Liver
   B. Stomach
   C. Kidney
   D. Appendix

2. What is most important to note while taking a history of abdominal injury?
   A. Location of trauma
   B. Velocity of contact
   C. Wearing of protective equipment
   D. All of the above

3. Ecchymosis in the periumbilical area is known as _____:
   A. Tinnel's sign
   B. Cullen's sign
   C. Turner's sign
   D. Kehr's sign

4. An injury to the spleen should be suspected with a blow to the _____:
   A. Left upper quadrant
   B. Right upper quadrant
   C. Left lower quadrant
   D. Right lower quadrant

5. Blood in the urine is called _____:
   A. Hemoccult
   B. Hematuria
   C. Hemaurine
   D. None of the above

6. Injuries to the pancreas are _____:
   A. Common
   B. Always life threatening
   C. Easy to diagnose
   D. Rare

7. A diagnosis of appendicitis is based on _____:
   A. Radiology tests
   B. Laboratory results
   C. Clinical picture
   D. A and B

8. A fertilized ovum implanted outside the endometrial wall is _____:
   A. An ectopic pregnancy
   B. A healthy pregnancy
   C. In its third trimester
   D. Common among young women

9. Localized pain to the abdominal wall is most commonly _____:
   A. A rib fracture
   B. Serious in nature
   C. A sign of internal damage
   D. A contusion

10. Kehr's sign is _____:
    A. Pain in the flank
    B. Pain in the shoulder
    C. Pain in the right upper quadrant
    D. Not seen in women

■ *Case Study 1*

A hockey player comes to you after practice and complains that he just noticed blood in his urine. His vital signs are stable and he has no pain on palpation of the abdomen. He has no previous history and does not remember getting hit recently.

Case Study 1 Questions

1. What should your initial management include?
2. What are the possibilities for the cause?
3. What other information would be appropriate to know?

■ *Case Study 2*

A female soccer player complains of fatigue and nausea. She tells you she has missed her last period, which she relates to her nausea, poor diet, and stress of school. She relates a vague history of abdominal discomfort over the past week.

Case Study 2 Questions

1. What are the possible causes for such symptoms?
2. What would be important to know regarding her past medical history?
3. What information would lead you to refer her to a physician?

References

1. Bergovist D, Hedelin H, Karlsson G, et al. Abdominal injury from sporting activities. Br J Sports Med. 1982;16(2):76–79.

2. Wan J, Corvino TF, Greenfield SP, et al. Kidney and testicle injuries in team and individual sports: Data from the National Pediatric Trauma Registry. J Urol. 2003;170:1528–1532.

3. Ryan JM. Abdominal injuries and sport. Br J Sports Med. 1999;155–160.

4. Foley RW, Harris LS, Pilcher DB. Abdominal injuries in automobile accidents: Review of care of fatally injured patients. J Trauma. 1977;17:611–616.

5. McAnena OJ, Moore EE, Marx JA. Initial evaluation of the patient with blunt abdominal trauma. Surg Clin N Am. 1990;70(3):495–515.

6. Mackersie RC, Tiwary AD, Shackford SR, et al. Intra-abdominal injury following blunt trauma. Arch Surg. 1989;124:809–814.

7. Davis JJ, Cohn I, Nance FC. Diagnosis and management of blunt abdominal trauma. Ann Surg. 1978;183: 672–680.

8. Rifat SF, Lilvydis RP. Blunt abdominal trauma in sports. Curr Sports Med Reports. 2003;2:93–97.

9. Bergman RT. Assessing acute abdominal pain: A team physician's challenge. Phys Sports Med. 1996;24:72–82.

10. Hill AC, Schecter WP, Trunkey DD. Abdominal trauma and indications for laparotomy. In Mattos KL, Moore EE, Feliciano DV, eds. Trauma. Norwalk, CT: Appleton & Lange; 1988:401–414.

11. Moore EE. Resuscitation and evaluation of the injured patient. In Zuidema GG, Ballinger W, Rutherford R. Management of trauma. Philadelphia: WB Saunders; 1985:1–10.

12. Colucciello SA, Plotka M. Abdominal trauma. Occult injury may be life threatening. Phys Sports Med. 1993;21:33–43.

13. Murphy CP, Drez D. Jejunal rupture in a football player. Am J Sports Med. 1987;15:184–185.

14. Rawls DE, Monford DC. Pancreatic trauma: An unusual soccer injury. South Med J. 2001;94:741–743.

15. Riviello RJ, Young JS. Intra-abdominal injury from softball. Am J Emerg Med. 2000;18:505–506.

16. Aherene NJ, Kavangh EG, Condon ET, et al. Duodenal perforation after a blunt abdominal sporting injury: The importance of early diagnosis. J Trauma Injury Infect Crit Care. 2003;54:791–794.

17. Dupuy DE, Raptopoulos V, Fink MP. Current concepts in splenic trauma. J Intensive Care Med. 1995;10:76–90.

18. Brown RL, Irish MS, McCabe AJ, et al. Observation of splenic trauma: When is a little too much? J Ped Surg. 1999;7:1124–1126.

19. Shackford SR, Molin M. Management of splenic injuries. Surg Clin North Am. 1990;70:595–620.

20. Schlater DC, Bui T, Shita T. Delayed rupture of the spleen. Ann Emerg Med. 1990;19:399–403.

21. McGahan JP, Richards JR. Blunt abdominal trauma: The role of emergent sonography and a review of the literature. Am J Radiol. 1999;172:897–903.

22. Siniluoto TM, Paivansalo MJ, Lanning FP, et al. Ultrasonography in traumatic splenic rupture. Clin Radiol. 1992;46:391–396.

23. Lynch JM, Meza MP, Newman B. Computed tomography grade of splenic injury is predictive of the time required for radiographic healing. J Ped Surg. 1997;32: 1093–1096.

24. Nelson ED, Holliman CJ, Juell BE, et al. Computerized tomography in the evaluation of blunt abdominal trauma. Am J Surg. 1983;146:751–757.

25. Ochsner MG. Factors of failure for non-operative management of blunt liver and splenic injuries. World J Surg. 2001;25:1393–1396.

26. Goettler CE, Stallion A, Grisoni ER, et al. Delayed hemorrhage after blunt hepatic trauma: Case report. J Trauma Injury Infect Crit Care. 2002;52: 556–559.

27. Carrillo EH, Platz A, Miller FB, et al. Non-operative management of blunt hepatic trauma. Brit J Surg. 1998;85:461–468.

28. Pal JD, Victorino GP. Defining the role of computed tomography in blunt abdominal trauma. Use in the hemodynamically stable patient with a depressed level of consciousness. Arch Surg. 2002;137:1029–1033.

29. Sahdev P, Garramone RR, Schwartz RJ, et al. Evaluation of liver function tests in screening for intra-abdominal injuries. Ann Emerg Med. 1991;20:838–841.

30. Karaduman D, Sarioglu-Buke S, Kilic I, et al. The role of elevated liver transaminase levels in children with blunt abdominal trauma. Injury. 2003;34:249–252.

31. Moore EE, Cogbill TH, Jurkovich GJ, et al. Organ injury scaling: Spleen and liver (1994 revision). J Trauma. 1995;38:323–324.

32. Cianflocco AJ. Renal complications of exercise. Clin Sports Med. 1992;11:437–453.

33. Margenthaler JA, Weber TR, Keller MS. Blunt renal trauma in children: Experience with conservative management at a pediatric trauma center. J Trauma. 2002;52:928–934.

34. Meng MV, Brandes SB, McAninch JW. Renal trauma: Indications and techniques for surgical exploration. World J Urol. 1999;17:71–77.

35. Boone AW, Haltiwanger E, Chambers RL. Football hematuria. JAMA. 1955;158:1516–1517.

36. Abarbanel J, Benet AE, Lask D, et al. Sports hematuria. J Urol. 1990;143:887–890.

37. Berkovich GY, Ramchandani P, Preate DL, et al. Renal vein thrombosis after martial arts trauma. J Trauma. 2001;50:144–146.

38. Aherne NJ, Kavanagh EG, Condon ET, et al. Duodenal perforation after a blunt abdominal sporting injury: The importance of early diagnosis. J Trauma. 2003;54:791–794.

39. Brooks AJ, Boffard KD. Current technology: Laparascopic surgery in trauma. Trauma. 1999;1:53–60.

40. Murphy CP, Drez D. Jejunal rupture in a football player. Am J Sports Med. 1987;15:184–185.

41. Hunt A, Dorshimer G, Kissick J, et al. Isolate jejunal rupture after blunt trauma. Phys Sports Med. 2001;29:39–46.

42. Rawls DE, Custer MD. Pancreatic trauma: An unusual soccer injury. South Med J. 2001;94:741–743.

43. Worobetz L, Gerrard D. Gastrointestinal symptoms during exercise in endurance athletes: Prevalence and speculations on the aetiology. N Z Med J. 1985;98:644–646.

44. Keefe E, Lowe D, Goss J, et al. Gastrointestinal symptoms of marathon runners. West J Med. 1984;141:481–484.

45. Fogoros RN. "Runner's trots": Gastrointestinal disturbances in runners. JAMA. 1980;243:1743–1744.

46. Scobie BA. Gastrointestinal emergencies with marathon type running: Omental infarction with pancreatitis and liver failure with portal vein thrombosis. N Z Med J. 1998;111:211–212.

47. Claus C, Majeus B. Acute hemoperitoneum caused by rupture of omentum adhesions after running. Surg Endosc. 2001;15:413.

48. Baril L. Pubic pain after a marathon. Lancet. 1998;351:642.

49. Rasmussen OO, Hoffmann J. Assessment of the reliability of the symptoms and signs of acute appendicitis. J R Coll Surg Edinb. 1991;36:372–377.

50. Dixon JM, Elton RA, Rainey JB, et al. Rectal examination in patients with pain in the right lower quadrant of the abdomen. BMJ. 1991;302:386–388.

51. Anderson REB. Meta-analysis of the clinical and laboratory diagnosis of appendicitis. Br J Surg. 2004;91:28–37.

52. Horton MD, Counter SF, Florence MG, et al. A prospective trial of computed tomography and ultrasonography for diagnosing appendicitis in the atypical patient. Am J Surg. 2000;179:379–381.

53. Malone AJ Jr, Wolf CR, Malmed AS, et al. Diagnosis of acute appendicitis: Value of unenhanced CT. AJR Am J Roentgenol. 1993;160:763–766.

54. Flum DR, McClure TD, Morris A, et al. Misdiagnosis of appendicitis and the use of diagnostic imaging. J Am Coll Surg. 2005;201:933–939.

55. Cobben LP, de Van Otterloo AM, Puylaert JB. Spontaneously resolving appendicitis: Frequency and natural history in 60 patients. Radiol. 2000;215:349–352.

56. Barnhart K, Esposito M, Coutifaris C. An update of the medical treatment of ectopic pregnancy. Obstet Gynecol Clin North Am. 2000;27:653–667.

57. Gracia CR, Barnhart KT. Diagnosing ectopic pregnancy: Decision analysis comparing six strategies. Obstet Gynecol. 2001;97:464–470.

58. Pisarka MD, Carson SA, Buster JE. Ectopic pregnancy. Lancet. 1998;351:1115–1120.

59. Seeber BE, Barnhart KT. Suspected ectopic pregnancy. Obstet Gynecol. 2006;107:399–413.

Chapter 11

Thoracic Injuries

Robert O. Blanc, MS, ATC, EMT-P

KEY TERMS

Adventitious

Crackles

Flail segment

Hemothorax

Hyperresonant

Hyporesonant

Nasal flaring

Needle thoracentesis

Pneumothorax

Pulmonary embolism

Rhonchi

Subcutaneous emphysema

Tracheal tugging

Wheezing

 EMERGENCY SITUATION

The star center from your basketball team reports to the athletic training room after practice. He describes a sudden onset of sharp chest pain just after the conditioning portion of practice. He is short of breath and says he feels like he can't take a deep breath. He states that he felt fine during practice and hasn't had any other problems. As you are questioning him he appears to become more anxious and uncomfortable. As you continue your evaluation you note that he has a pulse rate of 110 beats per minute, his blood pressure is 128/82, and his respirations are 24 per minute and shallow. You have difficulty hearing breath sounds on his left side, but sounds seem normal on the right side.

The vital organs of the thoracic cavity—the heart, lungs, and major vessels—are well protected by the rib cage (Fig. 11-1). It takes high energy and velocity forces to cause injury to these structures. In the athletic setting it is uncommon for those energies to be experienced because protective padding is worn and because humans are not typically able to generate such forces. Still, it is not impossible for athletes to suffer significant thoracic injury. Early suspicion and detection of symptoms are paramount to the survival of an individual with injuries to the contents of the thoracic cavity.

Assessment

Assessment of an athlete with suspected thoracic trauma must be thorough, efficient, and focused on the mechanism of injury. A systematic approach to evaluating the athlete will ensure that nothing is overlooked. First, observe the athlete's general appearance while determining his or her level of consciousness and evaluating the ABCs (airway, breathing, circulation). Take immediate action to correct any life-threatening condition as it is found.

Much can be learned from taking a thorough history. Although dyspnea may not be present in all cases of respiratory injury, it is present in most cases. Asking the athlete the proper questions may be valuable in rapidly identifying the injury. The rapid onset of symptoms versus a more chronic onset is more ominous, especially if the mechanism of injury is unknown. General observation of the athlete should continue while obtaining the history. Noting the athlete's

demeanor, level of anxiety, and ability to speak in full sentences will provide valuable information regarding the severity of the condition. Any athlete with difficulty breathing and who is unable to speak in full sentences needs emergent referral to a hospital. The mental status of the athlete is also important to determine because alterations in mental status are the first signs of hypoxia.

✪ *STAT Point 11-1. Dyspnea may not be present in all cases of respiratory injury, but it is present in most cases.*

✪ *STAT Point 11-2. Any athlete with difficulty breathing and who is unable to speak in full sentences needs emergent referral to a hospital.*

Vital signs are measured, including blood pressure, pulse oximetry, pulse rate and quality, skin color and temperature, and quality and frequency of respirations. In evaluating the quality of respirations be alert for the following: **nasal flaring** (the nostrils opening wide on inhalation), **tracheal tugging** (the Adam's apple is pulled upward on inhalation), retraction of the intercostal muscles on inhalation, use of the diaphragm and neck muscles to assist inhalation, use of abdominal muscles on exhalation, and cyanosis. Cyanosis is a late sign of hypoxia.

Auscultation of the lungs will determine the quality of respirations and efficiency of air movement (Fig. 11-2). The

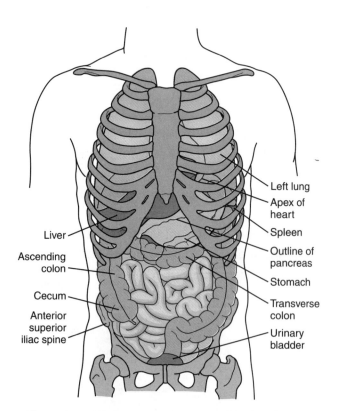

Figure 11-1. Vital organs are protected by the rib cage.

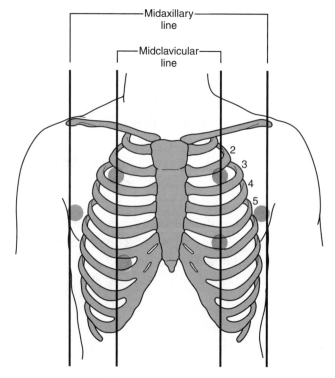

Figure 11-2. Proper auscultation sites.

examiner should listen at each site during expiration and inspiration for air movement. Identifying abnormal or **adventitious** sounds can help to characterize respiratory disorders (Table 11-1). A snoring sound would be indicative of an upper airway obstruction by the base of the tongue, and the use of an airway maneuver will most often clear the airway and allow normal breathing. *(See Chapter 3 for more information on managing airways.)* Stridor is a harsh, high-pitched sound heard on inhalation and is associated with a tight upper airway obstruction similar to the "seal bark" sound of a child suffering from croup. **Wheezing** is noted as a whistling sound resulting from the narrowing of the airways by constriction from bronchospasm, asthma, edema, or foreign body obstruction. **Rhonchi** are a rattling noise in the bronchi and most often result from partial obstruction of the larger airways by mucus. **Crackles** are a fine moist sound similar to a crackling or bubbling associated with fluid in the smaller airways as in pulmonary edema. Rubbing your hair between your fingers next to your ear produces a sound similar to crackles. Diminished or absent lung sounds unilaterally would indicate hypoventilation as a result of obstruction or lung collapse. Wheezing secondary to asthma is the most common adventitious lung sound heard in the athletic arena, whereas absent sounds are the most serious. Rhonchi and crackles are most commonly heard in patients with congestive heart failure or pneumonia and are not generally seen in an athletic population.

Next, palpate the chest by gently placing hands on the rib cage and feel for the rise and fall during breathing; it should be equal in motion, rate, and rhythm. Palpate the bony structures, looking for deformity of the ribs, unstable segments, and congruency of the sternoclavicular and costosternal joints. Also, the presence of swelling, crepitus, or crackling of **subcutaneous emphysema** (air under the skin) should be noted. The presence of subcutaneous emphysema is indicative of air escaping from the respiratory system and is a serious sign. Pain elicited by compressing the thorax front to back or inward from the sides indicates the possibility of a fracture to the ribs. Motion of the chest wall during respiration should be monitored closely. The rise and fall of the chest should be smooth and equal bilaterally. Motion of an unstable segment will be paradoxical. Because of acute muscle spasm this movement will be limited initially, but as the intercostal muscles fatigue this paradoxical movement will be exaggerated. Deformity of the ribs or sternum including sternoclavicular dislocation should also be assessed.

The final step in evaluating thoracic injury is to percuss the chest, noting whether it sounds normal, **hyperresonant,** or dull. These sounds indicate the density of the underlying tissue. Place the third finger of one hand flat against the chest wall and strike it with the tip of the third finger of the other hand (Fig. 11-3). If the result is a resonant sound equal bilaterally, then it should be considered normal. A hyperresonant or echoing response is indicative of excessive air accumulating in the thorax as would be present in the case of a **pneumothorax,** defined as air between the parietal and visceral pleurae. This hyperresonance would be noted over the

Table 11-1 **Adventitious Lung Sounds**

Term	Sound	Cause	Note
Snoring	Like the snoring of a sleeping person	Upper airway obstruction near the base of the tongue	—
Stridor	Harsh, high-pitched sound on inhalation	Tight upper airway obstruction	Similar sound to cough associated with croup
Wheezing	Whistling sound	Narrowing of airways from bronchospasm, edema, or foreign body obstruction	Wheezing secondary to asthma most common adventitious sound in athletics
Rhonchi	Rattling noise in the bronchi	Partial obstruction of larger airways, usually by mucus	Most common secondary to congestive heart failure or pneumonia
Crackles	Fine, moist sound similar to crackling or bubbling	Associated with fluid in smaller airways (pulmonary edema)	Similar to noise made by rubbing hair between fingers; most common secondary to congestive heart failure or pneumonia
Absent	None	Complete obstruction or collapsed lung	—

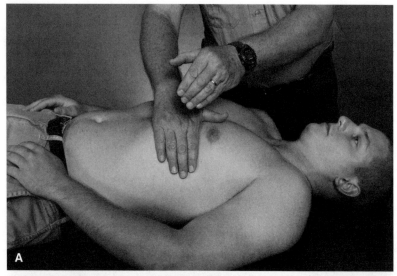

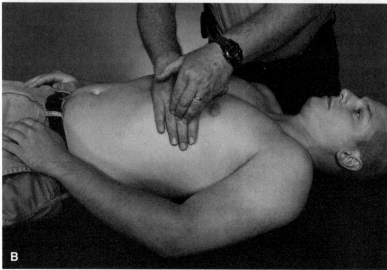

Figure 11-3. Proper hand placement for percussing the chest wall. **A:** Third finger of one hand flat against a chest wall. **B:** Strike with tip of third finger of other hand.

side of the pneumothorax because of the lack of lung tissue following the collapse of the lung. A dull sound would indicate the presence of fluid in the lung such as in the case of a **hemothorax,** defined as an accumulation of blood in the pleural cavity.

If blunt trauma to the thoracic cavity is suspected, the chest wall must be directly observed. Notice should be taken of any erythema, ecchymosis, deformity, or paradoxical movement. Alignment of the trachea in the midline of the throat should also be observed (Fig. 11-4). Injury to the lateral chest wall is likely to involve the lungs, whereas impact to the central chest wall is likely to involve the heart or great vessels. Note intercostal or suprasternal retraction or distention of the jugular veins, indicative of a tension pneumothorax.

In the case of an open wound it is important to determine if air movement in and out of the wound is present. This would be indicative of an open pneumothorax and should be addressed immediately. Determining the presence of an exit wound would also be important if the

mechanism of injury indicates this possibility. The incidence of an open chest wound in athletics is rare, but it must be mentioned nonetheless. Any injury to the thoracic cavity may lead to shock either acutely or over time. Observation of the athlete's skin color may be informative in identifying the onset of shock. The general presence of pale, ashen, or cyanotic coloring would be indicative of respiratory collapse, whereas red, dark-red, or blue coloring of the head and neck would be indicative of traumatic asphyxia. Continual observation and evaluation of the athlete and emergent transport to the hospital by emergency medical services (EMS) is crucial.

Assessment of injuries of the thorax requires constant monitoring. Any change in vital signs over time must be noted and considered immediately including respiratory rate; depth, quality, and symmetry of breaths; lung sounds; blood pressure; pulse; skin color and temperature; and level of consciousness. When changes are noted, treatment, including early activation of EMS, should be initiated without delay (Box 11-1).

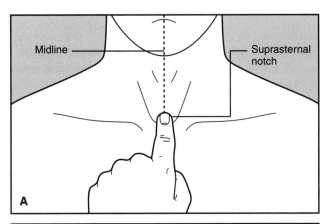

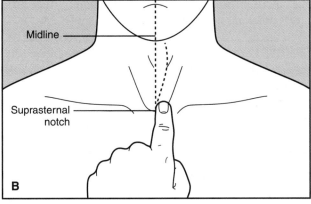

Figure 11-4. Normal **(A)** and abnormal **(B)** alignment of the trachea.

Box 11-1 Overview of the Assessment Process

1. Observe general appearance of athlete, determine level of consciousness, and check ABCs if necessary.

2. Obtain a history if possible.

3. Measure vital signs.

4. Auscultate lungs for adventitious sounds.

5. Palpate chest wall.

6. Percuss chest wall.

7. Directly observe chest wall.

8. Continue to monitor vital signs.

⭐ *STAT Point 11-3. When changes in vital signs are noted, treatment, including early activation of EMS, should be initiated without delay.*

Management

When caring for an athlete with a potentially significant injury to the thorax all treatment should be focused on maintaining adequate oxygenation for the athlete. *(See Chapter 3 for more information on airway management.)* High-flow supplemental oxygen by either simple face mask or non-rebreather face mask should be administered to any athlete complaining of difficulty breathing no matter what the underlying pathology. A common misconception is that people with chronic obstructive pulmonary disease (COPD) will stop breathing if given high-flow oxygen. This is only a remote possibility and should not preclude the use of high-flow oxygen in this population.

⭐ *STAT Point 11-4. When caring for an athlete with a potentially significant injury to the thorax all treatment should be focused on maintaining adequate oxygenation.*

Serious injuries to the thorax are life threatening, and anything other than early recognition, constant evaluation, and administration of oxygen is generally beyond the scope of practice for an athletic trainer. Prehospital treatment by paramedics may include intravenous administration of fluid for shock and endotracheal intubation for severe respiratory distress.

Types of Injuries

Fractures

The mechanism of injury for rib fractures in athletics is primarily either direct or indirect force. A direct force can result in a fracture or other injury at the site of force application. Indirect forces act to cause an injury at a site away from where the force is applied; for example, an athlete may suffer an anterior rib fracture as a result of a blow to the back. Significant force is required to fracture a rib; it also allows for the possibility of further internal injury. Fractures of ribs 10 through 12 may injure abdominal organs such as the liver or spleen, whereas upper rib fractures may injure the lungs. Rib fractures present with localized pain that increases on compression of the rib cage. Crepitus at the fracture site may also be felt with deep inspiration. Respiratory effort is limited because of pain, which typically prevents the athlete from being able to take a full breath (Fig. 11-5).

Although painful, a single rib fracture with no internal injury does not constitute an emergency and can be treated with rest, ice, and medication for pain. X-rays are required for a definitive diagnosis.

Fractures of the sternum require a significant amount of force and can be life threatening because the force may be transmitted to the heart, lungs, or great vessels of the chest. Severe dyspnea, point tenderness, and sternal deformity all

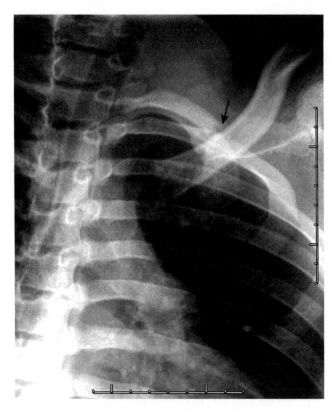

Figure 11-5. Radiograph of a rib fracture

indicate an emergency situation and require immediate transport to the hospital.

Sternoclavicular Dislocation

Posterior dislocation of the sternoclavicular joint may cause respiratory distress from the clavicle, placing pressure on the trachea and surrounding structures. If the athlete is in respiratory distress, immediately treat with basic airway maneuvers and supplemental oxygen. If improvement is not noted quickly, then reduction of the dislocation should be attempted. This may be accomplished by placing the athlete in a supine position with a sand bag or towel roll between the scapulae in line with the spine (Fig. 11-6). This technique allows the shoulders to be retracted, therefore pulling the head of the clavicle laterally and anteriorly. You may also be able to pull the clavicle laterally and anteriorly by grasping the clavicle with your fingertips. Because of the high forces typically involved in causing a dislocation, a cervical spine injury may also be suspected. Remember that a compromised airway always takes precedence. Take as many cervical spine precautions as seems reasonable, but the airway must be quickly managed.

Flail Chest

Fractures of two or more adjacent ribs in two or more places can create a condition known as **flail chest** and can cause the chest to move in a paradoxical manner during respiration

(Fig. 11-7). When the **flail segment** collapses during inhalation, the underlying tissue may be contused or also may collapse from the pressure of the unsupported chest. For this reason, a flail chest should increase suspicion of a pneumothorax because the two are often associated. Isolated flail chest injuries may be treated by placing the athlete on the affected side and transporting him or her to a trauma center. The athlete's own body weight on the affected side will act to splint and support the flail chest. If C-spine precautions are necessary, then the use of manual pressure or placement of a large bulky dressing directly over the flail segment may be beneficial in acting as a splint. High-flow oxygen therapy, vital sign monitoring, and rapid transport are crucial. If dyspnea increases, endotracheal intubation and positive pressure ventilations must be considered.

> ✪ *STAT Point 11-5. Flail chest should heighten suspicion for a collapsed lung because the two are often associated.*

Pneumothorax: Simple, Tension, Open

Simple Pneumothorax

A pneumothorax is defined as air between the parietal and visceral pleurae. This is normally a potential space filled with a small amount of fluid for lubrication. Air entry into the pleural space causes the lung to collapse as a result of the pressure imbalance that develops (Fig. 11-8). A pneumothorax may occur from the interior because of a laceration or rupture of the lung tissue by a fractured rib or from the exterior through an open wound in the chest wall. When this occurs, for whatever reason, the lung is compressed, preventing proper expansion.

A simple pneumothorax may be spontaneous or result from trauma. A spontaneous pneumothorax may be seen in young, tall, thin males. The athlete will present with a sudden onset of a sharp chest pain and difficulty breathing after exercising, strenuous coughing, or even air travel. Regardless of the cause, the athlete will have diminished lung sounds on the side of the collapsed lung.

> ✪ *STAT Point 11-6. A simple pneumothorax may occur spontaneously.*

Treatment of a simple pneumothorax is based on the severity of the symptoms. If marked respiratory distress is noted and tachycardia or hypotension is present, then rapid chest decompression may be required. Placement of a chest tube at the hospital is the definitive treatment for any pneumothorax greater than 15% of normal lung volume, associated rib fracture, or significant dyspnea. For a stable athlete without breathing difficulty and whose vital signs are within normal limits, transportation to a medical facility in a position of comfort with continual monitoring is acceptable.

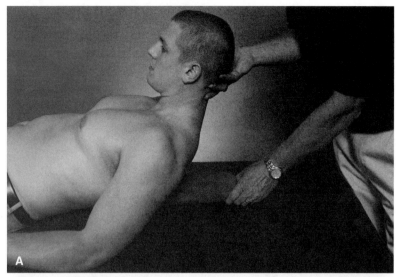

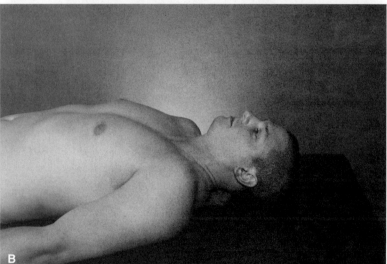

Figure 11-6. Reduction technique for posterior dislocation of the sternoclavicular joint. **A and B:** Place the athlete supine with a sandbag or towel roll between the scapulae in line with the spine and transport.

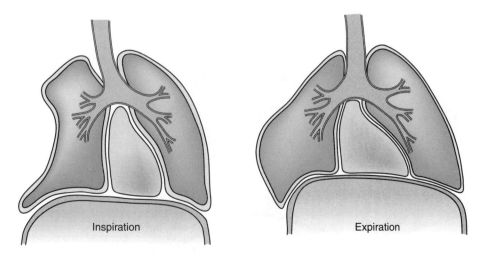

Figure 11-7. As a result of fracture of two or more ribs, the lungs function in a paradoxical motion.

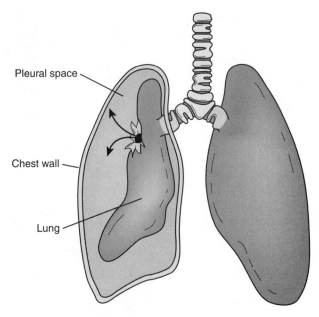

Figure 11-8. Simple pneumothorax. Pneumothorax occurs when air enters the pleural space, causing the lung to collapse.

Tension Pneumothorax

A pneumothorax that expands to the point where it compresses on the aorta, heart, and superior and inferior vena cava is called a tension pneumothorax and is a life-threatening injury (Fig. 11-9). Because of a buildup of pressure, the mediastinum and trachea are pushed away from the affected side. Compression of the superior vena cava results in jugular vein distension, whereas compression of the aorta and heart decreases cardiac output and results in both a drop in blood pressure and an altered mental status (Fig. 11-10).

✪ *STAT Point 11-7. A pneumothorax that expands to the point where it compresses on the aorta, heart, and superior and inferior vena cava is called a tension pneumothorax and is a life-threatening injury.*

If breathing sounds are absent on the affected side and severe dyspnea and jugular vein distension are present, then a tension pneumothorax should be immediately suspected. Tracheal deviation away from the affected side is a very late sign. Affected athletes will appear anxious and restless, hypotensive with a rapid and thready pulse, and on the verge of circulatory collapse. Percussion will result in hyperresonance on the affected side. Rapid recognition and treatment are essential, and this should be treated as an extreme emergency because this condition may be fatal within minutes. If the athlete is able to breathe adequately, give supplemental high-flow oxygen and call EMS immediately. Monitor the athlete closely and watch for deterioration in his or her condition. If the athlete is unconscious or unable to breathe adequately, then assist respirations with a bag-valve mask. If the symptoms still do not improve, **needle decompression** must be performed rapidly (Box 11-2).

Open Pneumothorax

An opening in the chest wall that allows air to enter the pleural space is an open pneumothorax (Fig. 11-11). The severity of this condition is dependent on the size of the opening in the chest wall and the causative agent such as a bullet, knife, or javelin. If the wound is the result of an assault, athletic trainers must first ensure their own safety by determining the location of the assailant and calling for police and EMS before treating the injured.

Management of an open pneumothorax includes administration of high-flow oxygen and monitoring of vital signs, especially respiratory effort and efficiency. Treatment of an open pneumothorax involves creating a one-way valve with a dressing. Covering the opening with a sterile occlusive dressing (Fig. 11-12) sealed on three sides will allow air to leave the thorax on exhalation but will seal off the opening so that air does not enter the chest cavity on inhalation. In doing this the open pneumothorax is converted into a closed pneumothorax by not allowing air to enter the thorax through the wound. If significant improvement is not seen, endotracheal intubation is indicated. This should also be

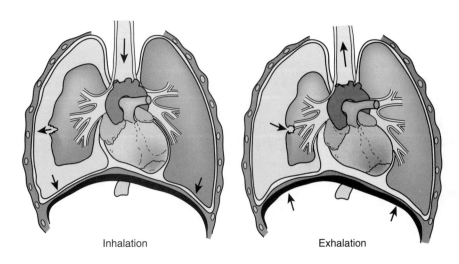

Inhalation   Exhalation

Figure 11-9. Tension pneumothorax. Because of a buildup of pressure, a tension pneumothorax causes the trachea to be pushed away from the affected side.

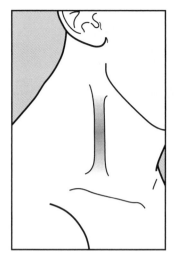

Figure 11-10. Jugular vein distension results from compression of the superior vena cava.

Box 11-2 Emergency Decompression for Tension Pneumothorax

Although outside of the scope of practice for athletic trainers, the procedure for performing an emergency decompression is presented here for the sake of informing the student.

An emergency **needle thoracentesis** is performed by placing a long 14-gauge intravenous catheter into the second intercostal space at the midclavicular line on the side of absent breath sounds. Attach a syringe filled with sterile saline or water to the catheter. Pass the needle just superior to the third rib because the intercostal artery, vein, and nerve pass just below each rib and may be injured if the needle is too high. Advance the needle until a pop is felt and air bubbles are seen in the syringe. At this point advance the catheter and remove the needle and syringe. Secure the catheter in place, and create a one-way valve by cutting the finger off of a latex glove, secure it to the hub of the catheter, and place a small opening in the end. If symptoms persist, place another catheter in the same manner in a slightly different location. Occasionally the catheter may clog or kink. If this should occur, the catheter may need to be replaced. Rapid transport to a trauma center for continued treatment is essential.

---

considered if the athlete's dyspnea increases, breath sounds decrease on the affected side, and jugular vein distension becomes apparent. Removal of the occlusive dressing is indicated at this time. If on removal of the dressing a rush of air is heard and the symptoms improve, replace the dressing and continue to monitor the athlete. If improvement is not noted, suspect that a tension pneumothorax is present and treat accordingly.

Hemothorax

Blood entering the pleural cavity results in a **hemothorax,** and the mechanism is the same as a pneumothorax (Fig. 11-13). As more blood is accumulated, there is less room for the lung and eventually the lung is unable to function. If the lungs become compromised, the athlete will develop dyspnea and chest pain and the jugular veins will become distended. The pleural cavity on each side of the thorax can hold 2 to 3 liters of blood so shock will quickly develop. Symptoms of a hemothorax are the same as for a pneumothorax except percussion will produce a dull **hyporesonant** sound.

Effective treatment of a hemothorax includes oxygen supplementation and respiratory support. Intravenous fluid resuscitation is undertaken with great care because an overload of fluid may result in significant pulmonary edema and difficulty in ventilation during the hospital course of treatment. Adequate oxygenation and ventilation will most likely require endotracheal intubation and positive pressure ventilation. Rapid transport to a trauma center is essential.

Pulmonary Embolism

A blood clot that enters the venous system and lodges in the lung results in a **pulmonary embolism.** The clot may come from any source and is not always related to trauma. Fat cells from a long bone fracture may also result in a pulmonary embolism. Females taking birth control pills are also at greater risk for pulmonary embolism. The clot blocks pulmonary circulation, and dead space in the lung increases. Left untreated, death of lung tissue will result. Symptoms of an acute pulmonary embolism include a sudden onset of chest pain, dyspnea, tachycardia, and bloody sputum. Lung sounds may reveal wheezing, although normal lung sounds are common. Treatment includes early recognition, oxygen administration, and rapid transport to the hospital.

Identifying the signs and symptoms of thorax injuries is not a skill that athletic trainers practice on a regular basis. The signs and symptoms that may present do not always clearly lead one to suspect such injuries and may appear to indicate a less serious condition. Constant monitoring of the injured athlete and a clear understanding of the mechanism of injury and potential effects will decrease the chance of missing an injury that may be life threatening.

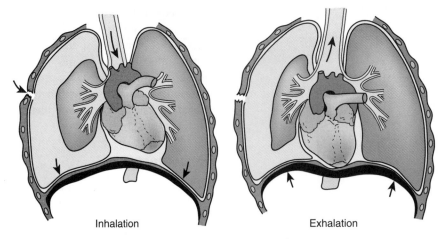

Inhalation

Exhalation

Figure 11-11. Open pneumothorax.

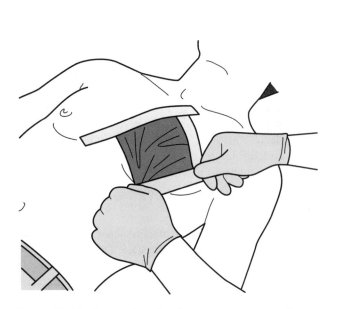

Figure 11-12. Proper dressing for an open pneumothorax.

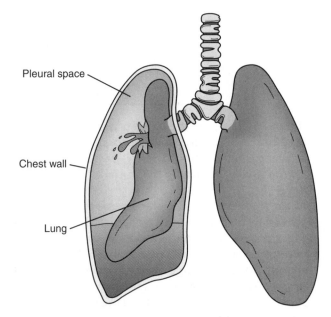

Pleural space

Chest wall

Lung

Figure 11-13. In a hemothorax, blood fills the pleural space.

 EMERGENCY ACTION

Because of the diminished left side breath sounds and the absence of an injury, the athletic trainer suspects a spontaneous pneumothorax. Oxygen is administered, the emergency action plan is initiated, and EMS is called. While awaiting the arrival of EMS the athletic trainer places the athlete in a position of comfort and monitors his vital signs and breath sounds every 5 minutes. EMS arrives and transports the athlete to the local hospital.

CHAPTER HIGHLIGHTS

- The rapid onset of symptoms is more ominous than a more chronic onset of symptoms, especially if the mechanism of injury is unknown.

- Auscultation of the lungs will determine the quality of respirations and efficiency of air movement. Auscultation should be performed anteriorly and posteriorly at the apexes and bases of the lungs bilaterally.

- Wheezing secondary to asthma is the most common adventitious lung sound heard in the athletic arena, whereas absent sounds are the most serious.

- If the result of percussing the chest wall is a resonant sound equal bilaterally, then it should be considered normal. A hyperresonant or echoing response is indicative of excessive air accumulating in the thorax as would be present in the case of a pneumothorax. A dull sound would indicate the presence of fluid in the lung, such as in the case of a hemothorax.

- If blunt trauma to the thoracic cavity is suspected, the chest wall must be directly observed. Notice should be taken of any erythema, ecchymosis, deformity, or nonparadoxical movement. Alignment of the trachea in the midline of the throat should also be observed.

- High-flow supplemental oxygen by either simple face mask or non-rebreather face mask should be administered to any athlete complaining of difficulty breathing no matter what the underlying pathology.

- Fractures of ribs 10 through 12 may injure abdominal organs such as the liver or spleen, whereas upper rib fractures may injure the lungs.

- Fractures of the sternum require a significant amount of force and can be life threatening because the force may be transmitted to the heart, lungs, or great vessels of the chest.

- Posterior dislocation of the sternoclavicular joint may cause respiratory distress as a result of the clavicle placing pressure on the trachea and surrounding structures. If the athlete is in respiratory distress, immediately treat with basic airway maneuvers and supplemental oxygen.

- Fractures of two or more adjacent ribs in two or more places can create a condition known as flail chest and will cause the chest to move in a paradoxical manner.

- Isolated flail chest injuries may be treated by placing the athlete on the affected side and transporting him or her to a trauma center.

- The athlete with a spontaneous pneumothorax will present with a sudden onset of a sharp chest pain and difficulty breathing after exercising, strenuous coughing, or even air travel.

- If breathing sounds are absent on the affected side and severe dyspnea and jugular vein distension are present, then a tension pneumothorax should be immediately suspected.

- An opening in the chest wall that allows air to enter the pleural space is an open pneumothorax.

- Treatment of an open pneumothorax involves creating a one-way valve with a dressing. Covering the opening with a sterile occlusive dressing sealed on three sides will allow air to leave the thorax on exhalation but will seal off the opening so that air does not enter the chest cavity on inhalation.

- Effective treatment of a hemothorax includes oxygen supplementation and respiratory support.

- Symptoms of an acute pulmonary embolism include a sudden onset of chest pain, dyspnea, tachycardia, and bloody sputum. Lung sounds may reveal wheezing, although normal lung sounds are common. Treatment includes early recognition, oxygen administration, and rapid transport to the hospital.

Chapter Questions

1. Altered mental status in conjunction with respiratory distress indicates _____.

   A. Hypoxia

   B. A head injury

   C. Nothing of significance

   D. A and B

2. Wheezing heard on auscultation of the lungs may indicate _____.

   A. Pneumonia

   B. Asthma

   C. Hypertension

   D. Pneumothorax

3. Rib fractures should be suspected with _____.

   A. A hard hit to the stomach

   B. Shortness of breath

   C. Localized tenderness on palpation

   D. Both B and C

4. When the superior vena cava is compressed, the result is _____.

   A. Low blood pressure

   B. Cyanosis

   C. Pain

   D. Jugular vein distension

5. A pneumothorax results when _____ enters the pleural space.

   A. Blood

   B. High pressure

   C. A foreign body

   D. Air

6. A _____ results when blood enters the pleural space.

   A. Pneumothorax

   B. Tension pneumothorax

   C. Hemothorax

   D. Blood clot

7. A tension pneumothorax is _____.

   A. A life-threatening injury

   B. Easily treated

   C. An open wound to the thorax

   D. Not an emergency

8. A sudden onset of chest pain and bloody sputum may indicate a(n) _____.

   A. Asthmatic attack

   B. Tension pneumothorax

   C. Pulmonary embolism

   D. Bronchitis

9. A fracture of two or more adjacent ribs in two or more places indicates a _____.

   A. Pneumothorax

   B. Hemothorax

   C. Pulmonary embolism

   D. Flail chest segment

10. An open chest wound should have a _____ dressing applied.

    A. Dry

    B. Occlusive

    C. Bulky

    D. Loose

■ *Case Study 1*

A wide receiver is hit in the lateral chest after making a catch in football practice and does not get up. The athletic trainer quickly determines that the athlete is unconscious and activates the emergency action plan. Evaluation of ABCs shows the athlete to be unresponsive and in significant respiratory distress. The athlete's cervical spine is kept in a neutral position and his face mask is removed. An oral airway is inserted and respirations are assisted with a bag-valve mask. Examination of the chest shows paradoxical motion of the left chest wall along with swelling and discoloration. His pulse rate is 120 beats per minute, blood pressure is 90/50, pulse oximetry is 96% with bag-valve mask and oxygen, skin is pale and moist, and spontaneous respirations are 36 per minute. Temperature is not obtained. Recognizing the critical nature of the injury, the athletic trainer and staff immobilize the athlete to a long spine board and continue to monitor vital signs until EMS arrives. On EMS arrival the athletic trainer gives a thorough report of the nature of the injury, vital signs, and interventions performed. The paramedics start an IV and administer medications to relax the patient so the airway may be secured by endotracheal intubation. The athlete is then quickly transported to the nearby trauma center.

Case Study 1 Questions

1. Based on the information given, what pathology do you suspect?
2. Is it possible that more than one pathology exists? If so, what are some other possibilities?
3. Is there anything you would have done differently in managing this athlete prior to arrival of EMS?

■ *Case Study 2*

A 19-year-old female gymnast comes into the training room complaining of difficulty breathing. She denies injury and states the dyspnea started suddenly a few hours ago while she was in class. She states the dyspnea is not bad, but she does not feel she can practice. She denies medical problems and takes no medications other than birth control pills. Examination shows a young female in no acute distress. Lung sounds show wheezing on the left side but it is clear on the right. Vital signs are pulse 100 beats per minute, blood pressure 110/50, respiratory rate 24 per minute, temperature 98.4°F, and pulse oximetry 98% on room air. She denies coughing up any blood-tinged sputum. Suspecting a pulmonary embolus the athletic trainer recommends that the athlete be evaluated at the hospital. The team physician is called to meet the athlete and the athletic trainer at the emergency room, and the athlete is transported to the on-campus hospital by the university police.

Case Study 2 Questions

1. What is a pulmonary embolism?
2. What other conditions might present with wheezing?
3. Because the athlete did not appear to be in any acute distress, why do you think the athletic trainer decided she should be taken to the hospital?

Suggested Readings

1. Baley EW, Turcke SA. A comprehensive curriculum for trauma nursing. Boston: Jones and Bartlett; 1992.

2. Bense L, Wiman LG, Hedenstierna G. Onset of symptoms in spontaneous pneumothorax: Correlations to physical activity. Eur J Resp Dis. 1987;71:181–186.

3. Hubble MW, Hubble JP. Principles of advanced trauma care. Albany, NY: Delmar; 2002.

4. Bledsoe BE, Porter RS, Cherry RA. Pre-hospital trauma life support, 3rd ed. St. Louis: Mosby-Year Book; 1994.

5. Sahn SA, Heffner JE. Spontaneous pneumothorax. New Engl J Med. 2000;342:868–874.

Chapter 12

Spine Boarding in Challenging Environments

Matthew Radelet, MS, ATC, CSCS

KEY TERMS

Diving towers

Diving wells

Front bun

Head-splint turnover

Panel mats

Pole vault crossbar standards

Pole vault landing pit

Scoop stretcher

Soft foam landing pits

Split litter backboard

Vault box

Waveless water entry

 EMERGENCY SITUATION

During a routine track practice, several pole vaulters are working with their coach. A vaulter plants her pole in the box, takes off from the runway, and inverts her body as the pole begins to bend normally. Suddenly, the pole breaks, and the athlete lands on her head and neck in the box. She is unmoving with her head and shoulders in the box and the rest of her body lying on the elevated surface of the front bun of the landing pit. As the athletic trainer, what should you do?

Since 1990 approximately 11,000 spinal cord injuries per year have been reported in North America. It is estimated that approximately 7% of these are the result of sports participation.[1] A study published in 1998 stated that the overall incidence of spinal cord injuries in the United States was approximately 4 per 100,000 people; of these, 5% to 10% were the result of sports participation.[2]

Certain sports may present the athletic trainer or other caregiver with a difficult emergency care situation because of the unusual environments in which they take place. Emergency care is always a demanding undertaking and particularly so when it involves a potentially catastrophic injury. When a caregiver is faced with having to extricate an injured athlete from an unstable surface or from the water, the level of difficulty for the rescuer and the potential risk to the injured athlete increase significantly.

There can be little doubt that improper immediate management of a potential cervical spine injury can worsen, or even cause, such an injury. It has been reported that an estimated 25% of cervical spine injuries happen during, or are aggravated by, emergency extrication and transport; approximately 40% of these injuries result in permanent neurological deficit.[3] In a worst-case scenario, improper management of a cervical spine injury could result in compromise of cardiac and respiratory function. Athletic trainers who have a duty to athletes involved in sports such as gymnastics, pole vault, diving, and ice hockey must be prepared to effectively respond to emergency situations in these particularly challenging environments.

✪ *STAT Point 12-1. Improper management of a cervical spine injury can worsen the injury, sometimes resulting in a catastrophic outcome.*

The Soft Foam Pit in Gymnastics

It is not surprising that the sport of gymnastics has among the highest rates of spinal cord injury. During the period 1973 to 1981, 50 cases of spinal cord injury resulting from gymnastics accidents in the United States were reported.[4] A study looking at the 10-year period from 1988 to 1998 found 325 spinal cord injuries suffered by gymnasts across all skill levels.[2] This significant increase in injury numbers is likely reflective of the increased popularity of the sport during this time and the subsequent higher numbers of participants. At least one published study notes that compared to football, gymnastics has a higher rate of cervical spine injuries per 100,000 participants.[5]

✪ *STAT Point 12-2. Gymnastics may have a higher rate of cervical spine injuries per 100,000 participants than football.*

A soft foam pit typically serves two purposes in gymnastics. One is to provide a soft environment into which the gymnast can land while learning new and more difficult skills, thus sparing the gymnast from repetitive falls onto a harder landing surface. The second purpose is to provide a means by which overuse injuries may be minimized by providing a landing surface that is significantly more energy-absorbent compared with other types of landing mats. As gymnasts perfect their skills through repetition, this benefit in terms of injury prevention cannot be overstated. Clearly, the chances of injury during the learning phase of any gymnastics skill are high. Even after the skill has been mastered, the risk of injury still exists, and it is usually during landings that many gymnasts will be injured. Landing into a soft foam pit does not eliminate the chance for injury.

✪ *STAT Point 12-3. Landing into a soft foam pit does not eliminate the chance for injury.*

Soft Foam Pits

Soft foam landing pits are analogous in some ways to swimming pools. Like pools, they can either be above-ground or in-ground. Above-ground pits may be constructed of a variety of materials and are essentially "containers" for the soft foam blocks that fill them, just as an above-ground swimming pool "contains" the water. These types of pits are often found in facilities that were not originally built with gymnastics in mind or when the gym is not on the ground floor of a building. These types of pits will generally have some kind of apparatus at their edge, typically a high bar. In some cases, there may also be an elevated runway adjacent to the pit, which will allow gymnasts to vault into the soft foam. Access to these pits is generally through the use of a ladder or stairs. If access is via a ladder, the athletic trainer will need to plan in advance a safe method of lowering an athlete secured to a spine board down to ground level. One potential method might involve the use of stacked mats to create a "stairway" down from the elevated pit edge.

In-ground pits are generally dug into the foundation of a facility and are therefore found in buildings that were designed specifically with gymnastics in mind (Fig. 12-1). A high bar usually is suspended over the pit or at one edge. If the pit is large enough, there may be more than one high bar. Gyms may also be arranged so that gymnasts can vault, tumble, and/or dismount off one end of a balance beam into these pits (Fig. 12-2).

Whether the pit is above-ground or in-ground, they will be filled with soft foam blocks that are generally 6 to 12 inches square. Pits will vary considerably in size and are square or rectangular in shape. They are generally at least 6 feet deep. In some cases, a trampoline may be at the bottom, beneath several feet of foam blocks.

Typical Injury Mechanisms

Injuries may occur to athletes in a number of ways using these types of landing pits. Direct contact with the sides of the pit, or with apparatus adjacent to or over the pits, can result in trauma. For example, improper technique could result in an athlete striking his or her head or neck on the high bar, vaulting table, or end of the beam before landing in

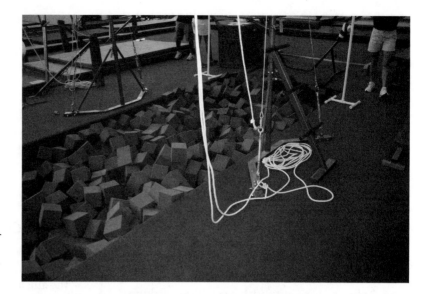

Figure 12-1. In-ground foam pit in a building designed specifically for gymnastics. Note the fixed high-bar standards on either side of the pit. This kind of equipment is considered semi-permanent because it is bolted to the floor, making it time consuming and sometimes difficult to remove.

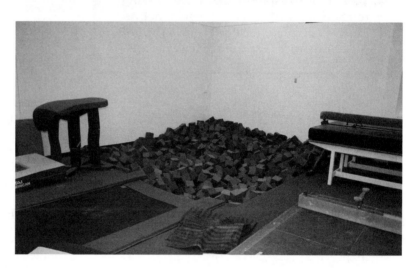

Figure 12-2. In-ground foam pit where gymnasts can vault into the pit off the vault table (*far left*), tumble into the pit from the tumbling runway (*lower left*), or dismount into the pit from the beam (*far right*). All of the equipment in this photo, including the mats in the foreground, is easily moveable to facilitate extrication of an injured athlete from the pit.

the pit. If many athletes are using the same pit, collisions with others could occur. In facilities where several athletes may be using the same pit at the same time, or in a facility where there are multiple pits, the athletic trainer or caregiver must plan in advance for the possibility of multiple injury victims that may require emergent care simultaneously. Improper entry into the foam itself could impart sufficient force to cause an injury. For example, landing headfirst in the foam, particularly if the cervical spine is flexed, could result in sufficient force transfer for a catastrophic injury to occur. If the athlete is falling from sufficient height and enters the foam headfirst, it is possible that momentum might carry him or her down through the foam to strike whatever is beneath, whether a trampoline or some other hard surface.

Suggestions for Extrication

Given the fact that every emergency situation is unique, it is not possible to describe in detail steps that will allow the athletic trainer or other caregiver to effectively manage every scenario, either involving a soft foam pit or any other

situation described in the following sections of this chapter. As such, the following information is meant to merely *suggest* sound principles for extrication of an athlete with a suspected cervical spine injury. This information is not intended as standards of care, but rather only as recommended guidelines.

It is assumed that all necessary equipment for this type of extrication is readily available in the facility and all of the staff, including the coaches, know where it is stored. It is also assumed that the equipment is in good repair and is appropriately sized. Many gymnasts, particularly females, are smaller than their same-aged peers and cervical stabilization collars must be available that will fit appropriately. College-aged gymnasts, for example, may require a pediatric-sized collar. It is also assumed that the facility has an emergency plan in place and that everyone, including the coaches, is familiar with it and understands the roles they may be asked to play during an emergency (Box 12-1). Clearly, any emergency plan will include emergency medical services (EMS) personnel. It is strongly recommended that athletic trainers establish a positive working relationship with their local

---

Box 12-1   Emergency Action Plan (EAP) Checklist

1. **Ensure that an EAP exists, is up to date, and is understood by all involved personnel, including the coaching staff.**

2. **Ensure that effective communication equipment is readily available and in working order at all times.**

3. **Ensure that all potentially necessary emergency equipment is readily available, is regularly checked and in good repair, and is appropriately sized for all athletes using the facility.**

4. **Take steps to establish a positive working relationship with local EMS personnel. As much as possible, include them in the EAP planning process and practice sessions.**

EMS personnel prior to any emergency. It is possible that EMS personnel will have had no prior experience with rescue from a soft foam pit, and regularly scheduled extrication practice sessions that include EMS personnel will be beneficial for all parties involved.

✪ *STAT Point 12-4. Appropriate and timely emergency care requires that a facility has an emergency action plan in place and that everyone, including the coaches, is familiar with it and understands the roles they may be asked to play during an emergency.*

The nature of the soft foam pit is that it is inherently unstable. Not only is the surface soft and yielding, but it is irregular. Motion will be transmitted across short distances. Foam pits that are suspended on trampolines tend to transmit motion across greater distances. For this reason, it is imperative that rescuers move slowly and carefully at all times when they are in the pit. A rescuer who jumps into a foam pit or moves recklessly near an injured athlete will cause significant motion of the head and neck of the injured athlete.

✪ *STAT Point 12-5. Rescuers must move slowly and carefully at all times when they are in a foam pit.*

Step 1: Communicate with the Athlete

If an injury is suspected for any reason, immediately stop any other activity into the pit and speak directly to the athlete. If the athlete is conscious and indicates there is a potentially serious injury, tell him or her to remain still and activate the emergency action plan for the facility. If the athlete is unresponsive, a cervical spine injury must be suspected and again the emergency action plan must be activated. In this situation, the primary concern is to confirm patency of the athlete's airway. In some cases, if the athlete is close enough to the edge of the pit, the athletic trainer may be able to observe for breathing or even reach out and perform a primary assessment without entering the pit. Keep in mind that the athlete may be facedown, or his or her head may be obscured by foam blocks, making clear communication difficult and possibly complicating the primary assessment (Fig. 12-3).

Step 2: Enter the Pit

If the unresponsive injured athlete is not close to the edge of the pit, the athletic trainer must *slowly* enter the pit and *carefully* move to the head of the athlete to perform the primary assessment (Fig. 12-4). The athletic trainer should enter the pit as close to the head of the athlete as possible.

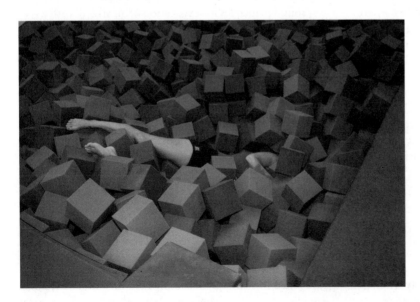

Figure 12-3. Gymnast in foam pit with face blocked by foam, making communication difficult. Communication will also be difficult if the athlete is prone. The fact that the athlete's head is also lower than her feet in this example may make management more challenging.

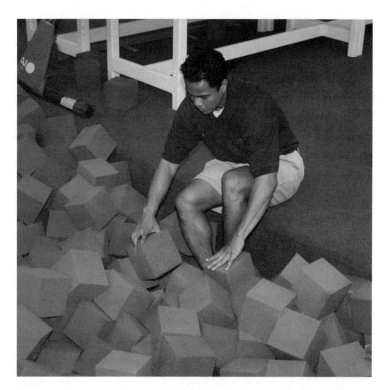

Figure 12-4. The highly unstable nature of a foam pit makes slow and careful movement essential. Some foam blocks may be carefully tossed out of the way, but this can become time consuming and probably will not significantly ease the difficulty of movement.

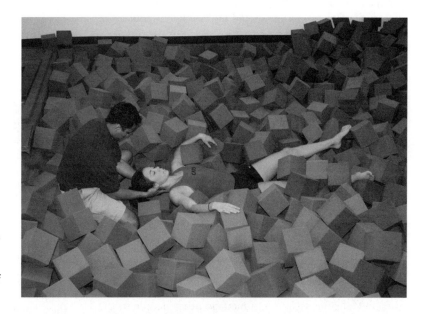

Figure 12-5. Establishing manual stabilization. The athletic trainer should already be considering from which direction other rescuers should enter the pit to minimize movement of personnel in the pit.

The objective is to move causing as little motion transfer as possible, while keeping in mind that an unresponsive athlete may not be breathing. Once at the head of the athlete, the athletic trainer should perform the primary assessment *(see Chapter 2 for more information)* and then establish manual stabilization (Fig. 12-5) *(see Chapter 6 for more information)*. This may involve carefully moving some foam blocks out of the way. Any blocks that are moved should be gently tossed out of the pit or some distance away to ensure that they do not later interfere with ongoing management of the injured athlete. Care must be taken when moving blocks because some may be helping to support the head of the athlete. The technique of choice for opening the airway in this situation is the jaw thrust maneuver *(see Chapter 3 for more information)*. If the athlete is not breathing and the athletic trainer cannot achieve an open airway for whatever reason while in the pit, the athlete must immediately be moved quickly out of the pit so that the airway can be opened. This may require the quick entry into the pit of additional rescuers, who should be standing by and ready to quickly enter the pit if directed to do so by the lead rescuer. Although every effort should be made to protect the cervical spine during a fast transfer out of the pit, the airway must be the primary concern in this situation.

✪ *STAT Point 12-6. Care must be taken when moving foam blocks because some may be helping to support the head of the injured athlete.*

✪ *STAT Point 12-7. When an athlete is not breathing, care should still be taken to protect the cervical spine, but quickly establishing an airway is the primary concern.*

If the athlete is conscious or it can be determined from outside the pit that the athlete is breathing, the athletic trainer can make a more careful and controlled entry into the pit and move to the head of the athlete. As the athletic trainer moves toward the athlete, he or she should already have begun to consider options for removal of the athlete from the pit, details such as which direction the athlete will probably be rolled if a spine board is to be used for extrication and to which edge of the pit the athlete will be moved once on the spine board. This is important because it will dictate from which direction the other rescuers approach. One objective for rescuers in the pit is to minimize risk to the athlete by moving around as little as possible, so efficiency in the initial approach is clearly indicated. Once at the athlete, the athletic trainer should immediately stabilize the head and reassure the athlete. If the athlete is unconscious and a primary assessment has not been performed, this must be done immediately. If the athlete is prone, foam blocks will likely need to be moved away from the face so that the airway and breathing can be assessed and monitored. Again, the athletic trainer must be cautious when removing foam blocks around the head of the athlete to prevent unintended motion of the head and neck. Once the head is stabilized and the primary assessment is completed, the first rescuer may choose to perform a quick secondary assessment for bleeding and obvious deformity in visible areas of the body. This information will then be conveyed to the other rescuers outside the pit so any additional necessary supplies (e.g., latex gloves, gauze, splints, and so on) can be gathered. During this time, members of the coaching staff and/or other rescuers should be moving any equipment at the edge of the pit that may interfere with the rescue. Members of the coaching staff may also be assigned to manage other people in the facility (e.g., athletes, parents, spectators), keeping them well away from the pit area.

As soon as the athletic trainer has stabilized the athlete's head and indicated that he or she is ready, the second rescuer can enter the pit and begin moving toward the head of the athlete. The second rescuer will bring a cervical collar and any other items that may be needed immediately. Once at the head, the second rescuer will apply the cervical collar, carefully moving any foam blocks that are in the way. Note that if the athlete is in a prone position with the head rotated to one side, the collar should *not* be applied until the athlete is rolled into a supine position. Of necessity, the athlete's head must be moved into a neutral position before a cervical collar can be properly applied; doing so while the athlete is prone means that rescuers will be unable to access the airway because the face would then be turned down into the foam. During this time, other necessary equipment and personnel should be assembled at the edge of the pit. If the athlete is conscious, he or she should be continually reassured. If the athlete is unconscious, breathing must be reassessed at regular intervals.

Step 3: Position Other Rescuers and Spine Board

Once the cervical collar has been applied (or, if the athlete is prone, once the second rescuer is in position), additional rescuers can begin entering the pit one at a time and moving into position. If at all possible, only one rescuer should be moving in the pit at any one time. This will dramatically help to limit motion transfer to the athlete. By this time, the athletic trainer will have decided (possibly in consultation with other rescuers) how the athlete will be placed onto the spine board and in which direction the spine board will be moved out of the pit. Considerations include position of the athlete, proximity to walls of the pit, and the closest unobstructed exit point from the pit. The athletic trainer will have communicated this plan to the other rescuers so that they can all enter the pit as close as possible to the side of the athlete where they will ultimately perform their roles. Rescuers should always carefully preplan their movement within the pit to minimize both the distance needed to reach the athlete and the need to reposition once they have arrived at the athlete. A rescuer should *never* attempt to step over any part of the injured athlete; the risk of falling on the athlete is high because of the unstable nature of the pit. Generally, the spine board is moved to the edge of the pit that is closest to the athlete, but this may not always be possible. For example, the closest edge may be blocked by immovable equipment. At least one rescuer should remain outside of the pit to assist in moving the spine board in and out of the pit (Fig. 12-6).

Step 4: Roll the Athlete and Secure Onto the Spine Board

Because of the soft and highly unstable environment within the pit, a "vertical lift" technique to allow spine board placement is not recommended. If any of the rescuers should lose their balance and fall while attempting the lift, the results could be disastrous for the injured athlete. The athletic trainer should decide which way the athlete will be rolled to allow for spine board placement and should direct positioning of the other rescuers accordingly (Fig. 12-7). Details of the logroll technique and techniques for securing the athlete to the spine board have been covered in Chapter 6. These techniques apply in a soft foam pit whether the athlete is prone or supine.

✪ *STAT Point 12-8. A vertical lift is not recommended in a foam pit because of the highly unstable environment.*

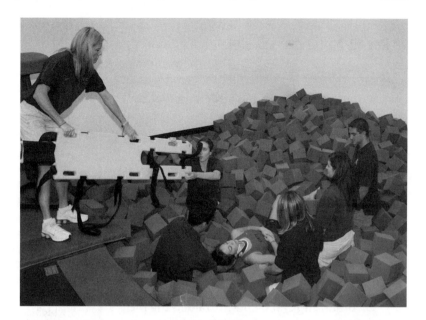

Figure 12-6. Passing the spine board into the pit. One rescuer should remain outside the pit to help with removal of the spine board. Note that a rigid cervical collar has been applied and that all rescuers are positioned before the spine board is passed into the pit.

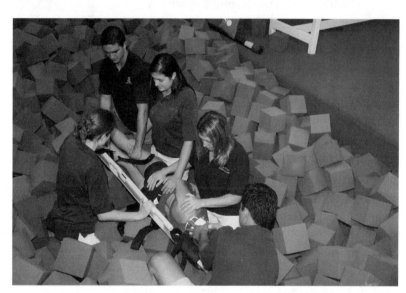

Figure 12-7. Log rolling the athlete for placement onto the spine board. The weight of multiple rescuers on one side of the athlete will compress the foam and often cause the athlete to sink. Because of this, the rescuer controlling the spine board will sometimes have to push the spine board down into the foam with some effort to achieve alignment of the spine board with the athlete's body.

It is possible for the injured athlete to end up sidelying and be supported in that position by the foam blocks. In this instance, it is likely that the rescuers will be able to clear most of the foam blocks from behind the athlete, place the spine board against the athlete's back, and then roll the athlete and the spine board together as a unit so the athlete comes to rest on the spine board in a supine position.

Step 5: Move the Spine Board Out of the Pit

If the athlete has landed close to the edge of the pit, it may be possible for the rescuers to simply lift the spine board and slide it onto the floor at the edge of the pit. Otherwise, it is recommended that the spine board be carefully pulled toward the edge until it is close enough to be lifted directly out. In this instance, placing **panel mats** or firm 4-inch landing mats to cover the foam between the spine board and the edge of the pit is recommended because it will make sliding

the spine board significantly easier. These types of mats are readily available in any gymnastics facility. It is *not* recommended that the board be lifted and carried by the rescuers because of the extremely unstable surface and the resultant high risk of falls (Box 12-2 and Fig. 12-8).

In many cases, the athletic trainer controlling the head and neck of the athlete will be unable to safely maintain this control *and* move with the spine board as it is transferred out of the pit. It is therefore very important that the head of the athlete be carefully immobilized to prevent any motion in the event that the rescuers decide to transfer the board without manual immobilization of the athlete's head and neck. If the athlete has been boarded at one edge of the pit, the athletic trainer controlling the head and neck may be able to maintain this control as the board is lifted out of the pit and placed onto the floor outside the pit. Control of the athlete's head and neck can then be transferred to a caregiver

---

Box 12-2   Steps for Athlete Extrication from a Soft Foam Pit

1. Communicate with the athlete; establish level of consciousness.

2. Carefully enter the pit, carefully move to the athlete, and check ABCs if necessary.

   a. Second rescuer enters pit with rigid cervical collar.

   b. If the athlete is prone and ABCs cannot be checked, or if the athlete is prone and is not breathing, the athlete must be quickly rolled.

   c. The airway can be opened and rescue breathing can be performed in the pit. If there is no pulse, or if the airway and/or breathing cannot be effectively managed in the pit, the athlete must be quickly moved out of the pit.

3. Apply cervical collar, if possible.

4. Direct movement of additional rescuers and equipment into the pit based on the most likely direction that the athlete will be rolled for placement onto the spine board and then removed from the pit.

5. Place athlete onto spine board. Cervical collar is now applied if not already in place.

6. Secure the athlete to the spine board. In some cases, manual stabilization cannot be maintained during movement of the spine board out of the pit; therefore, careful attention should be given to stabilization of the athlete's head on the spine board.

7. Carefully move the spine board out of the pit.

---

who is waiting there. Once the spine board is out of the pit, further assessment and transport can occur as with any "normal" spine boarding situation.

Alternate Methods and Suggestions

In addition to a long spine board, athletic trainers may also wish to consider a **scoop stretcher** or a **split litter back-board** as alternate equipment that may be used to extricate an injured athlete from a gymnastics pit. These devices are designed to separate along their length into two halves; each half is then inserted beneath the athlete, one from each side, and are then reconnected into a single piece. The athlete can then be secured and lifted in a fashion very similar to that of a traditional spine board. The advantage of this type of equipment is that it is not necessary to roll or lift the athlete to position them on a spine board. This can potentially simplify removal of an injured athlete from difficult environments such as a gymnastics pit. Anecdotally, some athletic trainers and emergency services personnel remain skeptical about the safety and efficacy of this type of equipment when managing athletes with a potential spine injury. There are concerns about the reliability of the fastening hardware that holds the halves together, along with concerns about the stiffness of these devices and their capacity to keep a secured victim from sliding during transfer. Athletic trainers should consider all of the pros and cons and practice with as many different types of equipment as possible before deciding which equipment they are most comfortable using.

Other methods for pit rescue have been suggested, including the use of a ladder.[6] A lightweight aluminum extension ladder can be kept near the pit; in the event a pit rescue becomes necessary, the ladder can be laid across the pit so that it is above the foam and passes near the head of the injured athlete. The athletic trainer can then move relatively quickly across the ladder to the head of the athlete and from a lying position stabilize the head and perform a primary survey from the comparatively stable platform the ladder provides. Although this may provide for faster initial access to the injured athlete, there are some potential drawbacks to this strategy. One is that if the head of the athlete has sunk down into the foam, the ladder may be too high above the foam to allow successful stabilization of the head and management of the airway. Another drawback is that it will be much more difficult for the athletic trainer to take part in rolling the athlete and moving with the spine board from a height that is higher than that of the other rescuers, who will be working down in the pit. This may necessitate transfer of control of the head to a rescuer in the pit. Finally, lying on a ladder may prove to be extremely uncomfortable for the athletic trainer for any length of time.

Another strategy, particularly in cases where the pit is very large and the injured athlete is not near the edge, is to use panel mats or firm 4-inch landing mats as a more stable surface to help rescuers move more quickly over the foam to the athlete (Fig. 12-9). These mats can be slid into position from the edge of the pit. If multiple mats are required, each subsequent mat can be positioned from the edge of the preceding mat. Although this surface will still be unstable and will require considerable caution to move across, it will be more stable and predictable than moving through the foam blocks. In the event that the injured athlete is not breathing and the airway cannot be managed in the pit, the athlete must be moved as quickly as possible out of the pit. Depending on the size of the athlete, the distance to the edge of the pit, and the number of rescuers immediately available, it may be possible to carefully lift the athlete directly out of the pit. In the event that the athlete cannot be lifted directly out of the pit, it may be helpful to have a piece of plywood readily available that is large enough to accommodate an athlete in unusual positions. The plywood can be quickly passed into the pit and the athlete can be carefully lifted up and onto the plywood in essentially the same position he or she was found in, no matter how contorted. The plywood can then be moved quickly to the edge and lifted out (Fig. 12-10). A spine board could be used for the same purpose, but because of the narrowness of spine boards, the athlete might need to be repositioned somewhat before the spine board could be moved. This will take time. Additionally, more care would need to be taken with an unsecured athlete on a narrow spine board to prevent "dumping" of the athlete off of the board during a fast transfer to the edge of the pit. Plywood could be cut to almost any size to ensure that there was adequate room for any size athlete in any position.

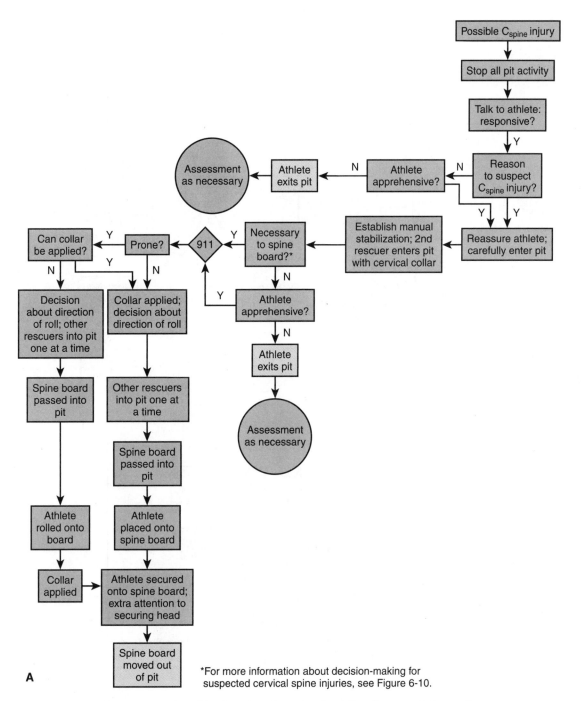

*For more information about decision-making for suspected cervical spine injuries, see Figure 6-10.

Figure 12-8. A and B: Flowchart for spine boarding from a soft foam pit.

(Continued)

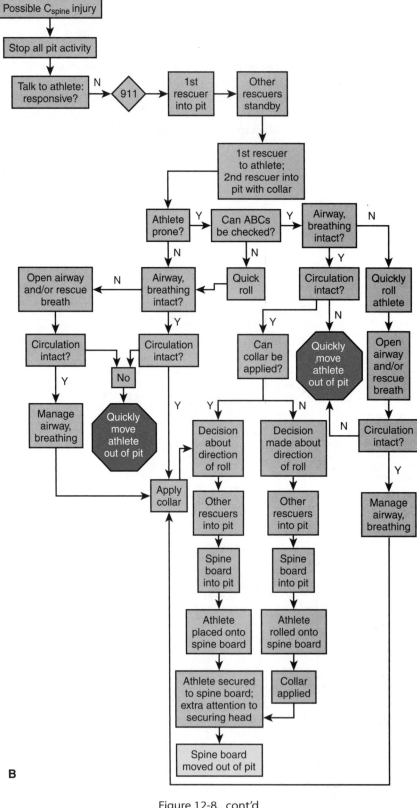

B

Figure 12-8. cont'd

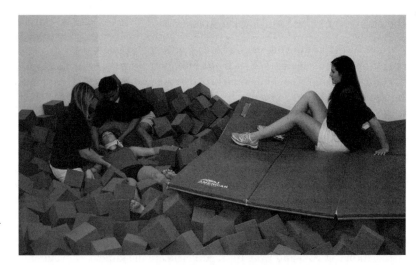

Figure 12-9. Use of a panel mat on top of the foam blocks to expedite movement of additional rescuers to the athlete. This method can be helpful when the athlete is far from the edge of the pit. Using panel mats can also facilitate moving the spine board out of the pit once the athlete is secured.

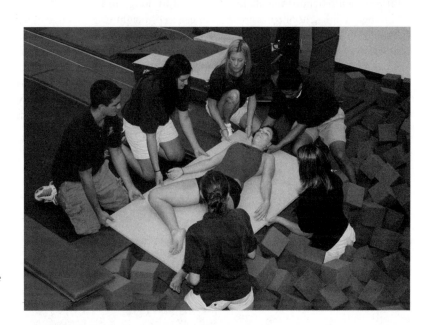

Figure 12-10. Using a piece of plywood to quickly move an athlete out of the pit. This method is used only in situations in which the athlete's airway cannot be managed in the pit or when the athlete does not have a pulse.

The Pole Vault Pit

The pole vault event in track and field is another sporting activity that, like gymnastics, involves a combination of height and an inverted body position. As a result, the risk of catastrophic head and neck injury is significant. Athletes will land on a padded surface from heights that range from around 10 feet above the ground to upward of 20 feet at the elite levels of competition. Research literature does not contain much information specifically regarding the epidemiology of catastrophic injuries in pole vault. Most of the injury data for pole vaulters focus on nonemergent injuries such as sprains, strains, and fractures.[7] One study examined catastrophic pole vault injuries in the United States that were reported to the National Center for Catastrophic Sports Injury Research from 1982 to 1998.[8] Thirty-two such injuries were reported; all but one involved head injuries, 16

of which were fatal. The other reported case involved a thoracic spine fracture that resulted in paraplegia. These data suggest that the annual overall incidence of a catastrophic pole vault injury is approximately 2.0 per year, with the rate of fatality being 1.0 per year.[8] However, participation in the pole vault by female athletes continues to grow. As the overall number of participating athletes increases, it is reasonable to expect that the annual incidence of catastrophic injury will increase as well. In 2002 alone, there were three well-documented fatalities during pole vault competitions. There has been some recent discussion among various sport governing bodies about mandating the use of helmets during this event, and several states now mandate the use of helmets during pole vault at the high school level.[8] Unlike sports such as football and ice hockey, it has not yet been clearly established that the use of helmets in pole vault will reduce the risk of catastrophic injury to the athlete.

Description of the Landing Pit Area

The **pole vault landing pit** area is made up of a large landing pad; a front pad called a *bun* or **front bun,** which usually slopes to the ground; two **pole vault crossbar standards** that support the crossbar, one on each side of the bun; and the **vault box,** where the tip of the pole is planted during takeoff (Fig. 12-11). The foundation beneath this equipment is typically concrete or asphalt; in some cases, the concrete or asphalt surrounds the pit area as well. Athletic trainers and coaches have a responsibility to ensure that the equipment that makes up the landing pit area for pole vault meets the minimum requirements as clearly defined by the sport governing bodies at the various levels of competition. The mat requirements as specified by the National Collegiate Athletic Association (NCAA) and USA Track and Field are the same: 19 ft 8 in. wide behind the standards, 20 ft 2 in. long, and 32 in. high. High school rules are the same, except height of the pit is 26 in. minimum. It should be kept in mind that these are *minimum* requirements for mat size. The base of each standard must be padded and standards cannot be closer than 13 ft 8 in. from each other. The back edge of the vault box must be within 14 in. of the front edge of the landing pad. Athletic trainers and coaches need to stay informed about the most recent standards regarding the equipment in the landing pit area, including mat sizes. Any exposed concrete or asphalt surface surrounding the landing pit area should be removed or padded to help protect vaulters who land off the edge of the pit.

 STAT Point 12-9. Any exposed concrete or asphalt surrounding the pole vault landing pit area should be removed or padded to help protect vaulters who land off the edge of the pit.

Typical Injury Mechanisms

The most commonly reported injury mechanism involves a vaulter who lands with the body near one edge of the landing mat or with the head and shoulders extending out over the edge of the mat; as the foam pit compresses, the athlete's head and shoulders then whip down over the edge to strike the ground or the hard foundation surface below the pit (Fig. 12-12).[8] In some cases, a vaulter releases the pole early or does not have enough forward momentum to carry him or her out over the padded landing surface and the vaulter may land on the head and neck on the unprotected hard runway

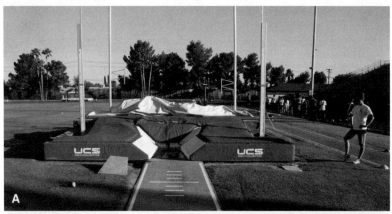

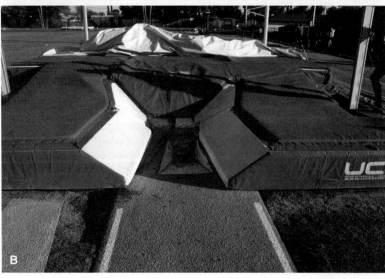

Figure 12-11. **A:** View of a typical pole vault pit with runway centered in the foreground. Note the standards on each side of the pit area. This particular pole vault pit is double-sided with a runway, vault box, and standards on each side of the pit. This allows vaulters to change direction of approach to the pit based on wind conditions. **B:** Close up of the sloped front bun and the vault box. The vault box itself is typically made of metal and usually set in concrete. Note that the pit itself has shifted slightly, and the vault box is no longer centered within the front bun. It is not unusual for pits to gradually shift over months of use. Eventually, the pit will need to be at least partially disassembled and shifted back into proper position.

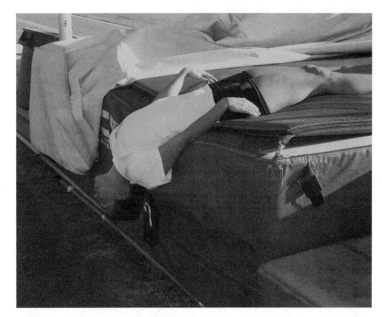

Figure 12-12. Common mechanism of head and neck injuries in pole vaulters. The force of the athlete's landing compresses the foam of the pit and allows the head, neck, and shoulders of the athlete to whip downward and strike the ground. Note the crossbars being stored along the base of the pit. Because of the potential for this injury mechanism, it is not recommended that equipment be stored along the sides of the pit. Any of the pit foundation that is not covered by the foam of the pit itself should be padded to help protect athletes who may land on the edge of the pit.

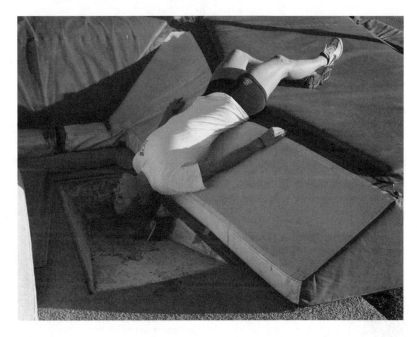

Figure 12-13. Athletes may land on the sloped front bun surface and may even come to rest with their heads in the vault box. Athletic trainers must be prepared to extricate athletes with potential cervical spine injuries from these difficult positions safely and efficiently.

surface at the front of the landing pit area. It is possible in these cases for a vaulter to actually land in the vault box (Fig. 12-13). It is also possible for vaulters to collide with the standards if their momentum carries them sideways during an attempt. In many cases poor technique is a major reason why a vaulter may not land safely in the proper landing area. Use of an inappropriately sized pole can also lead to injury. If an athlete is using a pole that is too small for his or her body weight, it may break during the bend, which could result in the athlete landing on his or her head in the box or on a hard surface in front of the bun. A pole that is too large for an athlete will be difficult for the athlete to bend and could result in insufficient momentum for proper penetration into the safe landing area. The practice of coaches, managers, or other athletes providing a "tap" or a push at the moment of takeoff should never be permitted because it encourages athletes to use poles that are too large for their body weight and natural speed. Coaches who are involved with the pole vault event should be experienced and well informed about current safe practice guidelines regarding technique and appropriate pole selection. Some states require pole vault coaches to be certified at the high school level.[8]

⭐ *STAT Point 12-10. A pole that is too large for an athlete will be difficult for the athlete to bend and could result in the athlete landing short of the pit area, either on the runway or in the box.*

Suggestions for Extrication

An injured athlete may come to rest in many potential positions after landing. In some cases, the athlete will land completely off the landing mat, which is probably the simplest of all potential situations that may involve spine boarding. All of the principles and techniques discussed in Chapter 6 will apply in these cases. As with extrication from the gymnastics pit, all of the possible injury situations and body positions cannot be covered here. Athletic trainers and other caregivers will at times need to be creative and resourceful while providing emergency care for an athlete who has suffered a potentially catastrophic head or neck injury while pole vaulting.

If the injured athlete is resting entirely on the landing mat, many of the considerations that were discussed regarding rescue from a gymnastics pit will apply. The landing mat is a soft surface and is therefore somewhat less stable than solid ground. It is, however, much more stable than a gymnastics foam pit. Rescuers will need to move slowly and carefully while on the landing pit to avoid unnecessary motion transfer to the athlete. If a standard is near enough to interfere with ongoing management of an injured athlete, it should be moved. If the athlete is right at the edge of the landing pit area, some consideration may be given to initially moving the athlete off of the pit and onto solid ground. Obviously, size of the athlete and the resting position will play a major role in this decision, made by the athletic trainer, possibly in consultation with other caregivers. Otherwise, the steps are very similar to that of a rescue from the gymnastics pit.

If the athlete comes to rest wholly or in part on the slanted surface of the front bun, other decisions will have to be made. If the athlete is entirely on the bun surface, it is possible that the spine boarding procedure can take place as usual. Some athletic trainers may decide to use a scoop stretcher or split litter backboard to move the athlete onto stable ground before securing him or her onto a spine board. It is more difficult if the athlete is partially on the bun and partially on the ground, particularly if the upper part of the athlete is on the ground. The same difficulty applies to injured athletes who are in the box, either partially or entirely. In some cases, the front bun sections of the landing pit, including the standards, may need to be moved to expedite the safe management of the injured athlete. In other cases, the athletic trainer may decide that the position of the athlete is such that they will need to be moved before safe and effective spine boarding can occur. In these instances, multiple rescuers should be positioned for a "vertical lift" style of transfer to a safer working environment, just a few steps away from the bun area. A piece of plywood could possibly be put to use at these times just as in some cases of gymnastics pit rescue. Whenever possible, a cervical collar should be placed on the athlete before moving him or her in this fashion. These types of transfers may also become necessary in instances where the injured athlete is not breathing and the airway cannot be managed in the position the athlete is found in or in cases of cardiac arrest.

Injuries from Broken Poles

As mentioned, it is possible for a potentially catastrophic head or neck injury to occur as the result of a broken pole. When a pole breaks, it will occur during the bend, and the pieces of the pole will snap back from the bent position with considerable force. Contusions and fractures can result if the pole strikes the athlete. Although extremely unlikely, the possibility does exist for an athlete who falls onto a sharp piece of broken pole to suffer an impalement injury. Athletic trainers must be prepared for this possibility. In other field activities, similar penetrating trauma could occur if an athlete, coach, or official is struck by a thrown javelin. Care for impalement injuries consists of leaving the impaled object in place whenever possible, unless the airway is compromised. The object should be stabilized as much as possible prior to transport. Bleeding should be controlled with direct pressure at the entrance and exit wounds (if an exit wound exists). If the impaled object is long enough to present significant obstacles to safe transport, it should be carefully cut down.[9] Some tool for cutting poles and javelins should be included as part of the emergency equipment in any facility where these events take place.

The Swimming Pool and Diving Well

Another challenging environment for extrication of an athlete with a potential cervical spine injury involves swimming pools and **diving wells.** Any swimming pool can be the site of a potentially catastrophic injury, typically occurring when an individual's head strikes the pool bottom as a result of a dive into water that is too shallow. Pool facilities also may include diving equipment, such as diving boards (springboards), or diving structures known as **diving towers.** At the collegiate and international levels of competition, facilities will include both 1- and 3-meter springboards; if there is also a diving tower, it will typically feature platforms at heights of 5, 7, and 10 meters (Fig. 12-14). These platforms are usually constructed of concrete. Diving towers are located at the edge of diving wells that are sometimes separate from the swimming pool itself; if there is a diving well, the springboards will also be located along one edge. These wells will be deep—12 feet or so beneath the springboards and perhaps 16 feet under the tower.

Prevalence of Diving Injuries

Diving is frequently mentioned as a leading cause of catastrophic cervical spine injuries. From 1973 to 1981, it was reported that 70% of the cervical spine injuries that were sport-related and resulted in quadriplegia happened during diving accidents.[4] In 1989 the U.S. Consumer Safety Commission Report stated that diving accidents accounted for approximately 700 spinal cord injuries every year.[10] Bailes and Maroon reported that diving injuries accounted for 10% of all injuries seen in large spinal cord injury treatment

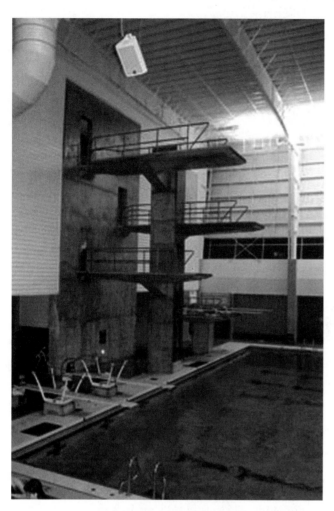

Figure 12-14. Diving facility. The diving well is separate from the pool and features a tower and springboards. The tower has cement platforms at 5-, 7-, and 10-meter heights above the water. The springboards are at 1- and 3-meter heights.

centers.[11] They also stated that 70% of diving accidents result in permanent neurological injury,[11] although this number is probably underestimated secondary to fatalities as a result of drowning. It is interesting that the populations involved in "diving injuries" are often not clearly defined. It is probable that these statistics include all diving injuries whether they were a result of organized sport participation or not. Other studies state that there has never been a reported catastrophic cervical spine or head injury from diving in a competition held in the United States.[4,12] It has been noted that although there has not been a reported fatality during a competition involving the USA Diving federation, there have been reports of paralysis that have resulted from diving accidents during practices.[13]

Typical Injury Mechanisms

Head and neck injuries in diving facilities have two main causes. A diver may strike his or her head or neck on the diving board or front edge of the tower platform during the execution of the dive. Head collisions with the bottom of the diving well are unlikely owing to the well's considerable depth. The other most common cause is an athlete striking his or her head on the bottom of the swimming pool following a dive from the pool deck. It is also possible for individuals to slip on the pool deck and strike their heads or necks on the edge of the pool or on the deck itself. Catastrophic injuries that occur from athletes striking their heads on the bottom of the pool typically involve an axial force to the top of the head with the cervical spine in a flexed position.

Suggestions for Extrication

Personnel who have a duty to render aid in this environment should have advanced training in water rescue. Rescue personnel must be strong swimmers and able to tread water for long periods. Rescuers who are not confident and capable in the water will likely be more of a hazard than a help during the extrication process. Athletic trainers and administrators should bear these points in mind during the formulation of the emergency action plan for these facilities.

It has been reported that in some cases, paraplegics whose paralysis resulted from water-related accidents indicated that they were able to tread water using their legs *after* the injury but *before* being extricated from the water.[14] This suggests that an existing cervical spine injury was worsened during extrication and underscores the need to pay strict attention to careful technique in protecting the stability of the spine during any rescue.

Any time that a potentially catastrophic injury occurs in the pool, all swimming and diving in that pool must be stopped immediately. Uninjured athletes in the water should carefully exit via the nearest edge to minimize wave generation. The emergency action plan for the facility should be activated. If the injured athlete is faceup in the water, the first rescuer should call out to the athlete to try and get information about the problem. If the athlete is unresponsive or is facedown in the water, it must be assumed that the airway is compromised and a rescuer must quickly reach the athlete to render care.

Two suggested methods of entry into the water will minimize wave generation (Fig. 12-15). The first method is for a shallow-water entry. Sit on the edge of the pool, support your weight on your hands, and slowly lower yourself into the water. Once in the water, slowly wade toward the injured athlete to avoid creating waves. The second method, used for deep-water entry or as an alternative method of shallow-water entry, is to sit on the edge and reach across your legs to the deck or pool gutter with one hand. Lower yourself into the water while turning your body 180 degrees. Carefully swim to the athlete using a breaststroke or other stroke that will minimize disturbance of the water.[10]

If the athlete is facedown, he or she must quickly be rolled into a supine position while protecting the cervical spine. One recommended method is the **head-splint turnover** (Fig. 12-16 and Box 12-3).[10] Move the individual's arms overhead, grasping at the elbows. Gently pull the body

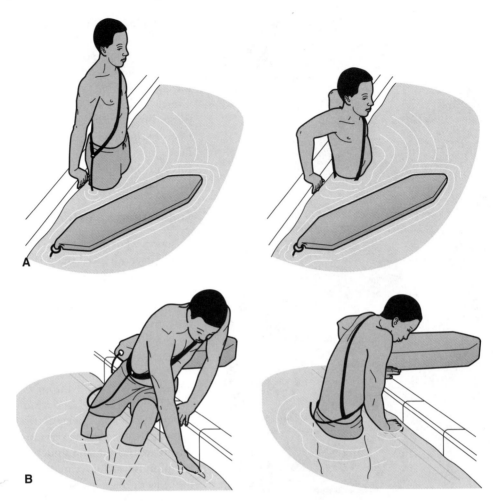

Figure 12-15. **Waveless water entry** techniques for shallow water **(A)** and for deep water **(B);** also an alternate technique for entry into shallow water.

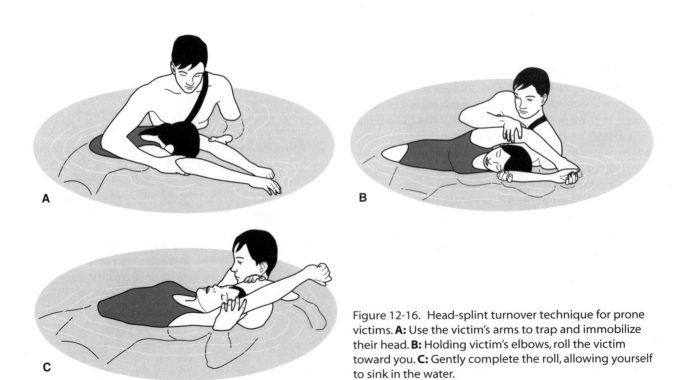

Figure 12-16. Head-splint turnover technique for prone victims. **A:** Use the victim's arms to trap and immobilize their head. **B:** Holding victim's elbows, roll the victim toward you. **C:** Gently complete the roll, allowing yourself to sink in the water.

Box 12-3   Head-Splint Turnover Technique Summary

1. Move the athlete's arms over his or her head. Their upper arms are now acting to stabilize the head and neck.

2. Holding the athlete's elbows to maintain stabilization of the head and neck, gently pull the athlete forward, causing the legs to rise toward the surface and making the turn easier to manage.

3. Roll the athlete toward you, keeping his or her arms against the sides of the head.

4. Gently complete the roll, allowing yourself to be pushed down in the water. Do not release the athlete's elbows.

5. Maintaining stabilization, carefully tow the athlete to the edge of the pool.

forward, which will cause the legs to rise in the water and make the turn easier. Roll the athlete toward you, keeping your forearm in contact with the athlete's upper arm as it rolls up out of the water. As you complete the turn, allow yourself to sink down into the water, gently lowering the

athlete into a supine position. Do not release the elbows because the athlete's upper arms are now stabilizing the head and neck. Move to the nearest edge of the pool, maintaining stabilization. Once at the edge, a second rescuer lying on the pool deck can reach down and take over stabilization of the head and neck, freeing the first rescuer to perform a primary survey (Fig. 12-17). Rescue breathing can be performed in the pool if necessary. If cardiopulmonary resuscitation (CPR) is indicated, the athlete must be quickly moved out of the pool and onto the deck.

⭐ *STAT Point 12-11. Rescue breathing can be performed while the athlete is still in the water, but CPR must be performed on the deck. Adequate chest compressions cannot be achieved while the athlete is in the water.*

If the athlete is floating supine, the **head-splint technique** of cervical stabilization can be used without the turnover and the athlete can be moved to the nearest pool edge, as described earlier. Another method of cervical stabilization is the **head-chin support technique** (Fig. 12-18). The rescuer places one forearm on the athlete's chest and grasps the chin; the other arm of the rescuer splints the athlete's upper back and the rescuer's hand stabilizes the back of the athlete's head.[15,16] The athlete can be moved to the edge of the pool using this technique as well.

Removing an injured athlete from the water can be accomplished using a spine board and multiple rescuers. The spine board ideally should be made of a buoyant material

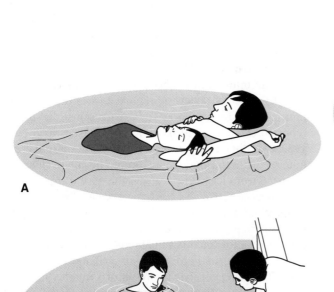

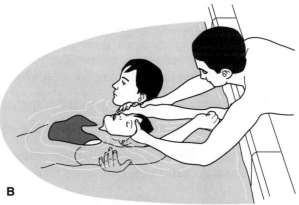

Figure 12-17. Head-splint technique for moving athlete to the edge. **A:** Perform the head-splint turnover if necessary; maintaining the splinted position, tow athlete to the edge of the water. **B:** Second rescuer on the deck takes over head splint. **C:** First rescuer can continue management in the water.

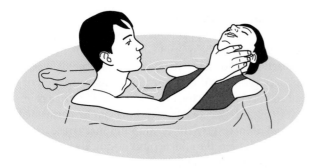

Figure 12-18. Head-chin support method of stabilization.

such as plastic or marine plywood and should have runners underneath to prevent the rescuers' fingers from being pinched when the board is placed on the pool deck. The runners will also make lifting the board from the pool deck significantly easier. Certain brands of spine boards are made specifically for water rescue.

Shallow-Water Rescue

In a shallow-water rescue in which the athlete is breathing, the head can be stabilized by a rescuer in the pool or by a rescuer lying on the pool deck. The board can be submerged by other rescuers and carefully floated to the surface beneath the athlete. A cervical collar can then be applied and the athlete can be secured to the spine board using traditional strapping techniques. If there are multiple rescuers, the board can then be lifted out of the water and up onto the edge of the pool deck.

A shallow-water rescue and removal from the pool can also be performed with only two rescuers, one in the pool and one on the deck. The rescuer on deck maintains cervical stabilization while the second rescuer submerges the spine board, floats it beneath the athlete, and then secures the athlete to the spine board and applies a cervical collar. The board is then tilted so that the end holding the athlete's head rises up out of the water and can be grasped by the rescuer on deck. The board is then pulled up onto the pool deck with assistance from the rescuer in the water (Fig. 12-19).[10] If this method is to be used, the rescuer who secures the athlete to the spine board will need to take special care with the strap placement and tightening to ensure that the athlete does not slide off the bottom end of the board when it is tilted up. The rescuer on deck should also keep this in mind and should try to tilt the board upward as little as possible.

Deep-Water Rescue

Deep water presents a significant challenge to removal of an injured athlete, and multiple rescuers will probably be required. The athlete should be moved to a corner of the pool where a rescuer lying on the deck can take over cervical spine stabilization using traditional hand placement. A spine board is floated beneath the athlete, who is then secured to the spine board with a cervical collar applied. Rescuers in the water should divide equally on each side of the spine board.

Each rescuer will place one hand on the pool gutter with the ipsilateral leg braced against the wall, giving leverage to help lift the board up out of the water. Ideally, there will be at least two rescuers on deck, one to maintain cervical stabilization and at least one other to help move the board up onto the deck (Fig. 12-20).

In the event that an injured athlete requires CPR, he or she must be rapidly moved out of the water while protecting the cervical spine. Once the athlete has been moved to the edge of the pool, he or she should be placed onto a spine board and lifted onto the deck as quickly as possible. Care must be taken not to dump the athlete off the spine board or lose control of the cervical spine. In this instance, taking time to strap the athlete to the spine board is not advised because time is critical. Rescue breathing can be performed while the athlete is still in the water.

The Ice Hockey Rink

Ice hockey is a collision sport played on an ice surface that will present challenges to the athletic trainer or other caregiver faced with managing a potentially catastrophic cervical spine or head injury during a practice or game. The incidence of such injuries in ice hockey has been reported to be higher than that of football. The actual number of these types of injuries is higher in football, but the overall number of football participants is significantly larger than that of ice hockey. One study reported that the incidence of nonfatal catastrophic injuries in high school ice hockey players in the United States to be approximately 2.56 per 100,000 participants; the incidence in high school football players is approximately 0.68 per 100,000, which is at least 3 times lower.[17] Another study examining spinal cord injuries in ice hockey players across all levels of play reported an incidence of 0.84 per 100,000 participants.[2]

A trend of interest has been that the vast majority of catastrophic injuries in ice hockey have occurred relatively recently. A study reviewing reported cases of spinal cord injuries related to ice hockey in Canada stated that the first reported case was in 1976, with 27 more cases reported by 1983.[4] Another study examined all cases of spinal cord injuries that were admitted to Toronto hospitals. None were reported from ice hockey during the period from 1948 to 1973. Between 1976 and 1987, there were 53 reported cases of spinal cord injury from ice hockey, with 42 of those victims suffering permanent deficits.[18] The generally agreed on causative factor for this sudden and dramatic increase in spinal cord injuries in ice hockey is a change in the style of play. This change in style is a result of a number of factors, foremost among them the introduction of the helmet and facemask as a more generally accepted or even required part of the protective equipment worn by the players. Players wearing this additional protective gear feel more of a sense of "invulnerability" and are therefore more aggressive on the ice.[4,17,19,20] Other factors that have been cited include referee leniency, a change in the strategies of play, a change in

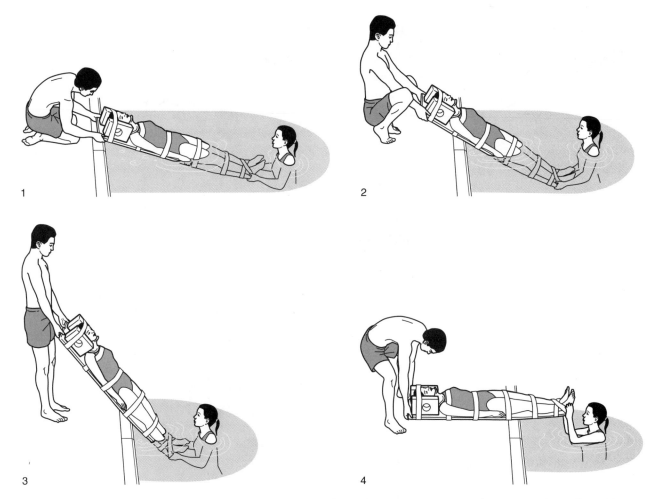

Figure 12-19. Two-person method of spine board removal from water. Except in unusual situations, there should be enough additional rescuers to make this method of spine board removal unnecessary.

societal attitudes toward aggressive play, and role modeling of older and more experienced players by younger players.[20]

Typical Injury Mechanisms

The most commonly cited mechanism for spinal cord injury in ice hockey is direct contact of the top of the athlete's head with the boards surrounding the ice surface. This impact, sometimes at high speeds, creates an axial load through the cervical spine with burst fractures and fracture–dislocations of the cervical spine resulting.[2,17–20] In some instances, the athlete's cervical spine is in some flexion at the moment of impact, greatly increasing the risk. In some cases, players may slide into the boards after falling on the ice. Because of the increase in aggressive play, more frequently contact with the boards is the result of being hit or pushed from behind during play along the boards. It is also possible for these types of injuries to occur following a collision with another player. In the late 1980s rule changes were enacted that made hitting another player from behind along the boards a major penalty, leading to an almost immediate significant decrease in the incidence of reported spinal cord injuries.[4] During the mid-1990s an initiative in youth hockey known as "Heads

Up Hockey" was started to help teach players at young ages the importance of not hitting other players or the boards with their cervical spines in a flexed position.[4] This effort is analogous to the work in football to prevent spearing (hitting an opposing player with the top of the helmet). The "STOP" campaign is another such effort in amateur ice hockey.[21] A "STOP" sign is printed on the upper backs of team jerseys to provide a visual reminder for players not to hit or push another player from behind.

Suggestions for Extrication

The biggest challenge in managing a potentially catastrophic cervical spine injury in ice hockey is the slippery ice surface, particularly early in the practice or game period when the ice is still relatively fresh. To prevent slipping while out on the ice, some athletic trainers choose footwear that features short spikes, or they may choose to use slip-on crampons that can be easily pulled on over the shoe. Athletic trainers who are approaching an athlete who is down on the ice need to be cautious to prevent falling on the athlete or falling on the ice and then sliding into the athlete. In some cases, uninjured players can provide assistance across the ice because they will

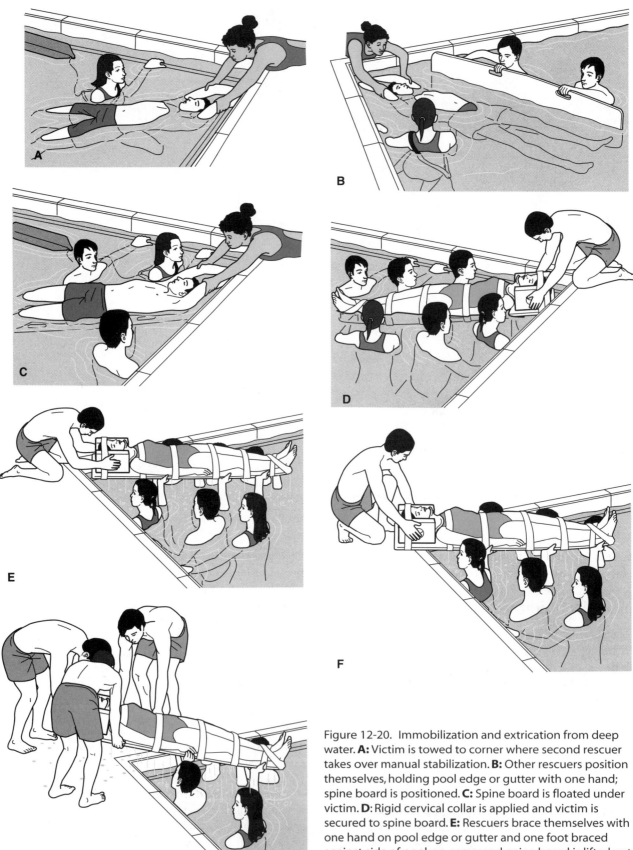

Figure 12-20. Immobilization and extrication from deep water. **A:** Victim is towed to corner where second rescuer takes over manual stabilization. **B:** Other rescuers position themselves, holding pool edge or gutter with one hand; spine board is positioned. **C:** Spine board is floated under victim. **D:** Rigid cervical collar is applied and victim is secured to spine board. **E:** Rescuers brace themselves with one hand on pool edge or gutter and one foot braced against side of pool; on command, spine board is lifted out of water. **F:** Lead edge of spine board is slid onto deck. **G:** Additional rescuers assist in pulling spine board completely onto deck.

be stable on their skates. Caregivers must never attempt to step over the injured athlete who is down on the ice.

In all other respects, management and spine boarding of the ice hockey player will be similar to the procedures for that of a football player. The hockey player will most likely be using a mouthpiece, which will need to be removed during airway management. The helmet and shoulder pads should be treated exactly as they are in football. It has been shown that removing the helmet of a hockey player but not the shoulder pads results in a significant alteration of cervical spine alignment.[22,23] Another study showed that appropriate spine boarding of helmeted ice hockey and lacrosse players effectively limited cervical spine movement during transport.[24] In collegiate hockey, the players are required to wear a full facemask. These are usually secured to the helmet with plastic snaps so that special equipment is not required to remove the facemask. If the athletic trainer is working with a team that uses helmets where the facemasks are secured using clips fastened to the helmet with screws, the athletic trainer will need to be prepared to remove these facemasks just as with football players. Professional hockey players wear a facemask that only covers the upper half of the face, leaving the airway easily accessible. Players at this level, however, are much more likely to wear the chinstrap of their helmet extremely loosely, which may have implications for securing the injured athlete's head to the spine board. If the head is not held securely in place by the helmet, the helmet will need to be removed (and therefore the shoulder pads as well) so that the injured athlete's head may be secured directly to the spine board.

Some additional concerns for spine boarding are unique to ice hockey (Box 12-4). The actual process will probably be somewhat slower because of the more cautious movements required on the slippery ice surface. Handling of the spine board itself will require more attention because it will easily slide on the ice during the procedure. As a result of the significant chance of a rescuer slipping on the ice, the vertical lift style of board placement is not recommended. In the event that the goalie requires spine boarding, athletic trainers and EMS personnel must be prepared with longer straps that will go over the bulky protective equipment that goalies wear. Once the athlete is secured on the board, it is recommended that the skate blades be covered to protect caregivers. A towel can be taped around the skates for this purpose. Once the athlete is secured to the board, thought can be given to moving the athlete off the ice. In some cases, the board is simply towed along the ice like a sled, which will certainly eliminate the chance for the spine board to be dropped as a result of a fallen caregiver.

Other Considerations for Emergent Injuries in Ice Hockey

High-Velocity Injuries from Pucks

Athletic trainers who cover ice hockey practices and events must be prepared for the types of injuries that might occur as a result of a player being struck by a driven puck. Hockey

---

> ### Box 12-4   Considerations for Spine Boarding an Ice Hockey Player
>
> 1. A slow, cautious approach to the athlete is emphasized to avoid falling onto the ice and sliding into the downed athlete.
> 2. Cautious movements throughout the spine boarding process will be necessary to avoid slips on the ice.
> 3. Extra attention will be required to prevent the spine board from sliding on the ice during the boarding process.
> 4. Extra-long straps may be required when securing a goalie to the spine board.
> 5. Once the athlete is secured to the spine board, cover the skate blades to protect rescuers.
> 6. Because of the slippery ice surface, extra care will be required during transport of the boarded athlete off the ice.

---

pucks are capable of causing fractures by striking an unprotected body part. Of particular concern in these instances is the exposed trachea. Although admittedly a remote possibility, a player who is struck in this area by a puck could suffer a severely compromised airway. The sports medicine team must be prepared to quickly and effectively manage this type of injury. (*See Chapter 3 for more information on airway management.*)

Lacerations from Skate Blades

The possibility for lacerations from skate blades also exists. Although rare because of the amount of protective gear worn by hockey players, these injuries can be life threatening. There have been well-publicized cases of skate blade lacerations occurring in the neck area of professional hockey players. Quick, effective actions on the part of the medical staffs for those teams are credited with saving those players' lives. Athletic trainers and the rest of the sports medicine team covering ice hockey practices and games must be prepared for the possibility of having to manage severe or even life-threatening lacerations.

Athletic trainers and other caregivers working in athletic environments may find themselves faced with managing potential cervical spine and/or head injuries that require athlete stabilization, immobilization, and extrication in extremely challenging environments. There are no "correct" strategies for management of these problems because each situation is highly unique. The soft foam pit in gymnastics requires considerable thought and care in positioning rescuers for athlete assessment and removal. Maneuvering through the soft foam blocks can be extremely difficult; the use of panel mats can be helpful in providing a more stable surface for rescuers. The pole vault pit area is another potentially difficult place for extrication, particularly in the box area because of its multiple planes of elevation and areas of unstable foam surfaces. Deep-water rescues may be the most challenging of all of these environments, requiring the rescuer to be adept at waveless water entries, rolling of a prone athlete in a safe manner, and stabilization and eventual extrication of the athlete from the water. Finally, the slippery ice surface found in ice rinks can be another environment that presents risks to the athlete with a potential cervical spine injury during stabilization and transport. Caregivers must take into account equipment and surface considerations when managing potentially catastrophic injuries on the ice.

EMERGENCY ACTION

The athletic trainer who arrives first at the injured pole vaulter must immediately perform a primary assessment, including level of consciousness. If indicated, the emergency action plan for the facility should be put into motion, including summoning nearby additional trained rescue personnel. If the athlete is not breathing, she must immediately be moved out of the box area so that her airway can be opened using the jaw-thrust method and rescue breathing can be initiated effectively if necessary. This move must be made quickly but with as much care as possible taken to stabilize the cervical spine. Subsequent management decisions should be made based on the ability of the rescuers to obtain satisfactory respiration and pulse patterns.

If the athlete in the vault box is breathing, but you, as the athletic trainer, decide it is necessary to take cervical spine precautions for removal and transport, the facility's emergency action plan should be activated. If there are not enough trained personnel to assist in extricating the athlete safely, simply stabilize the athlete's cervical spine while awaiting the arrival of EMS personnel. During this wait, the caregiver should continue to keep the athlete calm (if conscious), monitor vitals, and watch for signs and symptoms of shock. For the athlete to be safely and effectively placed onto a spine board for transport, she must first be moved out of the box area. One possibility for accomplishing this task is to carefully position the appropriate number of rescuers around the athlete, taking into account the unstable nature of the foam front bun. The athlete can then be lifted onto a level, stable surface adjacent to the runway and positioned for placement onto a spine board. Alternately, the athlete could be lifted and placed onto a piece of plywood, which could then be moved away from the pit to allow for more effective spine boarding. This strategy would eliminate the need for rescuers to carry the athlete in an awkward and potentially unsafe manner over even a short distance. In any event, the lift should be performed taking as much care a possible to protect the cervical spine and minimize movement of the athlete's body parts. Once the athlete has been moved out of the box area, management can proceed in a "traditional" fashion.

CHAPTER HIGHLIGHTS

- Soft foam pits present a major challenge for safe and effective spine boarding, particularly relating to rescuer movement within the pit and positioning the athlete for removal from the pit.

- Athletic trainers should consider various options for managing injured athletes in foam pits, including the use of panel mats, scoop stretchers, and plywood.

- Pole vault pits also present significant challenges, including the unstable pit surface, multiple planes of elevation around the box, and the presence of crossbar standards.

- Water rescues should be directed by personnel with advanced training in the water, such as lifeguards.

- Rescuers working in water environments should be strong swimmers themselves and competent in techniques such as waveless water entries, the head-splint turnover, and providing rescue breathing while in the water.

- Ice surfaces will require additional caution by rescuers to prevent slips that may endanger the injured athlete during assessment, spine boarding, and transport from the ice.

- Equipment worn by ice hockey players will create a need for additional considerations by the medical staff.

Chapter Questions

1. Improper management of an athlete with a cervical spine injury could result in _____.

   A. Inconvenience for the coaching staff

   B. Potentially catastrophic cervical spine injury

   C. Damage to rescue equipment

   D. Less accurate epidemiological research data

2. The soft foam pit in gymnastics practice facilities is designed to _____.

   A. Create a more challenging environment for gymnasts

   B. Eliminate the need for coaches to supervise practices

   C. Offer a soft landing surface for gymnasts to fall into while learning new skills

   D. Create more room in practice facilities for additional equipment

3. Possible strategies for approaching an injured athlete in a foam pit include _____.

   A. Using a "swim" technique to move through the foam

   B. Relying on EMS personnel because they will have much more experience in performing foam pit extrications

   C. Placing a panel mat or other firm landing mat on top of the foam blocks to provide a more stable surface to move on

   D. Slowly removing enough of the foam blocks from the pit so that rescuers can walk along the stable floor of the pit

4. Research examining catastrophic pole vaulting injuries suggests that the most common location of injury is

   _____.

   A. The head

   B. The thoracic spine

   C. The lumbar spine

   D. None of the above

5. If a pole vaulter is using a pole that is too large for his or her weight and skill level, the vaulter may not be able to bend the pole sufficiently. This could result in

   _____.

   A. Sanction from the governing agency overseeing that level of competition

   B. Damage to the box or crossbar standards

   C. Overuse injuries of the upper extremities

   D. A potentially catastrophic head and/or neck injury from the athlete landing headfirst in the box

6. Injuries that could result from a broken pole include

   _____.

   A. Fractures

   B. Contusions

   C. Penetrating trauma

   D. All of the above

7. The recommended method for a rescuer to enter a swimming pool or diving well is known as _____.

   A. The head-splint technique, which is designed to minimize movement of the head and neck of the injured athlete

   B. The waveless water entry, which is designed to minimize the movement of the head and neck of the injured athlete

   C. The marine rescue method, which is designed for a faster approach to the injured athlete

   D. There is no specific name or technique; the rescuer should simply get into the water carefully

8. An athlete who is floating facedown in the water should be managed by _____.

   A. First rolling the athlete's face out of the water using a head-splint turnover technique

   B. Quick towing to the edge of the pool and then being rolled

   C. Towing to the edge of the pool for immediate extrication and management

   D. Rolling the athlete as quickly as possible using whatever means necessary

9. Spine boarding techniques for injured ice hockey players are essentially the same as for injured football players with the exception of _____.

   A. Special consideration for spine board strap length when dealing with goalies and their large padding

   B. Special consideration for the slippery ice surface

   C. Protection for caregivers from sharp skate blades

   D. All of the above

10. The most commonly cited mechanism for head and neck injuries in ice hockey is _____.

    A. The athlete slipping and falling and striking the back of the head on the ice

    B. Being struck with a puck or another player's stick

    C. An axial load resulting from collision with the boards

    D. Colliding with the goal

■ *Case Study 1*

During a diving practice, one of the athletes strikes the back of his head on the edge of the 5-meter platform, falls into the diving well, and floats to the surface in a facedown position. Blood is in the water around the athlete's head and he is not moving.

Case Study 1 Questions

1. What should be the primary concern in this situation?

2. What techniques should caregivers use when entering the water and moving toward the athlete?

3. If rescue breathing is necessary, how could this situation be managed?

4. Regarding placement of the athlete onto a spine board, describe optimal positioning of rescuers in the water and on the pool deck.

■ *Case Study 2*

During a gymnastics practice, a gymnast is working on the high bar over an above-ground foam pit. The athlete misjudges a release move and lands on the top of his head on the bar. He falls into the pit on his side. When the athletic trainer arrives at the edge of the pit, he is partially covered by foam blocks and appears to be having a seizure. Access to this elevated pit from ground level is via an 8-foot ladder.

Case Study 2 Questions

1. Describe how the athletic trainer should enter the pit and move to the athlete.
2. What initial steps should be taken once the athletic trainer is next to the athlete?
3. Outline two different methods that might be used in moving the athlete out of the pit.
4. Once secured to a spine board, how can the athlete be moved from the elevated edge of the pit back to ground level for transport?

References

1. Cooper M, McGee K, Anderson D. Epidemiology of athletic head and neck injuries. Clin Sports Med. 2003;22(3):427–443.

2. Wilberger J. Athletic spinal cord and spinal injuries. Clin Sports Med. 1998;17(1):111–120.

3. Perry S, McLellan B, McIlroy W, et al. The efficacy of head immobilization techniques during simulated vehicle motion. Spine. 1999;24(17):1839–1844.

4. Clarke K. Epidemiology of athletic neck injury. Clin Sports Med. 1998;17(1):83–97.

5. Banerjee R, Palumbo M, Fadale P. Catastrophic cervical spine injuries in the collision sport athlete, part 2. Am J Sports Med. 2004;32(7):1760–1764.

6. Greaves I, Porter K, eds. Pre-hospital Medicine. The Principles and Practice of Immediate Care. London: Arnold; 1999.

7. Finkel C. Removal of a gymnast with suspected cervical injuries from a soft foam pit. Technique. 2001;Sept/Oct:5–39.

8. Boden B, Pasquina P, Johnson J, et al. Catastrophic injuries in pole vaulters. Am J Sports Med. 2001; 29(1):50–54.

9. Higgins G. Penetrating trauma: Managing and preventing javelin wounds. Phys Sports Med. 1994;22(4):88–94.

10. Forsten D, Murphy M, eds. On The Guard II. The YMCA Lifeguard Manual. Champaign, IL: Human Kinetics; 1994.

11. Bailes J, Maroon J. Management of cervical spine injuries in athletes. Clin Sports Med. 1989;8(1):43–58.

12. Rubin B. The basics of competitive diving and its injuries. Clin Sports Med. 1999;18(2):292–303.

13. Ferrell C. The spine in swimming. In: Watkins G, ed. The Spine in Sports. St. Louis: Mosby; 1996.

14. Campbell J. Basic trauma life support for paramedics and other advanced providers, 4th Ed. Upper Saddle River, NJ: Brady/Prentice Hall Health; 2000.

15. Prentice W. Arnheim's principles of athletic training, 11th ed. Boston: McGraw Hill; 2003.

16. Anderson M, Hall S, Martin M. Foundations of athletic training, 3rd ed. Philadelphia: Lippincott, Williams & Wilkins; 2004.

17. Reynen P, Clancy W. Cervical spine injury, hockey helmets, and face masks. Am J Sports Med. 1994;22(2): 167–170.

18. Bishop P, Wells R. Cervical spine fractures: Mechanisms, neck loads, and methods of prevention. In Castaldi C, Hoerner E, eds. Safety in ice hockey. Philadelphia: ASTM; 1989.

19. Deady B, Brison R, Chevrier L. Head, face and neck injuries in hockey: A descriptive analysis. J Emerg Med. 1996;14(5):645–649.

20. Murray T, Livingston L. Hockey helmets, face masks, and injurious behavior. Pediatrics. 1995;95(3):419–422.

21. Waninger K. Management of the helmeted athlete with suspected cervical spine injury. Am J Sports Med. 2004;32(5):1331-1350.

22. Stephenson A, Horodyski M, Meister K, Kaminski T. Cervical spine alignment in the immobilized ice hockey player: Radiographic analysis before and after helmet removal. J Athl Train. 1999;34(2):27.

23. LaPrade R, Schnetzler K, Broxterman R, et al. Cervical spine alignment in the immobilized ice hockey player. Am J Sports Med. 2000;28(6):800–803.

24. Waninger K, Richard J, Pan W, et al. An evaluation of head movement in backboard-immobilized helmeted football, lacrosse, and ice hockey players. Clin J Sport Med. 2001;11:82–86.

Suggested Readings

1. Banerjee R, Palumbo M, Fadale P. Catastrophic cervical spine injuries in the collision sport athlete, part 1. Am J Sports Med. 2004;32(4):1077–1087.

2. De Lorenzo R. A review of spinal immobilization techniques. J Emerg Med. 1996;14(5):603–613.

3. Del Rossi G, Heffernan T, Horodyski M, Rechtine G. The effectiveness of extrication collars tested during the execution of spine-board transfer techniques. Spine J. 2004;4:619–623.

4. Del Rossi G, Horodyski M, Heffernan T, et al. Spine-board transfer techniques and the unstable cervical spine. Spine. 2004;29(7):E134–E138.

5. Del Rossi G, Horodyski M, Powers M. A comparison of spine-board transfer techniques and the effect of training on performance. J Athl Train. 2003;38(3):204–208.

6. Stine R, Chudnofsky C, Aaron C, eds. A practical approach to emergency medicine, 2nd ed. Boston: Little, Brown and Company; 1994.

7. Stoy W. Mosby's EMT-basic textbook. St. Louis: Mosby–Year Book; 1996.

8. Swartz E, Boden B, Courson R, et al. National Athletic Trainers' Association Position Statement: Acute management of the cervical spine-injured athlete. J Athl Train. 2009;44(3):306–331.

9. United States Olympic Committee. Gymnastics pit removal for cervical injuries. Videotape. 1995. US Olympic Committee Productions. Colorado Springs, CO.

Chapter 13

The Psychological and Emotional Impact of Emergency Situations

Stephen A. Russo, PhD

KEY TERMS

Acute stress disorder

Cognitive-behavioral
  therapy

Compassion fatigue

Crisis interventions

Critical incident stress
  debriefing

Dissociation

Hardiness

Post-traumatic stress
  disorder

Psycho-education

Psychological debriefings

Psychological emergency
  response team

Psychological trauma

Resilience

Self-enhancement

Trauma intervention
  protocol

 EMERGENCY SITUATION

A group of athletes is participating in conditioning drills on an outdoor field when one player collapses. Teammates assist the fallen athlete to the sideline, and you, as the athletic trainer on duty, immediately rush to his aid. Although initially alert, the athlete becomes unresponsive. You check all vitals and find that the player is not breathing and has no pulse. Emergency personnel are summoned, but the player fails to respond to cardiopulmonary resuscitation (CPR) or the use of an automatic external defibrillator (AED). He is pronounced dead after being transported to a local hospital, with hypertrophic cardiomyopathy eventually identified as the cause of death. The player's teammates are shocked, upset, and confused over what has happened, but the athletes who assisted the fallen player are finding the situation even more difficult to bear. Over the next few days, these individuals have difficulty blocking out thoughts and images of what happened that day and are uncomfortable around the team, the coaching staff, and the practice facility. Their discomfort is also starting to interfere with their ability to concentrate in class and at practice. You are unsure how to help the team respond to this tragedy, and you are questioning whether you own reactions are "normal," given the situation. How should you and other medical staff respond?

Throughout this text, the authors have addressed the medical and physical aspects of emergency situations in sports, but what can be done about the emotional and psychological components of severe injuries, emergency situations, or other tragic events that can happen in sports? To what degree should we expect athletes to experience negative psychological effects as a result of catastrophic events that occur during sports, and to what degree can athletic trainers or medical support staff provide assistance? In addition to answering these questions, this chapter will also seek to provide an understanding of what constitutes psychological "trauma" and how it occurs in an athletic environment. As with the medical treatment of emergency situations, the psychological aspects of critical incidents require a specific mode of response. Given the inherent closeness that most athletic trainers and other medical personnel share with the athletes under their care, it behooves all who work in the field to have an understanding of what to expect cognitively and emotionally from athletes who have suffered major injuries and/or have witnessed other players experience serious threats to their body, their physical well-being, and their athletic careers.

Defining Psychological Trauma

Just as the term "trauma" in the medical community implies that a person is at serious risk for loss of life and/or significant areas of functionality, the psychiatric use of the term trauma implies that a person has experienced a significantly disruptive event. However, the difference in the medical and psychological use of the term can be easily confused. In medicine, trauma signifies that someone has a specific wound or injury that brings their physical well-being into risk. By contrast, in the most recent version of the *Diagnostic and Statistical Manual of Mental Disorders (DSM-IV),*[1] the American Psychological Association emphasized that, although one may experience an event that is life threatening, the subjective experience on the part of the person is ultimately what determines whether a person has experienced an emotional trauma. Thus, in psychology, one cannot be said to have experienced a traumatic event without a clear understanding of how one understood and interpreted the real, imagined, or anticipated stressor one has experienced.[2] According to this definition, it is conceivable that two athletes can experience the same physically "traumatic" injury, yet one can develop an emotional "trauma" reaction related to the incident, whereas the other can experience little or no emotional difficulty following the event.

Understanding the definition of **psychological trauma** is crucial to providing emotional assistance and support to athletes who suffer major and/or catastrophic events. In the *DSM-IV,* one can only be said to have experienced a traumatic event if one has encountered a situation that caused feelings of "fear, helplessness, or horror." However, this does not mean that every athlete who experiences or witnesses

these events will automatically have significant psychological symptoms that require treatment. In contrast, experience suggests that only a minority of individuals who experience potentially "traumatic" events actually develop significant emotional difficulties.[5,6]

⭐ *STAT Point 13-1. Psychological trauma is caused by feelings of fear, helplessness, or horror.*

Post-Traumatic Stress and Acute Stress Disorders

The most commonly known psychiatric disorder associated with extreme and/or traumatic experiences is **post-traumatic stress disorder** (PTSD). Individuals diagnosed with PTSD following a harrowing event typically experience significant interference in their social or occupational lives for more than a month after the event occurs. Symptoms can include nightmares and "flashbacks" about the event, concentration problems, extreme irritability, emotional fluctuations, insomnia, or attempts to avoid reminders of the event. A lesser known emotional reaction to trauma is what is known as **acute stress disorder** (ASD), which shares many of the same symptoms as PTSD but is used more to describe the extreme stress reactions that occur within the first month following a traumatic experience. Acute stress disorder also differs from PTSD in the emphasis it places on **dissociation,** which occurs when people experience ongoing emotional numbness or detachment from one's surroundings or an unexplained memory loss for events related to the trauma. Table 13-1 compares the two disorders.

The occurrence of emotional difficulties following extreme events is common, with rates of individual PTSD symptoms reported within the first month being as high as 100%. However, when PTSD and ASD are explored as formal disorders, their frequency is significantly lower. Based on a review of the literature on trauma, researchers estimate that only one third of the individuals who experience extreme situations are expected to suffer significant emotional difficulties during the first month after the event, suggesting that a formal diagnosis of ASD occurs at a significantly reduced rate.[3] Also, because the early studies into PTSD were historically conducted on those who endured trauma and subsequently sought treatment, original assumptions made about the widespread nature of PTSD were also grossly inflated.[5]

The National Institute of Mental Health[6] currently estimates that only 3.6% of U.S. adults between the ages of 18 and 54 have PTSD during the course of any given year, with this figure including victims of a variety of stressors. Other researchers have found that PTSD occurs in only 8% to 12% of individuals who experience noncombat trauma, and, despite perceptions to the contrary, even the majority of combat veterans (70%–92%) have endured their experiences with no significant long-term emotional distress.[6,7] Although the PTSD estimates represent a fairly large number of people (5.2 million), the proportion of people with PTSD is actually low when one looks at how many people experience potentially traumatic events, with some

Table 13-1   Diagnostic Criteria of Post-Traumatic Stress Disorder and Acute Stress Disorder

Post-Traumatic Stress Disorder	Acute Stress Disorder
A. The person is exposed to a traumatic event in which both of the following were present:	A. The person is exposed to a traumatic event in which both of the following were present:
■ The person experienced, witnessed, or was confronted with an event or events that involved actual or threatened death or serious injury or a threat to the physical integrity of self or others.	■ The person experienced, witnessed, or was confronted with an event or events that involved actual or threatened death or serious injury or a threat to the physical integrity of self or others.
■ The person's response involved intense fear, helplessness, or horror.	■ The person's response involved intense fear, helplessness, or horror.
B. The traumatic event is persistently reexperienced in one or more of the following ways:	B. Either while experiencing or after experiencing the distressing event, the individual has three (or more) of the following dissociative symptoms:
■ Recurrent and intrusive distressing recollections of the event, including images, thoughts, or perceptions.	■ A subjective sense of numbing, detachment, or absence or emotional responsiveness.
■ Recurrent distressing dreams of the event.	■ A reduction in awareness of his or her surroundings (e.g., "being in a daze").
■ Acting or feeling as if the traumatic event were recurring (including a sense of reliving the event, illusions, hallucinations, and dissociative flashbacks).	■ Derealization.
	■ Depersonalization.
■ Intense psychological distress at exposure to internal or external cues that symbolizes or resembles an aspect of the traumatic event.	■ Dissociative amnesia (i.e., inability to recall an important aspect of the trauma).
■ Physiological reactivity on exposure to internal or external cues that symbolizes or resembles an aspect of the event.	
C. Persistent avoidance of stimuli associated with the trauma and numbing of general responsiveness not present before the trauma, as indicated by three or more of the following:	C. The traumatic event is persistently reexperienced in at least one of the following ways:
■ Efforts to avoid thoughts, feelings, or conversations associated with the trauma.	■ Recurrent images.
■ Efforts to avoid activities, places, or the people that arouse recollections of the trauma.	■ Thoughts.
■ Inability to recall an important aspect of the trauma.	■ Dreams.
■ Markedly diminished interest or participation in significant activities.	■ Illusions.
■ Feeling of detachment or estrangement from others.	■ Flashback episodes.
■ Restricted range of affect (e.g., unable to have loving feelings).	■ A sense of reliving the experience.
■ Sense of foreshortened future (e.g., does not expect to have a career, marriage, children, or a normal life span).	■ Distress on exposure to reminders of the traumatic event.

(Continued)

Table 13-1   Diagnostic Criteria of Post-Traumatic Stress Disorder and Acute Stress Disorder—cont'd

Post-Traumatic Stress Disorder	Acute Stress Disorder
D. Persistent symptoms of increased arousal (not present before the trauma), as indicated by two or more of the following: ■ Difficulty falling or staying asleep. ■ Irritability or outbursts or anger. ■ Difficulty concentrating. ■ Hypervigilance. ■ Exaggerated startle response.	**D. Marked avoidance of stimuli that arouse recollections of the trauma (e.g., thoughts, feelings, conversations, activities, places, people).**
E. Duration of the disturbance (symptoms in Criteria B, C, and D) is more than 1 month.	**E. Marked symptoms of anxiety or increased arousal (e.g., difficulty sleeping, irritability, poor concentration, hypervigilance, exaggerated startle response, motor restlessness).**
F. The disturbance causes clinically significant distress or impairment in social, occupational, or other important areas of functioning.	**F. The disturbance causes clinically significant distress or impairment in social, occupational, or other important areas of functioning or impairs the individual's ability to pursue some necessary task, such as obtaining necessary assistance or mobilizing personal resources by telling family members about the traumatic event.**
	G. The disturbance lasts for a minimum of 2 days and a maximum of 4 weeks and occurs within the first 4 weeks of the traumatic event.

American Psychiatric Association, 1994.

estimates showing more than 70% of adults enduring at least one significant trauma over the course of their lifetime.[5,7,8] Also, although PTSD and ASD do not occur as often as once believed, these disorders do appear to be connected, with researchers finding that for a variety of traumatic experiences 72% to 83% of those diagnosed with ASD were diagnosed with PTSD at 6 months post-trauma and 63% to 80% of those same individuals remained positive for PTSD some 2 years following their traumatic experiences.[4]

Taken together, these findings highlight several important factors regarding traumatic reactions. First, some people who experience immediate and severe psychological problems following traumatic events can be expected to develop long-term psychological problems post-trauma. Second, not all people who develop long-term psychological problems (i.e., PTSD) will necessarily demonstrate poor adjustment immediately after their experiences. Thus, although ASD may be a good predictor of who may develop

PTSD in the future, studies also suggest that some individuals will develop a PTSD diagnosis slowly over time. Irrespective of the nature of trauma, however, one can also expect that a large number of people who experience potentially traumatic events will either handle the situation remarkably well or will recover from any emotional distress that occurs relatively quickly. This is demonstrated in that at least half of the trauma survivors who initially experience psychological discomfort eventually undergo a spontaneous remission to their symptoms in the months that follow their traumatic experiences.[3]

Trauma Characteristics, Individual Responsiveness, and Resilience

The fact that every occurrence of trauma does not automatically lead to pathological distress in victims and observers has led researchers and clinicians to investigate the characteristics that promote healthy and unhealthy functioning following significantly aversive events. Although some have looked into the characteristics of the individuals involved in traumatic situations, others have examined the nature of the traumatic event itself when attempting to understand human reactivity. In many ways, both avenues have yielded success in creating a better understanding of what qualities contribute to psychological reactivity to trauma.

When researchers have looked to predict long-term traumatic reactions (i.e., PTSD) based on individual characteristics and risk factors, factors such as lack of education, previous trauma, and general childhood adversity were found to influence diagnosis to some extent. However, other factors such as psychological difficulties prior to exposure, reported childhood abuse, and family psychiatric history were found to have slightly more influence over the development of PTSD symptoms. The most influential characteristics regarding PTSD were factors that were operating during or after the trauma itself because researchers have noted that trauma severity, lack of social support following the event, and more subsequent life stress carried the strongest risk of PTSD for survivors of trauma experiences. More specifically, people who felt their life was in danger, especially during noncombat trauma, were significantly more likely to develop emotional problems following these events as were people who experienced dissociative symptoms or intense negative emotions during and/or immediately after the event. Thus, for athletes and teams who endure physically or emotionally traumatic events outside the normal range of athletics, the presence of one or more of these characteristics might predict the development of emotional problems as a result of their experience (Box 13-1).

Whereas some authors have focused their energy on predicting PTSD and other traumatic reactions through risk factors and individual characteristics, others have looked at the event itself as a predictor of psychological reactivity.[2] Working on the principle that subjective interpretation is key to understanding traumatic reactions, many suggest that emotional difficulties following extreme experiences are a function of how one "interprets" the subjective severity of the event. More specifically, they maintain that traumatic reactions and maladaptive coping attempts often begin when an event violates some of the "core" beliefs that people instinctively hold true, such as a belief in a fair and just world, the need for physical safety, and the need for a positive view of oneself and one's abilities. In this line of thought, a person is likely to view an event as traumatic if he or she interprets the result as being especially unfair or unjust. Traumatic reactions are also more likely to persist when individuals conclude that they (or those around them) are no longer safe or when an experience challenges their self-worth or their ability to positively influence or control their life. Because physically traumatic injuries could jeopardize any and all of the basic human assumptions about the world, indeed, they too could be viewed as traumatic experiences by an athlete. Moreover, one can easily see how the death of a teammate might disrupt an athlete's value system or

---

Box 13-1   Individual Characteristics and Risk Factors Associated with Traumatic Reactions

Mild Risk Factors:
- Lack of education
- Family history of psychiatric problems
- General childhood adversity

Moderate Risk Factors:
- Positive psychiatric history in victim/witness
- Poor psychological functioning in victim/witness prior to event
- Reported child abuse
- Severe trauma
- Perceived life threat during event
- Extreme emotion during/after trauma

Significant Risk Factors:
- Lack of social support
- Extreme dissociation during/after trauma
- Subsequent life stress

---

alter his or her view of the sport or how he or she views the future.

Although both avenues of PTSD prediction have added significantly to the understanding of what leads to posttraumatic responses, neither explains why a significant portion of individuals show little or no ill effects after encountering life-threatening situations. The **resilience** or ability to recover quickly demonstrated by many suggests that protective psychological factors must be present to allow them to overcome difficulty with greater ease.[5,7,9] What characteristics contribute to these resilient reactions? Through an analysis of this question, experience has identified three characteristics that lead to successful coping in adverse situations and may be particularly influential in athletic populations: **hardiness, self-enhancement,** and the presence of positive emotion. Not only do social support, laughter, and the ability to experience genuine positive emotion in the wake of adverse events counteract negative emotion, but these qualities have also been shown to be associated with positive adjustment for survivors of both recent and distant traumatic events. Similarly, the ability to view oneself in a positive fashion (i.e., self-enhancement) has also been associated with resiliency following negative experiences in that these individuals have been shown to experience less stress, use social networks more effectively, and adjust with less difficulty when confronted with extremely negative events. It is interesting to note that most athletes tend to exhibit these traits as part of their psychological makeup.

⭐ *STAT Point 13-2. Three characteristics that lead to successful coping are hardiness, self-enhancement, and positive emotion.*

The personality trait of hardiness is also key to an individual's response to adversity because it is has been shown to be related to confidence, positive attitude, the ability to use social support and active coping, and the capacity to see difficult situations as less threatening.[5,10] Individuals high in hardiness tend to experience less distress because they believe they can have a positive influence on their surroundings, have a sense of commitment and purpose in their daily lives, and believe they can learn from both the positive and the negative events they encounter.[10–12] Because of the hardy individual's capacity to absorb greater levels of stress without suffering debilitating effects, individuals high in hardiness would also be expected to react to trauma and/or extreme events in a positive manner. Not only have elite-level athletes been found to have higher levels of overall hardiness when compared to lower-level athletes and the general population,[13,14] but also hardy athletes have been found to respond to stressful situations in a more positive, calm, and confident manner,[10,15] suggesting that athletes (and particularly athletes high in hardiness) are more prepared to endure physically traumatic injuries or experience critical incidents with less likelihood of experiencing significant emotional difficulties.

As more in the field have recognized, it is no longer a reasonable conclusion to assume that everyone who experiences grave situations or devastating injuries will automatically experience long-term psychological problems.[16] To the contrary, the research suggests that it is natural to expect most individuals who encounter or witness these situations will recover with minimal or no long-term psychological problems. However, as an athletic trainer or other member of the medical staff who serves athletes, it is important to understand that characteristics of the event and the athlete in question may determine whether long-term problems are more likely. Treatment providers who are aware of the athletes' personal and family histories and recognize how individuals react to traumatic events are better prepared to address potential emotional reactions prior to them causing significant interference in an athlete's athletic, social, educational, or occupational functioning. An awareness of these key characteristics not only places an athletic trainer or other medical staff member in a position to make predictions about whether psychological assistance may be necessary in the future, but this working knowledge also allows them to respond more readily at the first signs of ineffective coping.

Psychological Interventions in Crisis Situations

Because much of the research, policy development, and understanding of how to provide support in emergency and/or disaster situations have come from the world of trauma, many have come to equate **crisis interventions** with trauma resolution.[17] Although it is easy to see how these two intervention strategies have become synonymous, it is important to highlight the differences here because intervention strategies in crisis situations are fundamentally different than the manner in which one would treat someone with long-term psychological trauma reactions. It bears repeating that short-term acute stress reactions are, in many ways, a normal and expected response to an event that falls outside the range of "normal" everyday occurrences. Also, because not all who experience critical events will automatically develop severe traumatic responses, crisis intervention and trauma resolution work should be viewed as separate endeavors with separate goals. Whereas trauma work is meant to help individuals resolve emotional reactions and integrate critical events into one's experiential history, crisis intervention strategies are typically applied as a way to prevent the development of pathological difficulties in the first place.[17] Reyes and Elhai[17] highlight the aim of crisis intervention succinctly, stating that the strategies applied during a crisis are typically deemed a success if "a greater proportion of the survivors receiving these treatments . . . exhibit a relatively rapid return to 'normal' functioning" (p. 402) than they would if no intervention strategies were administered.

As people have become more aware of the emotional consequences of crisis situations, interest in potential intervention strategies has grown.[6,16–18] Although some strategies have garnered more empirical support and others have generated controversy, the unifying goals of these intervention techniques are to reduce immediate distress for survivors while attempting to prevent the development of long-term psychological problems.[17,18] Crisis intervention, **psycho-education, psychological debriefings,** and short-term cognitive therapy have all been used in various forms (and with varying success) following extreme events. Each of these strategies will be discussed in the following sections (Box 13-2).

Box 13-2 **Psychological Interventions in Crisis Situations**

- ■ **Crisis interventions**
- ■ **Educational interventions**
- ■ **Psychological debriefing interventions**
- ■ **Cognitive therapy interventions**

⭐ *STAT Point 13-3. The goals of intervention are to reduce immediate distress and try to prevent long-term problems.*

Crisis Intervention

Crisis intervention is often the first step in dealing with the emotional consequences of emergency situations and is the psychological equivalent to triage work in medicine where the primary goals are ensuring the safety of the individual while helping them reestablish an adequate level of independence and post-crisis functioning.[17] Crisis intervention techniques include, but are not limited to, assessing an individual's personal and interpersonal resources, establishing a supportive relationship, developing an understanding of the client's primary and secondary needs, coordinating referrals to specialized treatment providers and/or assistance organizations, and monitoring the client's progress and follow-through on an outlined recovery plan (Box 13-3).[17] Crisis intervention attempts to stabilize chaos and serve as the beginning of the recovery process for victims of critical incidents. Individuals who perform crisis intervention work function less like a therapist and operate more like an empathetic consultant whose aim is to reduce distress, ensure basic survival needs, and reconnect individuals to service providers and community resources that will establish a positive and hopeful outlook for long-term recovery.[17] Although the discussion of crisis intervention strategies is generally reserved for severe or large-scale traumas, it remains relevant when talking about serious physical injuries or extreme events in sport. In fact, athletic trainers often inherently serve in a crisis intervention role, considering the interconnection they share with the team, the coaching staff, and other medical providers. In this capacity, the management of an athlete's basic necessities becomes a backdrop to any other intervention attempts made following a traumatic injury.

Box 13-3 Crisis Intervention Techniques

- **Assess an individual's personal and interpersonal resources**

- **Establish a supportive relationship**

- **Develop an understanding of the client's primary and secondary needs**

- **Coordinate referrals to specialized treatment providers and/or assistance organizations**

- **Monitor the client's progress and follow-through on an outlined recovery plan**

⭐ *STAT Point 13-4. Individuals who perform crisis intervention work function less like a therapist and operate more like an empathetic consultant whose aim is to reduce distress, ensure basic survival needs, and reconnect individuals to service providers and community resources that will establish a positive and hopeful outlook for long-term recovery.*

Educational Interventions

Although not meant to serve as a treatment form, educational interventions are often used as a means of reducing psychological difficulties following trauma by informing and preparing people for the general consequences of traumatic situations.[17] Educational methods including brochures, media portrayals, and public seminars that can be used both before and after traumatic events to reduce the confusion and perceived helplessness that often accompany critical incidents and crisis situations. Educational interventions have been used in a variety of trauma situations and have been found to have both a direct and an indirect impact on recovery.[19] These strategies often include general messages about expected response patterns, but they can also be used as a means to provide contact information to survivors for support services. Using recognizable spokespeople, tailoring information and presentation forms for specific target audiences, and delivering messages through formal institutional avenues helps make this intervention strategy more effective. By providing accurate information and empowering others to care for themselves, it is hypothesized that educational endeavors help people feel more confident in their ability to endure difficult situations while also providing a sense of empathy, social support, and a willingness to ask for assistance.[17]

Psychological Debriefing Interventions

Psychological debriefing began as an intervention when **critical incident stress debriefing** (CISD) was introduced in the early 1980s.[20,21] Evolved from work with firefighters, CISD was developed with two basic intentions: to alleviate the distress that emergency personnel experience following grave situations in the line of duty and to help expedite the recovery from "normal" distress in people who endure abnormal and/or extreme situations.[21] The CISD process began as a formal, group-based intervention strategy for members of high-risk occupational groups such as emergency medical services workers, law enforcement officers, or disaster response personnel, but it quickly gained acceptance into occupational settings where industrial accidents are common or where life and death situations can occur. Presently, psychological debriefing techniques are often used as a single-session intervention strategy in groups that encounter situations that surpass the psychological threshold for what they would be expected to encounter.[17] These group debriefing sessions are often led by specially trained peers. Debriefing strategies operate on the assumption that processing the events and reactions of a potentially traumatic event shortly after it occurs will promote adjustment in victims while also preventing the development of long-term psychological problems. It is this basic assumption that led to the popularity and proliferation of debriefing strategies, which have now been used as an early intervention technique in countless work-related tragedies and numerous national and international disasters.[21] Over time, CISD response "teams" and organizations promoting the use of CISD have expanded, lending more credence to the intervention strategy. Despite the widespread use of psychological debriefing, and in particular CISD, the intervention form has become embroiled in a debate over its efficacy, with many studies showing inconclusive or even contraindicative results regarding the prevention of long-term psychological symptoms.[17,22,23] Although the CISD procedure will be described here, the depiction is meant to be used as an example of psychological debriefing strategies and is not intended to be an exhaustive exploration of the CISD process. For those interested in a more detailed accounting of CISD or other variations of psychological debriefing, many books and journal articles are devoted to the topic.[20,21,24,25]

Although some have depicted CISD and psychological debriefing as a form of therapy, it is important to understand that the procedure was originally designed to prevent PTSD and diminish the mental impact of trauma.[21] Although the structured format promotes the expression of emotion and an active exchange between group members, it also has educational and informative components where participants can process their experiences in a straightforward and nonthreatening manner. As people sort out what transpired, they also come to understand their own personal reactions and recognize that their peers or fellow co-workers are experiencing similar phenomena. Because the developers suggest that a formal CISD should be conducted between 3 and 5 days following the total completion of the traumatic event, when individuals within the CISD group are identified as having more significant emotional difficulties, they typically receive referrals for individual psychological care in a timely and efficient manner.

The various forms of psychological debriefing have both critics and supporters. The International Critical Incident Stress Foundation, Inc. (ICISF) reports that not only has CISD prevented the development of PTSD in a variety of groups, but the procedure was also found to be particularly helpful for intact groups who endured a wide range of potentially traumatic experiences.[18,28] Support for the CISD process is shown through the reduction of depression, anxiety, anger, and alcohol or drug use following traumatic experiences; the maintenance of high morale in these groups; and a decreased amount of sick days lost, employees lost, and medical claims filed in groups that have endured traumatic experiences. In addition, the ICISF (and critics of the psychological debriefing process) report that a consistent finding in the CISD literature was a subjective report on the part of participants that the process was helpful.[18,26,27]

> ✪ **STAT Point 13-5. Despite a debate over its efficacy, participants report that CISD is helpful.**

Support for psychological debriefing is countered by many experts who suggest that the CISD process provides little benefit beyond what is considered a "normal" recovery from traumatic events and, in some cases, has been shown to produce worse outcomes. Many researchers have claimed that single-session, early intervention strategies such as CISD were not only ineffective in reducing symptoms of PTSD, but also were less likely to produce improvements than when having no intervention at all.[22,23] Suggestions as to why the psychological debriefing in a variety of trauma situations failed to show significant long-term improvements center on the facts that these interventions may have been offered too early or for an insufficient length of time and the possibilities that the intervention may have increased peoples' expectation for having difficulties while inhibiting the normal interpersonal processing that occurs with one's primary social support group.[29]

The ICISF and other supporters of CISD note that the studies showing negative results for the procedure are often flawed in both their understanding of the procedure and in the application of the technique. Instead of using the intervention in homogenous groups of secondary survivors (i.e., a previously formed group that witnessed or encountered the effects of the event), many of the negative studies of CISD are conducted on an individual basis, with groups that have no prior relationship, or with individuals who are in active distress because they were directly affected by the traumatic event.[18] Negative CISD studies also make the mistake of analyzing the intervention as a unique, stand-alone treatment form instead of seeing it as part of a multifaceted traumatic stress management plan. As such, they expect that CISD will eliminate or treat PTSD symptoms rather than serve as a primary prevention technique. Ultimately, devotees of psychological debriefing maintain that when the procedure is used as a part of a comprehensive treatment plan in response to a group-based traumatic exposure, it has proved effective. Moreover, when the goals are the prevention of long-term difficulties and the promotion of normal recovery, CISD and other psychological debriefing strategies appear to be an effective and well-received early intervention approach, provided that they are carried out according to their outlined protocol and used with ongoing monitoring, follow-up after the initial meeting, and appropriate referrals to additional treatment providers when necessary.

> ✪ **STAT Point 13-6. CISD is part of a multifaceted traumatic stress management plan.**

Cognitive Therapy Interventions

Given the impact of perception and cognitive processes in the development and maintenance of post-traumatic reactions, clinicians in the disaster, trauma, and critical incident fields have begun to explore cognitive approaches as early intervention strategies.[3,30] In fact, many of the researchers in the field have begun to recommend an early course of cognitive-behavioral psychotherapy instead of psychological debriefing based on the accumulation of research showing the effectiveness of cognitive interventions.[3,22]

Examinations into **cognitive-behavioral therapy** (CBT) as an early intervention strategy started in the mid-1990s and have included a variety of clinical populations.[30–33] Trauma victims typically begin a CBT trial within the first few weeks following the traumatic event and undergo a training regimen that can include some or all of the following: cognitive restructuring; education about reactions to trauma; breathing and relaxation training; imagined exposure to the memory of traumatic events; and/or the actual confrontation of a feared, but safe, situation (Box 13-4). CBT interventions often seek to specifically address changes in a person's thinking patterns as a result of his or her traumatic experience while also encouraging people to return to many of the same behavior patterns that were present prior to their trauma experience. A treatment schedule in CBT is typically done on an individual basis and may last for up to 6 weeks, with most individuals completing the intervention program within the 3 months that immediately follow their traumatic experience. When used with victims from various trauma situations, CBT has been shown to reduce PTSD and depressive symptoms at a faster rate than when no intervention strategy was used.[31] In addition, people who participated in at least four sessions of CBT found that the benefits they received from the intervention were maintained for more than a year following the completion of treatment.[32] The success of CBT in trauma victims has also been demonstrated when compared to other treatment strategies. Using a number of survivors from "civilian" traumas such as industrial or motor vehicle accidents, investigators have found that CBT is more effective in reducing psychological difficulties when compared to supportive counseling or the use of a self-help booklet. Individuals who participated in CBT were consistently found to experience less depression, anxiety, and PTSD symptoms immediately after treatment and at 6-month and 12-month follow-up appointments.

Although the use of CBT as an early intervention strategy is somewhat new, its success in ameliorating the effects of trauma is well documented. Primarily, CBT has been championed as an efficient and effective means of resolving traumatic reactions because it directly addresses the cognitive features that maintain the disorder.[34] Over time, repeated exposure to trauma experiences promotes recovery in survivors because the emotionality connected to the event diminishes. In addition, fears about the world being a chaotic, unsafe, and threatening place can be restructured, and feelings of helplessness, inappropriate or misplaced blame, and beliefs that one can no longer live a meaningful or purposeful life can be challenged. It is natural to think that extending CBT's use into an early intervention role would further reduce the frequency of PTSD because the cognitive benefits from a CBT trial would occur before ineffective cognitive patterns have become crystallized, thus relieving initial difficulties more quickly, promoting more rapid recovery, and reducing the percentage of individuals likely to experience long-term problems.[30–33] Because CBT interventions occur over the course of a multiple-session format, some researchers suggest they are more likely to promote resolution of potential PTSD reactions than psychological debriefings, which are often carried out in single-session formats.[32] However, it is important to note that CISD and other debriefing strategies are not meant to be stand-alone treatments and CBT seems to make more intuitive sense when dealing with individuals who are direct victims of trauma, whereas psychological debriefings are designed to be implemented with intact groups who witnessed the traumatic experiences of others. It is worth noting that the primary role of the athletic trainer in these instances is to ensure that there is a plan in place and that it is followed. The role of the athletic trainer does not include conducting sessions or treatments that have been previously described. Indeed, it is possible that the athletic trainer will have also been affected by the catastrophe and will therefore be seeking assistance just as athletes and other affected staff.

Psychological Trauma in Athletic Environments

Although the death of an athlete or a severe athletic injury typically garners a tremendous amount of media attention, there has been relatively little written about these situations from a psychological treatment perspective. Currently, few articles center on traumatic experiences in athletic populations and even less focus on any type of formal intervention strategy. The earliest narratives on the subject appear in the 1990s and document the extreme and lasting impact that traumatic events can have on individual athletes and the team on which they play.[35–39] In articles focusing on the deaths of various athletes, authors cite parallels between PTSD symptoms, describing an initial reaction of shock and disbelief and noting that nightmares, vivid memories, and other reexperiencing phenomena were common experiences for the athletes

---

Box 13-4   Components of Cognitive-Behavioral Therapy

■ Cognitive restructuring

■ Education about reactions to trauma

■ Breathing and relaxation training

■ Imagined exposure to the memory of traumatic events

■ Confrontation of feared, but safe, situations

and teams who witnessed these events.[36–39] Moreover, the earliest entries into this topic area noted that traumatic events seemed to carry additional significance when they occurred within the confines of an athletic team. They and many of the clinicians who have been faced with the aftermath of trauma in sporting environments maintain that not only were witnesses unprepared for the extreme emotions that were attached to the event itself, but also the close and multilayered relationships that witnesses and survivors had with the victim only added to the emotional impact of these extreme events (D. Yukelson, personal communication, May 3, 2006).[35,38]

The sports psychology literature contains few articles that focus specifically on intervention attempts following the traumatic death or injury of an athlete. In most situations, the intervening professional was a performance consultant who found himself or herself in the unique situation of having to deal with the aftermath of a crisis that occurred on a team he or she was trying to help perform more effectively. Specifically, Vernacchia and his colleagues[38] described the assistance they provided to a men's university basketball team following the death of a player from myocardial infarction, whereas Buchko[40] outlined the intervention she conducted within a women's university basketball team following the suicide of a team member. In both situations, intervention strategies were implemented in a reactionary fashion, where the psychology consultants relied heavily on clinical intuition, collaborations with psychologists outside the athletic environment, and a basic understanding of crisis intervention and CISD techniques.

Although Vernacchia et al.[38] used CISD and several grief models as a backdrop to their intervention approach, there was no formal CISD intervention sessions and the application of both the CISD and grief models during the post-trauma time period was done in a "modified version."[38] Vernacchia provided an understanding of the grieving process to the team through a series of individual and small-group meetings and consulted with the coaching staff in an attempt to normalize the bereavement issues that the team members and coaches were experiencing. The first consultation with the coaching staff occurred approximately 36 hours after the player's death, and, although a team meeting occurred within 12 hours of the event, no CISD session was conducted at that time. Instead, the intervening professional attended the first practice after the player's death, which was almost 48 hours later. A team competition prevented any formal memorial service from being held prior to the game. When the game was completed and a formal memorial service was held, the intervention shifted to follow-up services, where Vernacchia and his colleagues[38] provided assistance to the players, coaching staff, athletic trainers, and the other support staff for the team. The coaching staff and sport psychology consultant held a series of individual and group meetings with players throughout the off-season and prior to the start of the next year's training, but the number of meetings and their exact format was unclear. Anniversary dates, formal tributes by the team, and the impact this event would have on new team members were addressed in individual and group meetings at the outset of the following season, but it appears that no formal intervention protocol was used in response to this tragic event.

Buchko[40] encountered a similar situation within a university women's basketball program after a team member committed suicide at the beginning of the season. Similar to the other example, she was forced to drastically alter her role as a performance consultant to implement an intervention strategy as a crisis counselor. Rather than implementing an informed primary prevention protocol designed for traumatic events, Buchko[40] found herself reacting to the extreme situation. She incorporated crisis intervention theory into the retrospective analysis of her intervention, but she also used a systems theory to account for the impact of traumatic experiences on an athletic team, viewing intervention as being aimed at the basketball team as a unit and its individual members.

Similar to other examples of trauma in sport, Buchko[40] met with coaches to determine action plans, identify athletes that may have potentially had greater difficulty adjusting to the traumatic event, and educated them about what to expect in terms of trauma resolution. Individual meetings with athletes, appropriate referrals to community and campus-based counseling resources, and meetings with the team before and during practices were conducted. Primary and secondary goals of treatment included identifying warning signs for PTSD and directly addressing trauma recovery and the grieving process by providing stress reduction techniques, assigning group homework, facilitating team-building activities, and drawing parallels for grief with the teams' sport performance knowledge base. Long-term follow-up throughout the season, preparation for anniversary reactions, and ongoing education and normalization of the trauma recovery process were critical components of Buchko's intervention as well, although it appears that much of these strategies were conducted in individual meetings.

Although both of these examples reported success in helping to promote recovery and prevent long-term difficulties in athletes following the unexpected death of a teammate, their commentaries highlight the current shortcomings of addressing mental recovery from trauma within a sport environment. One of the most glaring deficits remains the lack of a clear intervention protocol. Although this problem, in many ways, is a reflection of the state of early intervention strategies following disaster and trauma, it is even more glaring in athletic populations considering the paucity of attention the subject has received. As Vernacchia et al.[38] stated, "a sport-specific CISD protocol would have been extremely helpful" and one wonders if he and Buchko[40] would have been more effective and/or more efficient in their intervention had they been able to administer a standardized **trauma intervention protocol** instead of relying so heavily on clinical intuition. This point is even more important when one considers that neither of the authors who implemented the trauma intervention was actually working with the athletes they served in that capacity. Given the unpredictable nature of trauma and/or traumatic injury, it is important for athletic trainers, sport psychologists, and other members of the medical support staff of any athletic population to understand that they may be called on to respond to the intense emotional needs of an athlete or team without notice and that their prompt, appropriate reactions may be instrumental in avoiding long-term difficulties for these individuals. Not only should service providers have an awareness of what constitutes a "normal" reaction to an abnormal situation, but they must also know that a standard of care for these situations exists on both the physical and psychological end.

Treatment providers with an awareness of CISD and early intervention strategies may also recognize that the CISD protocol is ideally suited for use within an athletic environment. Whereas critics have questioned CISD's effectiveness in trauma situations, CISD proponents have argued that the group format in which the intervention strategy was designed is often abandoned in the studies that show it to be ineffective.[18] Not only has CISD been found to be consistently more effective in "homogenous" groups (i.e., groups that had a preexisting relationship prior to the occurrence of trauma), but CSID supporters also note that peer support interventions have been found to be even more effective in groups that view themselves as being unique, special, or somewhat different than the general population.[18,21] Given that athletic teams meet both of those unique characteristics, one would expect that a group-based CISD intervention approach would be a natural fit for an athletic team that experiences or is witness to a traumatic event. In this context, CISD-based interventions can allow team members to receive education, provide support to those around them, and capitalize on the strengths and resources available within the collective unit. This point is particularly relevant for support personnel who work closely with athletic teams because in the situations described by Vernacchia et al.[38] and Buchko,[40] both authors commented on the fact that the teams they served "closed ranks" and attempted to cope with the unusual situation on their own. Thus, athletic trainers and other medical staff who have an understanding of trauma, psychological debriefing interventions, and the signs of an ineffective response to traumatic events are better prepared to serve their athletes, particularly if the athletes or team decide to refuse assistance from sources outside the team environment.

⭐ *STAT Point 13-7. CISD is more effective in homogenous groups such as athletic teams than in nonhomogenous groups.*

Although Vernacchia et al.[38] and Buchko[40] used a CISD model as backdrop to their intervention attempts, it does not appear that either conducted a formal psychological debriefing session. Buchko reported that CISD was conducted by the university counseling center staff, but it is unclear how many of and in what manner these sessions were conducted. At this point, it is impossible to determine if CISD or psychological debriefing would be a more effective intervention strategy in athletic populations because there has not been a clear example of this reported in the literature. Although a more thorough analysis of psychological debriefing strategies in athletics must be conducted to resolve this question in the future, given the characteristics that athletic teams share with other intact groups that CISD has helped (i.e., police officers, firefighters, and emergency medical personnel), one could argue that CISD or other versions of psychological debriefing would be an appropriate intervention strategy following potentially traumatic experiences in this population.

The Psychological Emergency Response Team

When dealing with emergency situations or serious physical injury, proper training and thorough preparation help service providers respond more effectively to the complex and unpredictable situations they face on a regular basis. The parallels between physical and emotional trauma are relevant in this context as well, noting that training, preparation, and the development of a network of qualified service providers can be the difference between successful and unsuccessful resolution of a critical situation for both medical and psychological service providers. Because effective networking, clear communication, and referrals to equally adept and trained professionals can help expand a service provider's capabilities, professionals working within athletic environments should have an awareness of the types of professionals that will be needed when dealing with the effects of psychological trauma. Ideally, a team-oriented approach can be implemented where each qualified health professional addresses a key component of the situation to promote the most effective resolution possible. As mentioned by both Vernacchia et al.[38] and Buchko,[40] it is critical for members of the treatment team to be both on the "inside" and on the "outside" of an athlete's or team's immediate circle. The following is a description of the professionals that can be useful when responding to extreme emotional situations in sports and the role each can play in providing assistance. The list is divided into members who are presumably already within the team environment prior to the critical incident (i.e., "internal" team members) and those who may have been on the periphery prior to the critical event (i.e., "external" team members) but can be essential in helping athletes and teams recover (Box 13-5).

Internal Team Members

Athletic Trainer

A critical member of the sports medicine staff, the athletic trainer tends to serve as the point person in coordinating care and communicating with other treatment team members. Because of the closeness that many athletic trainers

---

Box 13-5 Psychological Emergency Response Team

Internal Members:
- Athletic trainer
- Team physician
- Sport psychologist
- Coaching staff
- Administrative staff

External Members:
- Counselors
- CISD "team"
- Staff psychiatrist

---

develop with their athletes, they may be more likely to recognize individual athletes who experience difficulties or they may be the person that athletes feel the most comfortable speaking to about emotional problems. The athletic trainer has an advantage over other sports medicine staff in that he or she tends to see athletes on a daily basis and is in the best position to compare their post-traumatic function to their level of functioning prior to the critical incident. As an internal team member, athletic trainers are generally trusted and respected by their athletes. Moreover, their role within the team is one of a caregiver, so questions about emotional status or difficulty coping would be seen as consistent with their role within the team. When physical injuries are part of the traumatic experience, athletic trainers are also in a position to gauge when an athlete's physical improvement is sufficient enough to allow treatment to address emotional ramifications of the event or when the emotional reactivity of an athlete is hampering physical recovery.

Team Physician

Team physicians, whether orthopedic specialists or general practitioners, are another invaluable member of an internal support team. They too are valued within an athletic environment as helpers and their position is often held in high regard. Not only can a team doctor monitor an athlete's physical recovery, but he or she can also conduct a basic psychiatric evaluation and thus serve as a person who can directly assess an athlete's emotional recovery. Evaluations of an athlete's mental status; prescriptions for both physical and emotional regulation; and basic education regarding PTSD, "normal" recovery, and what an individual athlete

can expect following a severe, traumatic injury all fall within the boundaries of a team physician's duties.

Sport Psychologist

Depending on whether a sport psychologist has been conducting ongoing consultation, he or she could be viewed as either an internal or external team member. For the purpose of this discussion, however, we assume that a sport psychologist is a known and frequently present influence on the team or athletes in question. Not only can a sport psychologist trained in CISD conduct debriefing sessions, but as with the other members of the sport medicine staff, his or her role also aligns closely with monitoring an athlete or group's emotional needs. Providing education about trauma reactions, assessing individual reactivity, meeting with affected athletes, and monitoring the long-term progress of an individual athlete or the entire team could fall under the responsibility of a team sport psychologist. In addition, sport psychologists can coordinate services with other members of the sports medicine group, communicate with administrative staff, and compare prior functioning to the post-traumatic presentation of the athletes within the group. A sport psychologist who has a close working relationship within a team will undoubtedly be of service in that athletes will feel comfortable asking for assistance from a known person and one who would be perceived to be helpful in facilitating their emotional recovery.

Coaching Staff

To the extent that they are capable and available, the coaching staff can provide tremendous assistance in helping an athlete and/or team overcome extreme events. A caveat to this comes with the knowledge that many coaches are often as equally emotionally affected by the events that unfold around them as the athletes in their charge. So, before enlisting the assistance of a coach or the entire coaching staff, it is imperative that the treatment team determine whether coaches are emotionally capable of helping others or, in turn, need emotional assistance themselves.

The coaches who are emotionally available for their athletes can help in numerous ways. Coaches can be yet another person to coordinate effective treatment and establish a referral network within the team, but because of the role as team leader, they are likely to be more influential in providing reassurance and perspective to their players while keeping a watchful eye on the daily reactions and emotional status of the team. Other helpful functions of a coach include modeling appropriate grief, concern, or positive expectations for the future and lending validation to intervention attempts through their own participation. Last, coaches can help athletes return to their pretrauma level of functioning by maintaining (or altering) a workout schedule to allow athletes the time they need to grieve without completely losing a sense of their pretrauma schedule and activities (Box 13-6).

Box 13-6   Roles of the Coaching Staff

■ Help to coordinate effective treatment and establish a referral network within the team.

■ Provide reassurance and perspective to the involved athletes.

■ Monitor daily reactions and emotional status of the involved athletes/team.

■ Model appropriate grief, concern, or positive expectations for the future.

■ Help validate intervention attempts through their own participation in the process.

■ Help athletes return to their pretrauma level of functioning by maintaining (or altering) a workout and/or practice schedule to allow athletes the time they need to grieve without completely losing a sense of their pretrauma schedule and activities.

Administrative Staff

Members of an athletic department and/or representatives of a university hierarchy or athletic organization can act as extended family members during times of crisis, and they can also be used to deflect attention away from affected athletes, allowing them the necessary time and space to start the recovery process. Interacting with media, arranging organizational functions such as memorial services or benefits, and providing institutional support to the members of the team in distress are critical functions for members of the administrative staff. Moreover, if organizational staff members are truly viewed as an extension of the team, it is likely that athletes will experience an increase in both perceived and actual social support. Given the importance that social support plays in the trauma recovery process, the reaction of the administrative/organizational staff is a crucial component in helping athletes and the team adapt after critical events.

External Team Members

Counselors

As mentioned earlier, the athletes within a team are not the only ones affected by the critical events that befall them. Many times the coaches, athletic training staff, and members within the organization are negatively affected as well. Counselors and/or psychologists outside the situation are

often needed in the weeks and months that follow a traumatic event to assist the athletes and the support staff within the team. Although these service providers may not necessarily be involved in psychological debriefings, in most cases they can provide crisis management and educational services. In addition, they can serve athletes and teams by working with individuals to help resolve traumatic reactions or by providing support and assistance to coaches and medical staff so they can be of service to those around them. Ultimately, counselors can provide a safe haven outside of the sporting environment and traumatic situation where individuals can help process, reorganize, and gain perspective, so they can eventually reenter the athletic world in a more emotionally stable mindset.

The CISD "Team"

When no professionals within the organization are qualified to conduct CISD, psychological debriefings, or other early intervention strategies for traumatic events, it may be necessary to bring professionals in from outside the system. Although introducing new people into an athletic team presents difficulties of its own, having a professional trained to conduct CISD meetings may have greater benefit than having someone within the organization attempt to conduct psychological debriefings with no prior experience. CISD teams and organizations exist throughout the United States and consist of a variety of professionals who are interested in helping to mitigate the effects of acute stress. Typically, a CISD "team" consists of both mental health professionals and peer support personnel who have an interest in helping the group in question.[21] Thus, when contacted by an athletic organization, a CISD organization will presumably assign professionals and support staff that have an interest or history in sports. With an eye toward accelerating the recovery process, CISD teams provide basic education about trauma and recovery; teach stress management and cognitive restructuring techniques; allow willing participants to discuss the events and their thoughts, fears, and concerns; and identify individuals who may experience difficulty recovering from traumatic events.

Staff Psychiatrist

Given that a percentage of individuals who experience traumatic events subsequently develop significant, long-term problems, the inclusion of a team psychiatrist seems a logical and warranted addition. Although orthopedic specialists or primary care physicians are also capable of prescribing medications for depression, anxiety, and other psychiatric conditions, a psychiatrist is better suited for handling medication management issues and more complex clinical presentations. Referrals to a psychiatrist may also be necessary when athletes or other individuals present with severe psychological impairment or when lethality or suicidality are part of the clinical picture.

Each athletic department or sport organization will have some, but perhaps not all, of the professionals listed previously. Where appropriate, it is recommended that service providers in a sport environment work to establish referral networks and develop professional relationships in areas of need, so that if team members outside of the organization are needed in an emergency, they understand their role and can be immediately contacted. Establishing a **psychological emergency response team** prior to a traumatic event will reduce the "reactive" nature of interventions that often follow extreme events. It will also help to establish clear roles and a more cohesive treatment team for when it is needed. Just as in emergency medical care, a more prepared treatment team leads to a more efficient response and reduces the likelihood that emergency situations will evolve into long-term problems. It is also recommended that once a treatment team is established, they conduct regular meetings prior to any emergency situation. Role playing how the team will handle emergency and/or crisis situations will help better prepare the members for an actual occurrence and will allow team members to interact in a nonpressure situation so that their interactions under duress are not confusing, inefficient, or misinterpreted. If an event has occurred, it is recommended that the entire treatment team meet on a regular basis (i.e., weekly or biweekly) to assess the effectiveness of intervention attempts; monitor the progress of the athletes, coaches, and support staff in question; and develop long-term plans for problematic situations before they arise.

✪ *STAT Point 13-8. A prepared treatment team reduces the likelihood of long-term problems.*

Psychological Intervention Recommendations

Sufficient evidence suggests that early intervention can be helpful in alleviating or avoiding severe long-term psychological consequences following emergency situations in a sporting environment. Because of the community-like atmosphere that is often present within an athletic team or an entire athletic department, it is important to recognize that catastrophic injuries, disastrous accidents, and deaths both on and off the playing surface can have a tremendous negative impact on the psyche of an individual, team, or large group of athletes. Moreover, these events may have complex and widespread consequences, where individuals and athletes far removed from the athletic team in question are deeply and dramatically affected. Ultimately, the desire to be helpful in these situations should be tempered with what has been shown to be successful rather than what has been shown to be popular or cost-effective. In addition, it is important to remember that the success of any intervention strategy is often dependent on its careful and precise implementation.

Psychological debriefing, in its various forms, has been used extensively when attempting to provide assistance to victims following disaster and traumatic events. Despite the fact that the procedure is generally viewed positively by the individuals who receive it, the empirical evidence related to the procedure does not support its use in isolation. Specifically, the psychological debriefing process has been shown to be more effective when used as a primary prevention tool in preexisting groups that are secondarily affected by traumatic experiences rather than when used with individuals who suffer traumatic experiences directly and are actively symptomatic. Taken separately, the findings supporting cognitive interventions and denouncing psychological debriefing in direct victims of trauma might suggest that CBT has a distinct advantage over CISD and other versions of psychological debriefing when used in response to crisis situations. However, this does not mean that psychological debriefing does not have a role in responding to the severe events that sometimes occur in sports. As some researchers have suggested,[22,32] it is more likely that a "stepped care" approach is the most effective way to prevent long-term difficulties following the occurrence of potentially traumatizing experiences. It stands to reason that a similar approach would be helpful for individual athletes and the athletic teams that experience these situations. Box 13-7 is a proposed step-based protocol for athletic organizations faced with the challenge of responding to emergency situations or critical events.

Step 1: Address Basic Needs

As mentioned earlier, the logical first step when responding to any emergency situation involves securing the physical safety of victims while helping them to reestablish a level of independence and adequate level of functioning. Because the majority of the potentially traumatic situations discussed throughout this book are physical in nature, the first step in serving direct victims of emergency situations or severe events must first address the physical needs or health ramifications of their injuries. Providing medical care and coordinating treatment modalities are undoubtedly the first necessary steps in helping victims of extreme situations—especially when physical injury is part of the clinical presentation. The importance of this point is exemplified by the finding of Bisson[22] that burn victims who received psychological debriefing closer to the time of their traumatic injury (and presumably before their physical injuries were sufficiently healed) actually fared worse than those same subjects who received the intervention at a later time. Thus, even when it is clear that psychological factors will play a role in an athlete's recovery, it is imperative that certain intervention strategies are initiated only after their physical injuries are treated or controlled. In addition to addressing athletes' physical concerns, activities of daily living must also be considered, with treatment providers assessing whether victims and/or witnesses of trauma are capable of caring for themselves during this critical time. Establishing a supportive social network, providing assistance when basic needs are not being met, and helping survivors develop a sufficient

Box 13-7 Fundamental Steps in Conducting Early Interventions Following Traumatic Events

Step 1: Address Basic Needs
Objectives:
- Provide necessary medical care.
- Coordinate treatment modalities.
- Assure successful achievement of activities of daily living.

Step 2: Anticipate Recovery, Screen for Ineffective Coping
Objectives:
- Recognize that "normal" distress is common.
- Identify individuals with signs of potential difficulty recovering.
- Monitor changes of identified individuals throughout the recovery process.

Step 3: Implement Early-Intervention Protocols
Objectives:
- Coordinate treatment interventions with other professionals.
- Implement individual and/or group-based interventions.
- Recognize the different needs of direct victims, witnesses, and significant others.
- Time intervention strategies in line with expected critical periods for post-trauma reactions.

Step 4: Termination, Referrals, and Follow-Up
Objectives:
- Foster independence in victims and survivors.
- Facilitate long-term care and monitor treatment progress for individuals in need.
- Address potential anniversary reactions through timing of follow-up meetings.

level of hope for recovery are essential goals throughout this phase of an intervention protocol.

✪ *STAT Point 13-9. Physical injuries must be treated before psychological interventions.*

Step 2: Anticipate Recovery, Screen for Ineffective Coping

Once the basic needs of an individual or group are stabilized, it is appropriate to begin addressing the psychological effects of the traumatic situation. During this time, treatment providers must be aware that many individuals will experience a level of distress that is proportionate to the magnitude of the trauma but will typically undergo a natural recovery to their previous level of functioning shortly after the incident (i.e., days or weeks). Thus, whereas rapid intervention in a crisis situation may affect survival for medical emergencies, there does not appear to be a direct psychological parallel for critical events, considering that resiliency and spontaneous "normal" recoveries are common for many following traumatic events. As athletic organizations coordinate an appropriate response to the traumatic injuries and emergency situations that occur within their institution, care providers should keep a watchful eye on individuals at greater risk of developing psychological problems. The risk factors discussed earlier in the chapter can guide treatment providers during this time, and when individual athletes show signs of ineffective coping, they should be identified during any early intervention program so that they can be referred for individual treatment and/or monitored during the weeks and months following the traumatic event. In particular, treatment team members should consider individuals and/or groups of athletes who were particularly close to the victim both emotionally and physically during their accidents. Roommates; training partners; and the athletes, coaches, and support staff members who share a close interpersonal relationship with victims should be monitored closely, as should individuals who personally witnessed the emergency situation or dramatic injury as it unfolded.

Step 3: Implement Early-Intervention Protocols

The next stage in a stepped-care approach to emergency situations in sports is the implementation of a number of early intervention strategies. The crisis intervention approach and the specific educational, psychological debriefing, and cognitive therapy protocols discussed earlier in this chapter are fundamental ways that treatment providers can assist the athletes in their care. Although the immediate implementation of emotional processing strategies (i.e., within the first 24–72 hours) does not appear to be as necessary as originally believed, some research has found that at the group and individual level, intervention strategies conducted within the first month following trauma have reduced the percentage of people who developed long-term psychological difficulties.[18,31,32] For survivors of traumatic events at both the team and individual level, successful prevention of significant long-term psychological problems involves providing people with a basic education about what to expect following their experience while also screening for the signs of unsuccessful or dysfunctional attempts at coping. Given the empirical findings in the area, however, early intervention treatment modalities should differ depending on whether the person providing psychological care is dealing with an athlete who was the direct victim of an emergency situation and/or severe injury or a treatment provider is assisting an individual or group of athletes that witnessed a tragic event.

For individuals directly affected by trauma, it is clear that cognitive interventions offer the most effective and straightforward treatment approach. When these athletes are identified as being at risk for developing long-term psychological difficulties, a referral to a professional psychotherapist with the expressed intent of conducting a multiple-session CBT intervention aimed at resolving traumatic stress symptoms is warranted, preferably within the first month following the traumatic injury or event. Based on the findings reported here, at-risk individuals should participate in a minimum of five individual sessions of a CBT-based intervention program where stress management training, the restructuring of cognitive distortions and dysfunctional perceptions, and imagined exposure and planned encounters of feared situations are included. Signs of effective treatment would include the gradual reduction of emotionality during repeated discussions of the traumatic experience; the reformulation of thoughts, beliefs, and perceptions concerning the events; and the reduction of negative emotions or reliance on ineffective coping strategies. Although individuals indirectly affected by emergency situations may also benefit from cognitive interventions, at the team level, providing basic education to survivors and screening for the signs of unsuccessful coping attempts can prove to be more difficult. This is where psychological debriefings can play a significant role in the recovery process if it is included as part of an all-encompassing trauma intervention program. Considering that "true" psychological care should be directed at those who demonstrate the highest risk in developing long-term problems, in many ways, debriefing sessions can provide an excellent opportunity to provide all willing participants or witnesses with a basic understanding of what they can anticipate following their experiences while also giving the crisis management team time to formally or informally screen individuals for the warning signs of potential long-term problems.

> ✪ *STAT Point 13-10. Signs of effective treatment include the gradual reduction of emotionality during repeated discussions of the traumatic experience; the reformulation of thoughts, beliefs, and perceptions concerning the events; and the reduction of negative emotions or reliance on ineffective coping strategies.*

If group debriefing sessions are to be used, careful attention should be paid to the timing, number, and context in which these sessions are framed. Noting that many have failed to recognize the recommendations that proponents of psychological debriefings have made regarding the initiation of this primary prevention strategy, it is important for sport organizations to understand that these processing meetings are meant to be held after the total completion of events related to the emergency situation. Thus, if emergency situations are ongoing and have complications without a clear conclusion, psychological debriefing sessions are not recommended. Ideally, processing meetings would follow memorial services or other "official" proceedings conducted by family members or organizations associated with the event. Considering that many people have found immediate intervention strategies disconcerting, it is also suggested that any scheduled psychological debriefings that occur during this time be voluntary in nature. Moreover, if group debriefing sessions are conducted, based on the findings in several studies, it is recommended that more than one session be administered, preferably at key time periods following the incident in order for treatment providers to truly monitor the progress of the collective group or the individuals identified as having problems adjusting.[18] Ideally, three psychological debriefing sessions should be conducted, with the first occurring within the 2-week period that follows the event and the subsequent meetings occurring at 1 month and 2 months after the incident. These times coincide with the ASD and PTSD diagnoses and the periods where one would expect to see the complete cycle of "normal" distress and a return to prior functioning that is typical of the post-trauma phase.

> ✪ *STAT Point 13-11. Group debriefing sessions should follow memorial services and should be voluntary.*

Step 4: Termination, Referrals, and Follow-Up

As mentioned earlier, it is important to recognize the difference between crisis intervention and trauma intervention. Professionals serving athletes and teams in a crisis intervention mode must understand that their primary goals should be to stabilize an emotionally chaotic situation, ensure the safety of the participants, and assist athletes and teams in reestablishing an adequate level of independence and post-crisis functioning. Thus, unless providing long-term psychological care is consistent with their professional role, individuals who serve athletes and teams following emergency situations must be prepared to make appropriate referrals outside of the athletic system in a timely fashion.

Despite the short-term and focal nature of crisis intervention work, the monitoring of a client's (or team's) progress and their adherence to an outlined recovery plan does fall within a crisis counselor's responsibility. For individuals negatively affected by severe injuries or emergency situations, regularly scheduled follow-up meetings are recommended to ensure that they have maintained any gains received through their participation in an intervention strategy. For athletes who complete a trial of CBT, sessions held at 6 months, 9 months, and 1 year following the conclusion of the traumatic would not only help with an individual's long-term transition, but also could be used to address anniversary reactions or any long-term situations that develop as a result of their experience. For groups that have participated in debriefing sessions after an emergency situation, a sport organization could choose from a number of ideal times to conduct follow-up meetings. Sessions held at the end of a competitive season or at the beginning of the subsequent competitive season could be used to establish closure or mark new beginnings for an athletic organization. Sessions timed in relation to the event itself could be conducted at either 6 months or 12 months after the incident and would be ideal times to address the incident, the team's collective recovery, and the anniversary reactions that are often an emotional time for survivors.

> ✪ *STAT Point 13-12. Follow-up debriefing sessions should be held at ideal times, especially anniversaries.*

Finally, athletic trainers and medical staff personnel must recognize the different needs of athletes directly affected by traumatic injuries/experiences and the teams that endure situations outside the normal range of experiences for an athlete. Although each organization has the ability to implement a variety of intervention strategies in response to these events, it is recommended that instead of focusing on any specific intervention approach, organizations prepare for these situations in advance by developing a clear trauma response protocol that can be put into practice when these tragic events occur. Although a number of the intervention strategies presented here have been shown to be effective, they should not be deemed as the entire range of possible intervention modalities for crisis resolution. Direct intervention approaches will be more effective if they are part of a multifaceted, multidisciplinary primary prevention program that includes a clear structure; ongoing support for athletes and monitoring for the signs of ineffective coping; and the coordination of services from athletic training, medical, and psychological service providers. With the prevention of long-term psychological problems as the primary goal, early intervention strategies should be viewed as an appropriate response on the part of an athletic organization to mitigate the effects of catastrophic injuries, disastrous accidents, or the death of an athlete.

> ✪ *STAT Point 13-13. Direct intervention approaches will be more effective if they are part of a multifaceted, multidisciplinary primary prevention program that includes a clear structure; ongoing support for athletes and monitoring for the signs of ineffective coping; and the coordination of services from athletic training, medical, and psychological service providers.*

Understanding Compassion Fatigue

No exploration of trauma or crisis intervention would be complete without a discussion of **compassion fatigue.**[41–43] Although the concept of compassion fatigue will not be fully explored here, it is important for athletic trainers to recognize the emotional and psychological toll that caring for victims of trauma can take. First described by Figley,[42] compassion fatigue represents a caregiver's diminished ability to feel empathy or interest in helping victims of trauma as a result of being exposed to the intense emotions associated with their experiences. Often linked to burnout and secondary traumatization, compassion fatigue can lead to emotional and physical exhaustion in caregivers, frequent reliving of their clients' personal narratives, a persistent emotional state, and a desire to avoid their clients or reminders of their clients' experiences. Ironically, it appears that the emotional connection and empathetic identification that allow professionals to be helpful to survivors is part of the underlying causes of compassion fatigue. Thus, the development of close interpersonal relationships with survivors of trauma combined with the high level of stress involved in their treatment leaves caregivers susceptible to their own emotional problems. Lack of social support, a personal history of trauma, and a diminished level of self-care on the provider's behalf have also been associated with higher levels of compassion fatigue.

> ✪ *STAT Point 13-14. Athletic trainers must recognize the risk of compassion fatigue.*

> ✪ *STAT Point 13-15. Lack of social support, a personal history of trauma, and a diminished level of self-care on the provider's behalf have also been associated with higher levels of compassion fatigue.*

In addition to therapists and social workers who work with trauma victims, a significant number of professionals conducting CISD sessions have developed compassion fatigue or were at serious risk of developing the syndrome.[44] Athletic trainers, medical support staff, coaches, athletic administrators, and anyone involved in helping athletes recover from traumatic events need to have an awareness of compassion fatigue not only to guarantee successful treatment of their athletes, but also to ensure their own successful recovery from these intense experiences. In addition to focusing on treatment successes rather than failures, caregivers are urged to focus on their own self-care to combat the effects of compassion fatigue. Therefore, caregivers are encouraged to separate their own emotional experience from their athletes' narratives and to structure their work in a way that allows time outside of the athletic environment. Moreover, sport organizations must recognize the level of stress associated with traumatic situations for members of the support staff and seek to provide outlets for these individuals. Ultimately, a caregiver's ability to model self-care and develop an appropriate perspective regarding traumatic experiences will have a positive influence on their athletes' emotional status, their team's morale, and their own emotional regulation.

Serious accidents and life-threatening injuries are an unfortunate and unavoidable part of sports. Over the course of their entire careers, those who care for athletes on a regular basis may find themselves in potentially tragic situations on but a handful of occasions. Although a caregiver's response during these situations is pivotal to ensuring a successful outcome, there are times when instituting an appropriate emergency action plan and providing the best possible medical care is not enough to avoid a disastrous and regrettable conclusion. Moreover, merely surviving a life-threatening illness or injury does not guarantee that individuals, or those who witness these extreme events, will be unaffected. In these situations, medical staff may have no other recourse than to address the consequent emotional and mental health of their athletes by understanding the "normal" effects of tragedy and recognizing the difference between traumatic reactions and natural grief or bereavement. Addressing the basic needs of athletes, screening for signs of ineffective coping, implementing early-intervention protocols, and making appropriate treatment referrals may seem like inconsequential attempts to provide help in the wake of such serious events, but these strategies can help ameliorate the short-term discomfort that individuals may experience following trauma while also serving to prevent the development of more serious long-term difficulties.

 EMERGENCY ACTION

Ideally, the athletic trainer's organization would have an emergency action plan in place to help initiate a coordinated response to the situation. The crisis management team would obviously be dictated by the professionals available, but the intervention protocol would determine how members of the coaching staff, counseling service, medical and athletic training staff, or other groups within the organization should respond. Although support services would naturally focus on all athletes, individuals deemed to be at a greater risk for the development of psychological difficulties would command more attention. In this situation, these people would include the athletes who carried the player to the sideline; anyone (including the athletic trainer) who witnessed his death; and, perhaps to a lesser degree, anyone who was present during the workout session. Once treatment providers determine that witnesses are capable of caring for themselves, early intervention strategies can be initiated at the group or individual level. If psychological debriefing sessions are implemented, the emergency action plan would outline what role each member of the crisis response team will fill, how referrals for individual treatment will be monitored, and how follow-up services will be conducted. Formal means of remembrance such as funerals, memorial services, and the institution of scholarships or memorial funds along with more informal modes of honoring the victim of this tragedy should be considered.

CHAPTER HIGHLIGHTS

- Whereas medical trauma indicates an injury that threatens a person's well-being, psychological trauma is based on the subjective experience of the person where fear, helplessness, or horror are part of an individual's reaction.

- Post-traumatic stress disorder is the psychological disorder most commonly associated with threatening or harrowing events, and the primary hallmarks of the disorder are reexperiencing phenomena, emotional numbing, behavioral avoidance, and increased physiological arousal that last longer than 1 month.

- Although dissociation is more heavily emphasized in the clinical presentation of acute stress disorder, ASD shares many of the same diagnostic criteria as PTSD, with the main difference being that the emotional distress is limited to 1 month following the traumatic experience.

- A significant proportion of people who experience psychological trauma develop "normal" emotional distress following the event, but not all of these individuals will develop long-term psychological problems and many will experience a spontaneous remission of their discomfort.

- Incidence and prevalence rates suggest that a large group of people may have PTSD at any given time, but the proportion of people who have PTSD compared to the number of people who experience events that could potentially cause traumatic reactions is relatively low.

- Individual characteristics that can lead to increased susceptibility to PTSD include experiencing prior trauma, having a family history of psychiatric problems, having poor psychological functioning prior to the trauma experience, feeling general life stress, and enduring a severe trauma in which the person believed his or her life was in danger and/or reacted with extreme levels of emotion or dissociation.

- The most significant predictor of PTSD for survivors of trauma was an actual or perceived lack of social support in the person's life.

- Events that violate a person's "core" beliefs, such as the belief in a fair and just world, the need for physical safety, and the need for a positive view of oneself and one's abilities, are more likely to cause traumatic reactions.

- Resiliency is demonstrated in that a significant proportion of individuals who experience traumatic events maintain relatively stable, healthy levels of psychological and physical functioning. Positive emotion, self-enhancing perceptions, and the personality trait of hardiness have been associated with resiliency.

- Individuals high in hardiness tend to experience less distress because they believe they can have a positive influence on their surroundings, have a sense of commitment and purpose in their daily lives, and believe they can learn from both the positive and the negative events they encounter.

- Trauma interventions are designed to help individuals resolve emotional reactions and overcome the problems related to traumatic experiences. Crisis interventions, however, are generally designed to prevent the development of psychological difficulties following trauma.

- Crisis intervention seeks to stabilize chaotic situations, reduce emotional distress, ensure basic survival needs, connect survivors with necessary resources, and initiate the recovery process so victims can return to a relatively normal level of functioning as quickly as possible.

- Educational interventions help reduce psychological difficulties by informing and preparing people for the general consequences of traumatic events. Educational interventions can include, but are not limited to, brochures, media portrayals, public seminars, and the coordination of support services.

- Psychological debriefings are structured, group-based intervention strategies that were initially developed to reduce distress in emergency personnel following grave situations and to help speed up the recovery process in everyday people who experience traumatic situations. Critical incident stress debriefing, the most popular debriefing form, was developed for high-risk occupational groups and other organizations where life and death situations are common.

- CISD has not been shown to be effective when used as a stand-alone treatment form for individuals who were directly affected by trauma. However, CISD has been shown to be a well-received primary prevention intervention when used as part of a comprehensive therapeutic response for homogenous groups following traumatic exposure.

- Cognitive behavioral therapy that focuses on cognitive restructuring, relaxation training, and the confrontation of safe but feared situations has become a successful early intervention for victims of trauma.

- CBT effectiveness is related to its ability to reduce fear reactions, work through the thoughts and fears that developed shortly after the traumatic event, and ultimately change cognitive patterns that contribute to the psychological difficulties following trauma.

- Although severe traumatic injuries or the accidental death of an athlete generally receive a tremendous amount of media attention, relatively little has been written about these situations from a psychological treatment perspective.

- Not only are athletes often unprepared for the extreme emotions associated with traumatic situations, but the relationships that witnesses and other athletes often have with the victims only add to the emotional impact of these situations when they occur within the context of sports.

- One of the most glaring deficits in the psychological treatment of athletes and teams following traumatic events is the absence of a clear intervention protocol.

- Training, preparation, and development of a network of multidisciplinary service providers can be the difference between the successful and unsuccessful resolution of critical incidents because athletes and teams often refuse assistance from professionals outside the sport community.

- A stepped-care approach is likely the most effective organizational response to critical incidents in a sport environment. However, early intervention treatment modalities should differ depending on whether care is being provided to a person directly affected by a traumatic event or given to an athletic team that witnessed a tragic event secondarily.

- A trauma intervention protocol should include the following steps: addressing basic needs; anticipating recovery while screening for signs of ineffective coping; implementing early intervention strategies; and coordinating appropriate termination, referral, and follow-up on the part of the treatment team.

- Individuals faced with providing emotional support to victims of trauma must be aware of compassion fatigue, which can result in a caregiver losing empathy or interest in caring for victims.

- Compassion fatigue is often a result of the intense emotionality involved in the treatment of survivors, but it can also be exacerbated when treatment providers have a personal history of trauma, lack social support, and fail to engage in proper self-care.

Chapter Questions

1. From a psychological perspective, what must be present for an event, injury, or situation to qualify as a traumatic experience?

   A. A significant amount of blood

   B. The subjective experience of pain by the victim

   C. A sudden or unexpected onset

   D. The subjective experience of fear, horror, or helplessness

2. For people who experience potentially traumatic events, approximately what percentage actually develop significant, long-term psychological or emotional difficulties?

   A. 40%

   B. 60%

   C. 10%

   D. 90%

3. A significant predictor of long-term difficulties following a traumatic experience is _____.
   A. Pain
   B. Lack of education
   C. A difficult childhood
   D. Lack of social support after the event

4. The use of posters and public service announcements to inform people about the potential impact of traumatic situations would best qualify as what form of intervention?
   A. Psycho-educational
   B. Psychological debriefing
   C. Crisis intervention
   D. Cognitive-behavioral therapy

5. Short-term acute stress reactions following the experiencing of extreme events can best be described as _____.
   A. A sign of certain long-term difficulties
   B. A warning for poor prognosis
   C. An indication of weak character
   D. A normal and expected response

6. Debriefing strategies operate on the basic assumption that _____.
   A. Irrespective of the nature of trauma, one can expect that a large number of people who experience potentially traumatic events will not handle it well
   B. Processing the events and reactions of a potentially traumatic event shortly after it occurs can promote adjustment and prevent the development of long-term psychological problems
   C. Subjective interpretation is key to understanding traumatic reactions because emotional difficulties following extreme experiences are often a function of how one "interprets" the subjective severity of the event
   D. Athletes are better prepared to endure traumatic injuries or critical incidents with less likelihood of having significant emotional difficulties because they respond to stressful situations in a more positive, calm, and confident manner

7. At the organizational level, the most effective way to mitigate the emotional effects of catastrophic injuries, disastrous accidents, or the unfortunate death of an athlete is to _____.
   A. Develop a clear trauma response protocol before events occur
   B. Train employees in critical incident stress debriefing techniques
   C. Refer all witnesses for cognitive-behavioral therapy
   D. All of the above

8. When responding to the needs of trauma victims, what should the first response of treatment providers be?
   A. Assume that most witnesses will inevitably develop long-term problems
   B. Ensure physical safety and help reestablish a level of independence
   C. Begin the immediate implementation of emotional processing strategies
   D. Make referrals to counselors, psychologists, or psychiatrists

9. For individuals who are directly affected by traumatic events and are experiencing significant emotional or psychological difficulties 1 month after the event, what is the best form of intervention?
   A. Psycho-educational
   B. Psychological debriefing
   C. Crisis intervention
   D. Cognitive-behavioral therapy

10. Some have suggested that compassion fatigue, or a caretaker's diminished ability to feel empathy or interest in helping victims of trauma, may actually be the result of _____.
    A. Their desire to avoid reminders of the event
    B. The seriousness of the event in question
    C. The empathy they feel and emotional connection they make with clients
    D. None of the above

■ *Case Study 1*

A college wrestler began having back pain and chills shortly after his 1:00 p.m. class. By 3:00 p.m. he presented at the athletic training office where, in addition to preparing a host of other athletes for their daily practices, the team athletic trainer and medical staff sought to determine what was causing his increasing fever, rash, and cold shivering. As his condition deteriorated over the next few hours, he was sent to a local emergency room for medical attention. Less than 12 hours later he died, succumbing to meningococcal septicemia, a bacterial bloodstream infection that can cause meningitis. By mid-morning of the following day, players on the wrestling team had heard about their teammate's death and were both shocked and dismayed about his sudden death. In addition, they, along with many other athletes who were present in the athletic training office that day, were concerned about whether the illness was contagious and if they were at risk for developing a potentially deadly disease.

Case Study 1 Questions

1. How does the situation described meet (or fail to meet) the criteria necessary for it to be considered a potentially traumatic experience?
2. Assuming that a psychological debriefing is conducted following this event, what information do you think is the most important to cover during such a meeting?
3. As part of the psychological emergency response team, what are your primary objectives during the period immediately following such an event?

■ *Case Study 2*

While competing in the conference championship, a collegiate pole vaulter suffered a dramatic and deadly fall while attempting to clear a height that was well below his personal best. In a shocking turn of events, as the vaulter swung upside down, he stalled in midair and tumbled backward, headfirst, into the metal box. Unconscious and bleeding profusely, he was treated by emergency medical technicians at the track and transported to a local area hospital. Despite the efforts of medical personnel, he was pronounced dead shortly after his arrival. In response to their teammate's death, the rest of the championship meet was canceled and news spread to members of the men's track and field team and to the athletes on the women's team, who were at their own conference championship at a different facility.

Case Study 2 Questions

1. What aspects of this accident cause greater concern for potential emotional reactions among teammates or witnesses?
2. What athletes would you expect to have more difficulty coping with this injury and death? Why?
3. What signs would you look for in individuals to suggest that their reaction to the situation described is atypical?

References

1. American Psychiatric Association. Diagnostic and statistical manual of mental disorders, 4th ed. Washington, DC: American Psychiatric Association; 1994.

2. Everly GS Jr, Lating JM. The defining moment of psychological trauma: What makes a traumatic event traumatic? In Everly GS Jr, Lating JM. Personality-guided therapy for posttraumatic stress disorder. Washington, DC: American Psychological Association; 2004:33–51.

3. Harvey AG, Bryant RA. Acute stress disorder: A synthesis and critique. Psych Bull. 2002;128:886–902.

4. Harvey AG, Bryant RA. The relationship between acute stress disorder and posttraumatic stress disorder: A prospective evaluation of motor vehicle accident survivors. J Consult Clin Psychol. 1998;66:507–512.

5. Bonanno GA. Loss, trauma, and human resilience: Have we underestimated the human capacity to thrive after extremely aversive events? Am Psychologist. 2004;59:20–28.

6. National Institute of Mental Health. Reliving trauma: Post-traumatic stress disorder (NIH Pub. No. 01-4597). Bethesda, MD: National Institute of Mental Health; 2001.

7. Ozer EJ, Best SR, Lipsey TL, et al. Predictors of posttraumatic stress disorder and symptoms in adults: A meta-analysis. Psych Bull. 2003;129:52–73.

8. Norris FH. Epidemiology of trauma: Frequency and impact of different potentially traumatic events on different demographic groups. J Consult Clin Psychol. 1992;60:409–418.

9. Brewin CR, Andrews B, Valentine JD. Meta-analysis of risk factors for posttraumatic stress disorder in trauma-exposed adults. J Consult Clin Psychol. 2000;68:748–766.

10. Allred KD, Smith TW. The hardy personality: Cognitive and physiological responses to evaluative threat. J Pers Soc Psychol. 1989;56:257–266.

11. Britt TW, Adler AB, Bartone PT. Deriving meaning from stressful events: The role of engagement in meaningful work and hardiness. J Occup Health Psychol. 2001;6:53–63.

12. Kobasa SC. Stressful life events, personality and health: An inquiry into hardiness. J Pers Soc Psychol. 1979;37: 1–11.

13. Golby J, Sheard M. Mental toughness and hardiness at different levels of rugby league. Pers Indiv Diff. 2004;37: 933–942.

14. Golby J, Sheard M, Lavalee D. A cognitive behavioural analysis of mental toughness in national rugby league football teams. Percept Motor Skills. 2003;96:455–462.

15. Hanton S, Evans L, Neil R. Hardiness and the competitive trait anxiety response. Anxiety Stress Coping. 2003;16:167–184.

16. Hamilton SE. Where are we now? A view from the Red Cross. Fam Sys Health. 2004;22:58–60.

17. Reyes G, Elhai JD. Psychological interventions in the early phases of disasters. Psychotherapy. 2004;41:399–411.

18. Mitchell JT. Crisis intervention and CISM: A research summary. From http://www.icisf.org/articles/cism_research_summary.pdf. Accessed February 18, 2009.

19. Dudley-Grant GR, Mendez GI, Zinn J. Strategies for anticipating and preventing psychological trauma of hurricanes through community education. Prof Psycho Res Pr. 2000;31:387–392.

20. Mitchell JT. When disaster strikes: The critical incident stress debriefing process. J Emerg Med Serv. 1983;8: 36–39.

21. Everly GS, Mitchell JT. Prevention of work-related posttraumatic stress: The critical incident stress debriefing process. In Murphy LR, Hurrell JJ Jr, Sauter SL, et al, eds. Job stress interventions. Washington, DC: American Psychiatric Association; 1995:173–183.

22. Bisson JI. Single-session early psychological interventions following traumatic events. Clin Psych Rev. 2003; 23:481–499.

23. Van Emmerik AAP, Kamphuis JH, Hulsbosch AM, et al. Single session debriefing after psychological trauma: A meta-analysis. Lancet. 2002;360:766–771.

24. Dyregov A. Caring for helpers in disaster situations: Psychological debriefing. Disaster Manage. 1989;2: 25–30.

25. Mitchell JT, Everly GS. Critical incident stress debriefing: an operations manual for the prevention of trauma among emergency service and disaster workers. Baltimore, MD: Chevron Publication Corporation; 1993.

26. Boudreaux ED, McCabe B. Critical incident stress management: Interventions and effectiveness. Psych Serv. 2000;51:1095–1097.

27. Kaplan Z, Iancu I, Bodner E. A review of psychological debriefing after extreme stress. Psych Serv. 2001;52: 824–827.

28. Boscarino JA, Adams RE, Figley CR. A prospective cohort study of the effectiveness of employer-sponsored crisis interventions after a major disaster. Inter J Emerg Mental Health. 2005;7:9–22.

29. Mayou RA, Ehlers A, Hobbs M. Psychological debriefing for road traffic accident victims. Brit J Psych. 2000;176:589–593.

30. Ehlers A, Clark DM, Hackmann A, et al. A randomized controlled trial of cognitive therapy, a self-help booklet, and repeated assessments as early interventions for posttraumatic stress disorder. Arch Gen Psych. 2003;60: 1024–1032.

31. Foa EB, Hearst-Ikeda D, Perry KJ. Evaluation of a brief cognitive-behavioral program for the prevention of chronic PTSD in recent assault victims. J Consult Clin Psychol. 1995;63:948–955.

32. Bisson JI, Shepard JP, Joy D, et al. Early cognitive-behavioral therapy for post-traumatic stress symptoms after physical injury: Randomized controlled trial. Br J Psych. 2004;184:63–69.

33. Bryant RA, Harvey AG, Dang ST, et al. Treatment of acute stress disorder: A comparison of cognitive-behavioral therapy and supportive counseling. J Consult Clin Psychol. 1998;66:862–866.

34. Foa EB, Kozak MJ. Emotional processing of fear: Exposure to corrective information. Psych Bull. 1986;99:20–35.

35. Heil J. Psychology of sport injury. Champaign, IL: Human Kinetics; 1993.

36. Henschen KP, Heil J. A retrospective study of the effect of an athlete's sudden death on teammates. Omega J Death Dying. 1992;25:217–223.

37. Karofsky PS. Death of a high school hockey player. Phys Sports Med. 1990;18:99–103.

38. Vernacchia RA, Reardon JP, Templin DP. Sudden death in sport: Managing the aftermath. Sport Psychologist. 1997;11:223–235.

39. Bauman NJ, Carr CM. A multi-modal approach to trauma recovery: A case history. Psychotherapy Patient. 1998;10:145–160.

40. Buchko KJ. Team consultation following an athlete's suicide: A crisis intervention model. Sport Psychologist. 2005;19:288–302.

41. Adams RE, Boscarino JA, Figley CR. Compassion fatigue and psychological distress among social workers: A validation study. Am J Orthopsychiatry. 2006;76:103–108.

42. Figley CR. Compassion fatigue as secondary traumatic stress disorder: An overview. In Figley CR, ed. Compassion fatigue: Coping with secondary traumatic stress disorder in those who treat the traumatized. New York: Brunner-Routledge; 1995:1–20.

43. Figley CR. Compassion fatigue: Psychotherapists' chronic lack of self care. J Clin Psych. 2002;58: 1433–1441.

44. Wee D, Myers D. Compassion, satisfaction, compassion fatigue, and critical incident stress management. Inter J Emerg Mental Health. 2003;5:33–37.

Suggested Readings

1. National Athletic Trainers' Association: www.nata.org

2. National Collegiate Athletic Association: www.ncaa.org

3. American Sports Medicine Institute: www.asmi.org

4. American Red Cross: www.redcross.org

5. American Psychological Association: www.apa.org

6. National Safety Council: www.nsc.org

7. National Center for Sports Safety: www.sportssafety.org

8. American College of Sports Medicine: www.acsm.org

9. National Institute of Mental Health. www.nimh.nih.gov

10. International Critical Incident Stress Foundation, Inc. www.icisf.org

abdomen   the part of the body between the pelvis and the thorax.

abdominal splinting   a rigid contraction of the muscles of the abdominal wall. It usually occurs as an unconscious reaction to abdominal pain. Abdominal splinting, in turn, may result in hypoventilation and respiratory complications.

acute compartment syndrome   usually secondary to trauma; increasing pressure within a fascial compartment as a result of swelling or bleeding can result in nerve damage and necrosis of muscle tissue (avascular necrosis).

acute mountain sickness   a syndrome associated with the relatively low concentrations of oxygen in the atmosphere at altitudes encountered during mountain climbing or travel in unpressurized aircraft.

acute stress disorder   a condition that develops soon after an individual experiences or witnesses an event involving a threat of or an actual death, serious injury, or physical violation and responds to this event with strong feelings of fear, helplessness, or horror.

adventitious   coming from an external source or occurring in an unusual place or manner. During auscultation of the chest or abdomen, adventitious sounds are those that are normally not heard.

agonal respirations   a type of breathing that usually follows a pattern of gasping followed by apnea.

airway obstruction   an abnormal condition of the respiratory system characterized by a mechanical impediment to the delivery or to the absorption of oxygen in the lungs.

airway patency   the condition of an airway being open or unblocked.

alignment   the association of long bone fracture fragments to one another; measured in degrees of angulation from the distal fragment in relation to the proximal fragment.

aneroid sphygmomanometer   a device using air pressure to measure arterial blood pressure. Aneroid refers to the absence of liquid, in this case the absence of a mercury column in the pressure gauge.

aneurysm   a localized weakening and swelling in the wall of a blood vessel. Can be caused by a number of factors, including hypertension, atherosclerosis, trauma, infection, or genetics.

angiogram   an x-ray of blood vessels that can be seen because the patient receives an injection of dye to outline the vessels on the x-ray. A coronary angiogram can be used to identify the exact location and severity of coronary artery disease (CAD).

anterograde amnesia   the inability to recall events of long ago with normal recall of recent events.

aortic dissection   a progressive tear in the aorta. When the inner lining of the aorta tears, blood surges through the tear, creating a new false channel, separating (dissecting) the middle layer from the outer layer of the aorta.

aortic stenosis   narrowing of the aortic valve and obstructing blood flow from the left ventricle into the aorta, resulting in decreased cardiac output.

apnea   an absence of spontaneous respiration.

apneic   pertaining or relating to apnea or affected with apnea.

apposition   when the edges of adjacent tissues meet; in a fracture, when fracture fragments are in contact with one another.

arrhythmogenic right ventricular dysplasia   a rare form of cardiomyopathy in which the heart muscle of the right ventricle is replaced by fat and/or fibrous tissue. The right ventricle is dilated and contracts poorly. As a result, the ability of the heart to pump blood is diminished. Patients with this condition often have arrhythmias, which can increase the risk of sudden cardiac arrest or death.

aspiration pneumonitis   inflammation of the lungs caused by inhaling foreign material, such as liquid or vomitus.

asthma   a respiratory disorder characterized by recurring episodes of paroxysmal dyspnea, wheezing on expiration as a result of constriction of the bronchi, coughing, and viscous mucoid bronchial secretions.

asystole   the absence of a heartbeat, as distinguished from fibrillation (in which electric activity persists but contraction ceases).

ataxia   an abnormal condition characterized by impaired ability to coordinate movement.

auscultation   the act of listening for sounds within the body to evaluate the condition of the heart, lungs, pleura, intestines, or other organs.

automated external defibrillator   also called an AED; a portable defibrillator designed to be automated such that it can be used by persons without substantial medical training who are responding to a cardiac emergency.

avascular necrosis   tissue death from lack of circulation; typically refers to bone death.

axial load   a force administered along the lines of an axis. Typically used to describe an injury in which there is compression of the spine from the head, such as when a person dives headfirst into shallow water and hits the top of his or her head on the bottom. This frequently causes fractures of the spine and possibly spinal cord injury.

bag valve mask (BVM) also known as an Ambu bag; a handheld device used to provide ventilation to a patient who is not breathing or who is breathing inadequately.

balance error scoring system (BESS) a postural-stability test commonly used as part of a concussion-assessment battery.

Ballone sign a fixed dullness in the left flank and shifting position dullness in the right flank.

Battle's sign an indication of fracture of the base of the posterior portion of the skull; may suggest underlying brain trauma.

beta-2 antagonists a class of drugs used to treat asthma and other pulmonary disease states.

bloodborne pathogens microorganisms in the blood or other body fluids that can cause illness and disease in people. These microorganisms can be transmitted through contact with contaminated blood and body fluids.

blood–brain barrier an anatomic–physiologic feature of the brain thought to consist of walls of capillaries in the central nervous system and surrounding glial membranes.

bradycardia generally defined as a heart rate of less than 60 beats per minute.

bradypnea an abnormally slow rate of breathing.

Brugada syndrome a genetic disease that is characterized by abnormal electrocardiogram (ECG) findings and an increased risk of sudden cardiac death.

capillary refill the process of blood returning to a portion of the capillary system after being interrupted briefly. Commonly used as a test of distal integrity of the circulatory system by applying pressure to a fingernail or toenail to interrupt capillary blood flow and then observing for return of blood to the nailbed after release of pressure.

cardiomyopathy the deterioration of the function of the myocardium (i.e., the actual heart muscle) for any reason. People with cardiomyopathy are often at risk of arrhythmia and/or sudden cardiac death.

cardioversion the restoration of the heart's normal sinus rhythm by delivery of a synchronized electric shock through two metal paddles placed on the patient's chest.

cerebral concussion a head injury with a transient loss of brain function. A concussion can cause a variety of physical, cognitive, and emotional symptoms.

cerebral contusions a form of traumatic brain injury; bruises of the brain tissue. Like bruises in other tissues, cerebral contusion can be caused by multiple microhemorrhages (small blood vessel leaks into brain tissue).

cerebral hematomas involves bleeding into the cerebrum, resulting in an expanding mass of blood that damages surrounding neural tissue.

cerebral infarction blockage of the flow of blood to the cerebrum, causing or resulting in brain tissue death. Blockage may be caused by a thrombosis, an embolism, a vasospasm, or a rupture of a blood vessel.

Cheyne-Stokes respirations an abnormal breathing pattern characterized by alternating periods of apnea and deep, rapid breathing.

cholinergic urticaria an abnormal and usually transient vascular reaction of the skin, often associated with sweating in susceptible individuals subjected to stress, strong exertion, or hot weather. The condition is characterized by small, pale, itchy papules surrounded by reddish areas; it is caused by the action of acetylcholine on mast cells.

cognitive functions intellectual processes by which one becomes aware of, perceives, or comprehends ideas. It involves all aspects of perception, thinking, reasoning, and remembering.

cognitive-behavioral therapy psychotherapy based on cognitions, assumptions, beliefs, evaluations, and behaviors, with the aim of influencing negative emotions that relate to inaccurate and maladaptive appraisal of events.

cold exposure and illness cold exposure can occur in weather that is not freezing. Wind, humidity, and moisture remove body heat, which can eventually lead to cold-related illnesses and pathology.

Colles' fracture fracture of the radius at the epiphysis within 1 inch of the joint of the wrist. It is easily recognized by the resulting dorsal and lateral position of the hand.

Combitube a device designed to facilitate the blind intubation of a patient. It consists of a cuffed double-lumen tube with one blind end. Inflation of the cuff allows the device to function as an endotracheal tube and closes off the esophagus, allowing ventilation and preventing reflux of gastric contents.

commotio cordis a sudden disturbance of heart rhythm observed mostly in young people during participation in sports. It occurs as the result of a blunt, nonpenetrating impact to the precordial region, often caused by impact of a ball, a bat, or other projectile.

compassion fatigue a gradual reduction of compassion over time. It is common among victims of trauma and individuals who work directly with victims of trauma.

consciousness a clear state of awareness of self and the environment in which attention is focused on immediate matters, as distinguished from mental activity of an unconscious or subconscious nature.

contrecoup injury an injury most often associated with a blow to the skull in which the force of the impact is transmitted to the opposite side of the head (*compare to coup injury*).

coronary artery anomalies a coronary artery is one of a pair of arteries that branch from the aorta, including the right and the left coronary arteries, and anomalies are deviations from what is regarded as normal.

coup injury occurs directly beneath the site of impact with an object (compare to contrecoup injury).

crackles fine bubbling sounds heard on auscultation of the lung. It is produced by air entering distal airways and alveoli that contain serous secretions.

crepitus the grating, crackling, or popping sounds and sensations that may be experienced under the skin and within joints.

crisis interventions therapeutic interventions to help resolve particular and immediate problems. No attempt is made at in-depth analysis. The goal is to restore the level of functioning that existed before the current crisis.

critical incident stress debriefing a specific technique designed to inform and assist others in dealing with the physical or psychological symptoms that are generally associated with trauma exposure. Debriefing allows those involved with the incident to process the event and reflect on its impact.

Critical Incident Stress Management (CISM) a technique to help people deal with their trauma one incident at a time by allowing the individual to talk about the incident when it happens without judgment or criticism.

Cullen's sign the appearance of faint, irregularly formed hemorrhagic patches on the skin around the umbilicus. The discolored skin is blue–black and becomes greenish-brown or yellow. It may appear 1 to 2 days after the onset of the severe, poorly localized abdominal pains that are characteristic of acute pancreatitis. It is also present in massive upper gastrointestinal hemorrhage and ruptured ectopic pregnancy.

cyanosis bluish discoloration of the skin and mucous membranes caused by an excess of deoxygenated hemoglobin in the blood.

defibrillation the termination of ventricular fibrillation by delivering a direct electric counter shock to the patient.

Destot sign the presence of a hematoma above the inguinal ligament or over the scrotum. Indicative of pelvic fracture.

diabetes mellitus a complex disorder of carbohydrate, fat, and protein metabolism that is primarily a result of a relative or complete lack of insulin secretion by the beta cells of the pancreas or of defects of the insulin receptors.

diabetic ketoacidosis a life-threatening complication in patients with diabetes mellitus. Near-complete deficiency of insulin and elevated levels of certain stress hormones increase the chance of a diabetic ketoacidosis episode. Typically occurs in patients with diabetes who do not take the prescribed insulin.

diastolic blood pressure the lowest pressure during the resting phase of the cardiac cycle.

diffuse brain injuries widespread injuries resulting from the brain forcefully hitting the inside of the skull in addition to being twisted.

dislocation the displacement of any part of the body from its normal position, particularly a bone from its normal articulation with a joint.

dissociation an unconscious defense mechanism by which an idea, thought, emotion, or other mental process is separated from the consciousness and thereby loses emotional significance.

diving towers structures that typically hold three levels 5-meter, 7-meter, and 10-meter heights. A tower can be found at both indoor and outdoor pools.

diving wells separate pools or a pool set off to the side of the competition pool. This pool has deeper water and diving boards/platforms.

documentation may refer to the process of providing evidence ("to document something") or to the communicable material used to provide such documentation.

dysphagia difficulty in swallowing, commonly associated with obstructive or motor disorders of the esophagus.

dyspnea a shortness of breath or a difficulty in breathing that may be caused by certain heart conditions, strenuous exercise, or anxiety.

echocardiography a diagnostic procedure for studying the structure and motion of the heart. Ultrasonic waves directed through the heart are reflected backward (or echoed) when they pass from one type of tissue to another. Also called ultrasonic cardiography.

ectopic pregnancy an abnormal pregnancy in which the fertilized ovum implants outside the uterine cavity.

electrocardiographic a procedure used to record the electrical impulses that immediately precede the contractions of the heart muscle. It allows diagnosis of specific cardiac abnormalities. The *device* used for this is an electrocardiograph (ECG). The *data* produced by this procedure are called electrocardiograms (EKG).

emergency action plan also called an EAP; a written plan to guide personnel and identify the role of each member of the emergency response team, emergency communications, the necessary emergency equipment, and the emergency protocol for various situations.

emergency medical services (EMS) a national network of services coordinated to provide aid and medical assistance from primary response to definitive care, involving personnel trained in the rescue, stabilization transportation, and advanced treatment of traumatic or medical emergencies.

endotracheal intubation   the management of the patient with an airway catheter inserted through the mouth or nose into the trachea.

epigastrium   the part of the abdomen in the upper zone between the right and left hypochondriac regions.

epiglottis   the cartilaginous structure that overhangs the larynx like a lid and prevents food from entering the larynx and the trachea while swallowing.

epistaxis   bleeding from the nose.

Essex-Lopresti fracture   an injury to the forearm consisting of a comminuted and displaced fracture of the radial head with subluxation or dislocation of the distal radioulnar joint. The radial shaft migrates proximally to a degree determined by the severity of the fracture, and disruption of the interosseous membrane occurs.

excursion   movement of one fracture fragment in relation to another.

exercise-induced anaphylaxis   a syndrome in which patients experience the symptoms of anaphylaxis, occurring only after increased physical activity.

exercise-related SCA   sudden cardiac arrest occurring in athletes during exercise.

first responder   a person who has completed training in providing prehospital care for medical emergencies.

flail segment   a life-threatening medical condition that occurs when multiple adjacent ribs are broken in multiple places, separating a segment, so a part of the chest wall moves independently. The flail segment moves in the opposite direction as the rest of the chest wall; because of the ambient pressure in comparison to the pressure inside the lungs, it goes in while the rest of the chest is moving out, and vice versa. This so-called "paradoxical motion" can increase the work and pain involved in breathing.

fluid challenge   a procedure in which a patient exhibiting signs and symptoms of hypovolemic or neurogenic shock is treated with a fluid infusion. If the patient's vital signs demonstrate improvement, additional fluid may be administered; if there is no improvement, a vasopressor may then be administered.

focal brain injuries   brain injuries that occur in a specific location in the brain. These localized injuries are often associated with symptoms corresponding to the part of the brain that was injured.

front bun   the sloped portion of a pole vault pit that surrounds the plant box.

frostbite   a freezing of the skin and superficial tissue resulting from exposure to extreme cold. The lesion is similar to a burn and may become gangrenous.

glottis   that part of the larynx associated with voice production.

golden hour   the first 60 minutes after the occurrence of multisystem trauma. It is widely believed that the victim's chances of survival are greatest if he or she receives definitive care in the emergency department within the first hour after a severe injury.

gravity (modified Stimson's) method   method of joint reduction using gravity and the weight of the limb to assist in the reduction of the dislocation.

hardiness   a personality trait measuring the positive capacity of people to cope with stress and catastrophe. It is also used to indicate a characteristic of resistance to future negative events.

head-splint turnover   method of cervical spine stabilization used to turn over an unconscious victim who is prone in the water.

heat cramps   any cramp in the arm, leg, or abdomen caused by depletion in the body of both water and salt. It usually occurs after vigorous physical exertion in an extremely hot environment or under other conditions that cause profuse sweating and depletion of body fluids and electrolytes.

heat exhaustion   collapse, with or without loss of consciousness, suffered in conditions of heat and high humidity largely resulting from loss of fluid and salt by sweating.

heat exposure and illness   prolonged exposure to high heat and possibly humidity that can eventually lead to heat-related illnesses and pathology.

heat index   an index that combines air temperature and relative humidity in an attempt to determine the human-perceived equivalent temperature—how hot it feels, termed the felt air temperature.

heat stroke   medical emergency in which a person's cooling systems have stopped working and core body temperature has become dangerously high. Immediate and heroic measures must be taken to cool the victim or death may occur.

hemothorax   blood in the pleural cavity.

high-altitude cerebral edema   a severe (frequently fatal) form of altitude sickness, resulting from swelling of brain tissue from fluid leakage. Symptoms can include headache; loss of coordination; weakness; and decreasing levels of consciousness including disorientation, loss of memory, hallucinations, irrational behavior, and coma. It generally occurs after a week or more at high altitude, but symptoms of mild high-altitude cerebral edema can sometimes show up even after few hours at higher altitudes.

high-altitude pulmonary edema a life-threatening form of noncardiogenic pulmonary edema that occurs in otherwise-healthy subjects at altitudes higher than 8200 feet. This occurs as a result of the shortage of oxygen caused by the lower air pressure at high altitudes. It remains the major cause of death related to high-altitude exposure with a high mortality in absence of emergency treatment.

hilum a depression on the surface of an organ where vessels, ducts, and the like enter and exit.

hypercapnia increased CO_2 tension in arterial blood.

hyperkalemia excessive potassium in the blood as occurs in renal failure; early signs are nausea, diarrhea, and muscular weakness.

hyperresonant higher than normal pitched sounds (resonance) in response to percussion of the chest wall; suggestive of a pneumothorax.

hypertension abnormally high tension, by custom abnormally high blood pressure involving systolic and/or diastolic levels; commonly defined as consistently elevated blood pressure higher than 140/90 mm Hg.

hyperthermia a much higher than normal body temperature. Body temperatures higher than 104°F are life threatening. This compares to normal human body temperature of 97°F to 98°F. At 106°F, brain death begins, and at 113°F, death is nearly certain.

hypertrophic cardiomyopathy a disease of the myocardium (the muscle of the heart) in which a portion of the myocardium is hypertrophied (thickened) without any obvious cause. It is perhaps most famous as a leading cause of sudden cardiac death in young athletes.

hyporesonant lower than normal pitched sounds (resonance), similar to a thud, in response to percussion of the chest wall; suggestive of a hemothorax.

hypotension an abnormal condition in which the blood pressure is not adequate for normal perfusion and oxygenation of the tissues.

hypothermia an abnormal and dangerous condition in which the temperature of the body is lower than 95°F, usually caused by prolonged exposure to cold.

hypovolemia oligemia; diminished total quantity of blood.

hypoxemia a diminished amount of oxygen in the arterial blood, shown by decreased arterial oxygen tension and reduced saturation.

hypoxia a diminished amount of oxygen in the tissues resulting from a deficiency of hemoglobin.

iatrogenic pathology or illness caused by treatment or diagnostic procedures.

ischemia deficient blood supply to any part of the body.

jaw thrust maneuver a technique used on patients with a suspected spinal injury and on a supine patient. The practitioner uses the thumbs to physically push the posterior aspects of the mandible. When the mandible is displaced forward, it pulls the tongue forward and prevents it from occluding the entrance to the trachea, helping to ensure a patent airway.

Kawasaki disease a poorly understood self-limited vasculitis that affects many organs, including the skin and mucous membranes, lymph nodes, blood vessel walls, and the heart. It does not seem to be contagious.

Kehr's sign the occurrence of acute pain in the tip of the shoulder as a result of the presence of blood or other irritants in the peritoneal cavity. Kehr's sign in the left shoulder is considered a classical symptom of a ruptured spleen. May result from diaphragmatic or peridiaphragmatic lesions, renal calculi, splenic injury, or ectopic pregnancy.

kidney a gland situated one on either side of the vertebral column in the upper posterior abdominal cavity. Its main function is secretion of urine, which flows into the ureters.

King laryngeal tube-disposable (King LT-D) a disposable supraglottic airway tool for emergency ventilation when direct laryngoscopy is not feasible.

Korotkoff sounds the sounds that medical personnel listen for when they are taking a blood pressure measurement.

laparotomy an abdominal surgical procedure involving a small incision in the abdominal wall allowing access to the abdominal cavity.

laryngeal mask airway (LMA) used in anesthesia and in emergency medicine for airway management. Consists of a tube with an inflatable cuff that is inserted into the pharynx. A standard laryngeal mask airway does not protect the lungs from aspiration, making the masks unsuitable for patients at risk for this complication. The device is useful in situations where a patient is trapped in a sitting position, when trauma to the cervical spine is suspected (where tilting the head to maintain an open airway is contraindicated), or when intubation is unsuccessful.

larynx the organ of voice situated below and in front of the pharynx and at the upper end of the trachea.

lateral flexion bending to one side. The term lateral flexion is used to describe motions of the trunk and neck.

legal need the legal basis for the development and application of an emergency action plan.

Lisfranc fracture a fracture and dislocation of the joints in the midfoot in the area of the base of the first and second metatarsals.

liver   the largest organ in the body, situated in the right upper section of the abdominal cavity. It secretes bile, forms and stores glycogen, and plays an important part in the metabolism of proteins and fats.

long QT syndrome   a heart condition associated with prolongation of repolarization (recovery) following depolarization (excitation) of the cardiac ventricles. It is associated with syncope (fainting) and sudden death from ventricular arrhythmias.

lucid   clear; describing mental clarity.

lymphadenopathy   any disease of the lymph nodes.

lymphocytosis   an increase in lymphocytes in the blood.

manual stabilization   refers to stabilization of the head and cervical spine of a victim by a rescuer.

Marfan's syndrome   a hereditary disorder of unknown cause, characterized by elongation of the bones, often with associated abnormalities of the eyes and the cardiovascular system. The disease can cause major pathological musculoskeletal disturbances, such as muscular underdevelopment, ligamentous laxity, and joint hypermobility. This syndrome is a risk factor for sudden cardiac death in athletes.

mental status   the degree of competence shown by a person in intellectual, emotional, psychological, and personality functioning as measured by psychological testing with reference to a statistical norm.

mitral valve prolapse   protrusion of one or both cusps of the mitral valve back into the left atrium during ventricular systole, resulting in incomplete closure of the valve and the backflow of blood.

mononucleosis   an acute herpes virus infection caused by the Epstein-Barr virus. It is characterized by fever, sore throat, swollen lymph glands, atypical lymphocytes, splenomegaly, hepatomegaly, abnormal liver function, and bruising.

morbidity rate   refers to either the incidence rate or the prevalence rate of a disease.

mortality rate   refers to the number of people dying during a given time interval divided by the total number of people in the population.

motor function   the ability to use and control muscles and movements.

mucosa   mucous membrane.

myositis ossificans   a rare condition in which muscle tissue is replaced by bone. Can occur secondary to intramuscular bleeding.

nares   the nostrils.

nasal cannula   a device for delivering oxygen by way of two small tubes that are inserted into the nares.

nasal flaring   the enlargement of the opening of the nostrils during breathing. It is often a sign that increased effort is needed to breathe.

nasopharyngeal (NP) airway   also known as a nasal trumpet because of its flared end; a tube that is designed to be inserted into the nasal passageway to secure an open airway. Nasopharyngeal airways can be used on patients in whom the oropharyngeal airway is contraindicated, such as patients who are conscious or patients with deformity of the oral cavity.

nasopharynx   the portion of the pharynx above the soft palate.

nebulizer   an apparatus for converting a liquid into a fine spray. It can contain medicaments for application to the skin, nose, or throat.

needle thoracentesis   an invasive procedure to remove fluid or air from the space between the lining of the outside of the lungs (pleura) and the wall of the chest for diagnostic or therapeutic purposes. A cannula, or hollow needle, is carefully introduced into the thorax, generally after administration of local anesthesia.

nephrectomy   the surgical removal of a kidney.

neuropraxia   the interruption of nerve conduction without loss of continuity of the axon.

neuropsychological testing   specifically designed tasks used to measure a psychological function known to be linked to a particular brain structure or pathway. Tests are typically administered following traumatic brain injury and are usually computer-based. Used to assess level of recovery in short- and long-term memory, reaction time, and information processing systems.

omental infarction   a localized area of necrosis in the peritoneum caused by an interruption in the blood supply to the area.

oropharyngeal (OP) airway   used to maintain a patent (open) airway. This type of airway prevents the tongue from either partially or completely covering the epiglottis, thereby obstructing the airway.

oropharynx   that portion of the pharynx below the level of the soft palate and above the level of the hyoid bone.

osmotic diuresis   increased urination caused by the presence of certain substances in the small tubes of the kidneys.

osteomyelitis   inflammation in the marrow of bone.

otorrhea   a discharge from the external ear.

Ottawa rules   a set of guidelines for deciding if a patient with foot or ankle pain should be offered x-rays to diagnose a possible bone fracture.

oxygen therapy   any procedure in which oxygen is administered to a patient to relieve hypoxia.

pancreas   a tongue-shaped glandular organ lying below and behind the stomach. Secretes the hormone insulin and pancreatic juice, which contains enzymes involved in the digestion of fat and proteins in the small intestine.

pancreatitis   inflammation of the pancreas. The lipase level of blood and urine is used as an indicator of pancreatitis.

panel mats   landing mats used in gymnastics that fold into numerous sections.

paraplegia   paralysis of the lower limbs, usually including the bladder and rectum.

parenchymal injury   injury to the functioning tissues of an organ, as distinguished from connective or supporting tissues.

paresis   partial or slight paralysis; weakness of a limb.

patent   open; not closed or occluded.

patient assessment   the process of evaluating and appraising a patient's condition.

perfuse   To force a fluid or a gas to flow over or through something, especially through an organ of the body.

pneumothorax   a collection of air or gas in the pleural cavity, causing the lung to collapse.

pocket mask   a device used to safely deliver rescue breaths during a cardiac arrest or respiratory arrest. Air is administered to the patient when the emergency responder exhales through a one-way filter valve. Modern pocket masks have either a built in one-way valve or an attachable, disposable filter to protect the emergency responder from the patient's potentially infectious bodily substances, such as vomit or blood.

pole vault crossbar standards   refers to the height-adjustable metal towers, one on each side of the pole vault pit, that hold the crossbar.

pole vault landing pit   the area of thick foam where the pole vaulter lands after a vault attempt.

polydipsia   excessive thirst characteristic of several conditions, including diabetes mellitus.

polyuria   the excretion of an abnormally large quantity of urine.

postconcussion syndrome   the persistence of any of a number of symptoms associated with concussion, which may be present in varying degrees for a considerable time after the head injury.

postictal state   any of a number of symptoms, such as feelings of exhaustion or mental confusion, that may follow a seizure.

post-traumatic stress disorder   an anxiety disorder characterized by an acute emotional response to a traumatic event or situation involving severe emotional stress.

priapism   prolonged penile erection in the absence of sexual stimulation.

primary survey   consisting of assessment of airway, breathing, and circulation; the purpose of the primary survey is to identify life-threatening problems that must be managed immediately.

psycho-education   refers to the education offered to people who live with a psychological disturbance. Frequently psycho-educational training involves patients with schizophrenia, clinical depression, anxiety disorders, psychotic illnesses, eating disorders, and personality disorders and includes patient training courses in the context of the treatment of physical illnesses.

psychological debriefings   a one-time, semi-structured conversation with an individual who has just experienced a stressful or traumatic event. In most cases, the purpose of debriefing is to reduce any possibility of psychological harm by informing people about their experience or allowing them to talk about it.

psychological emergency response team   a network of qualified service providers, including but not limited to athletic trainers, physicians, sport psychologists, coaching staff, administrative staff, counselors, a CISD team, and staff psychiatrists, who are prepared to respond to the needs of those involved in a traumatic event.

psychological trauma   a type of damage to the psyche that occurs as a result of a traumatic event. Damage may involve physical changes inside the brain and to brain chemistry, which affect the person's ability to cope with stress. One person may experience an event as traumatic, whereas another person would not suffer trauma as a result of the same event.

pulmonary embolism   the blockage of a pulmonary artery by foreign matter such as fat, air, tumor tissue, or a thrombus that usually arises from a peripheral vein.

pulse oximetry   a noninvasive method allowing the monitoring of the oxygenation of a patient's hemoglobin.

pulseless electrical activity   refers to any heart rhythm observed on the electrocardiogram that should be producing a pulse but is not. The condition may or may not be caused by electromechanical dissociation. The most common cause is hypovolemia.

pulsus paradoxus   arterial pulsus paradoxus is alteration of the volume of the arterial pulse sometimes found in pericardial effusion. The volume becomes greater with expiration. Venous pulsus paradoxus (Kusman's sign) is an increase in the venous pressure with inspiration—the reverse of normal.

quadriplegia   paralysis of all four limbs.

raccoon eyes   also known as periorbital ecchymosis; a sign of basal skull fracture. It results from blood tracking down into the soft tissue around the eye.

radial palsy a compression or entrapment neuropathy involving the radial nerve.

reservoir bag face mask also known as a partial rebreather face mask. Allows collection of part of the exhaled CO_2 in the attached bag, where it is mixed with oxygen from a tank; the CO_2 serves as a respiratory stimulant.

resilience ability to quickly recover from psychological stress or trauma.

retrograde amnesia the loss of memory for events occurring before a particular time in a person's life, usually before the event that precipitated the amnesia. The condition may result from disease, brain injury or damage, or a traumatic emotional incident.

rhabdomyolysis the rapid breakdown of muscle tissue resulting from trauma or chemical or biological factors. The rapid breakdown leads to the release of byproducts that can be harmful to the kidneys and can lead to kidney failure.

rhinorrhea the discharge of a thin nasal mucus or the flow of cerebrospinal fluid from the nose after an injury to the head.

rhonchi abnormal sounds heard on auscultation of a respiratory airway obstructed by thick secretions, muscular spasm, neoplasm, or external pressure. The continuous rumbling sounds are more pronounced during expiration, and they characteristically clear on coughing.

Romberg test a test in which the patient is asked to stand erect, with feet together and eyes closed, to check for a loss of balance or sense of position.

Roux sign a decrease in the distance from the greater trochanter to the pubic spine on the affected side in lateral compression fracture of the pelvis.

sagittal plane the anteroposterior plane or the section parallel to the median plane of the body.

sarcoidosis a granulomatous disease of unknown etiology in which histological appearances resemble tuberculosis. May affect any organ of the body, but most commonly presents as a condition of the skin, lymphatic glands, or the bones of the hand.

scoop stretcher a device used specifically for casualty lifting. It is a tubular structure that can be split vertically into two parts; blades are fixed to the tubes. The two halves are put on each side of the casualty and then clipped together; the blades go under the casualty and replace the hands of the first responders during lifting.

second impact syndrome occurs when an athlete who has recently sustained a traumatic brain injury (e.g., a concussion) sustains a second brain injury before the symptoms associated with the first injury have resolved. This syndrome most often results in fatal or catastrophic outcomes.

secondary survey following primary survey. Once resuscitation efforts are well established and the vital signs are normalizing, the secondary survey can begin. The secondary survey is a head-to-toe evaluation of the trauma patient, including a history and physical examination and the reassessment of all vital signs. Each region of the body must be fully examined. If at any time during the secondary survey the patient deteriorates, another primary survey is carried out because a potential life threat may be present.

self-enhancement generally accepted by social psychologists as a basic motive that drives the cognition, affect, and behavior of people. Additionally, social psychologists consider the tendency toward self-enhancement as a way for individuals to preserve stable emotions and mental well-being.

self-reduction technique technique of dislocation reduction where the victim performs the reduction, typically using some type of traction method.

sensory function ability of the nervous system to provide information related to sensation.

shock the circulatory disturbance produced by severe injury or illness and resulting in large part from reduction in blood volume.

sickle cell trait the way a person can inherit one of the genes of sickle cell disease but not develop actual symptoms of the disease. Sickle cell *disease* is a blood disorder in which the body produces an abnormal type of the oxygen-carrying substance hemoglobin in the red blood cells.

simple face mask a basic disposable mask, made of clear plastic, to provide oxygen therapy for patients who are experiencing conditions such as chest pain, dizziness, and minor hemorrhages. It is often set to deliver oxygen between 6 and 10 L per minute. This mask is only meant for patients who are able to breathe on their own but who may require a higher oxygen concentration than the 21% concentration found in ambient air.

Smith's fracture also sometimes known as a reverse Colles' fracture; a fracture of the distal radius caused by falling onto flexed wrists, as opposed to a Colles' fracture, which occurs as a result of falling onto wrists in extension. Smith's fractures are less common than Colles' fractures.

soft foam landing pit used in gymnastics to provide a safe landing area to facilitate teaching of advanced skills. The pit is typically filled with soft foam blocks that cushion landings and help protect from injuries.

spleen an organ immediately below the diaphragm, at the tail of the pancreas, behind the stomach, where it functions in the destruction of redundant red blood cells and holds a reservoir of blood. It is regarded as one of the centers of activity of the reticuloendothelial system (part of the immune system). It has been increasingly recognized that its absence leads to a predisposition to certain infections.

split litter backboard   a backboard that separates into two pieces.

sports medicine staff and emergency team   includes specialty physicians and surgeons, athletic trainers, coaches, or other personnel who are part of a team of people who put the emergency action plan into motion.

stridor   a high-pitched sound during inspiration and/or expiration. Stridor can be indicative of a medical emergency.

subcutaneous emphysema   the presence of free air or gas in the subcutaneous tissues. The air or gas may originate from the rupture of an airway or alveoli and migrate through the subpleural spaces to the mediastinum and neck of the victim.

subluxation   incomplete or brief dislocation of a joint.

sudden cardiac arrest   the abrupt cessation of normal circulation of the blood from failure of the heart to contract effectively during systole.

sudden cardiac death   refers to natural death from cardiac causes, heralded by abrupt loss of consciousness within 1 hour of the onset of acute symptoms.

supraventricular tachycardia   tachycardia whose origin is above the ventricles but usually cannot be specifically identified as arising from the sinoatrial (SA) node, atria, or atrioventricular (AV) node.

syncope   a sudden, and generally momentary, loss of consciousness caused by a lack of sufficient blood and oxygen in the brain. The first symptoms that have been reported prior to loss of consciousness include dizziness; a dimming of vision, or brownout; tinnitus; and feeling hot.

systolic blood pressure   the peak pressure in the arteries, which occurs near the beginning of the cardiac cycle when the ventricles are contracting.

tachycardia   generally defined as a heart rate of more than 100 beats per minute.

tachypnea   an abnormally rapid rate of breathing, as seen with hyperpyrexia.

thrombosis   an abnormal vascular condition in which thrombus develops within a blood vessel of the body.

trachea   a nearly cylindrical tube in the neck, composed of cartilage and membrane, that extends from the larynx at the level of the sixth cervical vertebra to the fifth thoracic vertebra, where it divides into the two bronchi.

tracheal tugging   an abnormal downward movement of the trachea during systole that can indicate a dilation or aneurysm of the aortic arch.

traction/external rotation procedure   method of dislocation reduction specific to the glenohumeral joint that uses a combination of traction and careful external rotation of the humerus.

transect   to sever or cut across.

trauma intervention protocol   a plan that guides how a psychological trauma intervention will be managed.

traumatic brain injury (TBI)   occurs when physical trauma injures the brain. TBI can result from either a closed or a penetrating head injury; damage may occur in a specific location or may be diffuse, occurring over a more widespread area.

Turner's sign   bruising of the skin of the flank in acute hemorrhagic pancreatitis.

tympanic   pertaining to a structure that resonates when struck; drumlike, such as a tympanic abdomen that resonates on percussion because the intestines are distended with gas.

vasoconstriction   a narrowing of the lumen of any blood vessel, especially the arterioles and the veins in the blood reservoirs of the skin and abdominal viscera.

vasodilation   a widening or distention of blood vessels, particularly arterioles, usually caused by nerve impulses or certain drugs that relax smooth muscle in the walls of the blood vessels.

vasopressor   pertaining to a process, condition, or substance that causes the constriction of blood vessels.

vault box   the area at the end of the runway where the pole vault pole is planted prior to an athlete's takeoff.

ventilation   the process by which air or gases are moved into and out of the lungs.

ventricular ectopy   type of arrhythmia resulting from disturbance of the electrical conduction system of the heart.

ventricular fibrillation   a cardiac arrhythmia marked by rapid, disorganized depolarizations of the ventricular myocardium. Blood pressure falls to zero, resulting in unconsciousness. Defibrillation and ventilation must be initiated immediately.

viral myocarditis   an inflammatory condition of the myocardium, caused by viral infection.

vital signs   measures of body systems function, including heart rate, respiration rate, temperature, and typically including blood pressure.

Volkmann's ischemic contracture   permanent claw-like flexion contracture of the hand and wrist, typically resulting from damage to the brachial artery.

waveless water entry a method of entering a swimming pool or diving well that minimizes disturbance of the water to protect a potential cervical spine victim.

wheezing a form of rhoncus, characterized by a high-pitched musical quality. It is caused by a high-velocity flow of air through a narrowed airway and is heard both during inspiration and expiration. Usually associated with asthma and chronic bronchitis.

wind chill factor expressed in degrees Celsius or Fahrenheit, the effective temperature felt by a person exposed to weather, taking into account wind speed, air temperature, and humidity.

Wolff-Parkinson-White (WPW) syndrome a syndrome involving disordered atrioventricular (AV) conduction patterns.

Suggested Readings

1. Como ND, ed. Mosby's Medical, Nursing & Allied Health Dictionary, 3rd ed. St. Louis, Mosby; 1990.

2. Roper N, ed. New American Pocket Medical Dictionary, 2nd ed. New York, Scribner Book Company; 1995.

Answers to Chapter Test Questions

Chapter 1

1. C; To check for life-threatening injuries
2. D; All of the above
3. D; All of the above
4. C; Direct EMS to the scene
5. A; Family contact information
6. B; As many times as possible
7. D; All of the above
8. D; A and C only
9. D; All of the above
10. C; Proximity to venue location

Chapter 2

1. E; All of the above
2. A; Minimum time to get the injured athlete to a trauma center
3. D; Body fat measurement
4. B; Airway compromise
5. D; Central venous pressure
6. B; Shock
7. C; 80%
8. A; 0–10 with 10 the worst
9. C; Tympanic
10. A; Further evaluation and possible assistance

Chapter 3

1. A; Tongue
2. B; Fluid
3. D; Snoring respirations
4. C; Jaw thrust maneuver
5. B; Ear and tip of nose
6. A; 40 to 60%
7. D; In a holder away from flame
8. C; E-C
9. A; About 16%
10. B; Endotracheal intubation

Chapter 4

1. C; Sudden cardiac arrest
2. A; Go to the person and assess him or her
3. C; Sudden cardiac arrest
4. D; Sudden fibrillation syndrome
5. B; Performs ECG rhythm analysis

6. A; Must be operated by professional medical personnel
7. D; Ventricular fibrillation
8. B; Interrupt chest compressions as little as possible
9. B; On-site EMS crew
10. A; Determine if any responders require CISM

Chapter 5

1. E; All of the above
2. E; All include information the clinician should obtain
3. C; An arterial bleed
4. C; Mental status deterioration and worsening symptoms
5. C; May produce brain stem failure
6. C; Focal and diffuse
7. C; He or she should be allowed to return whenever ready
8. B; Can be an indication of whether the injury is improving or worsening over time
9. C; Recognizing the injury and its severity, determining whether the athlete requires additional attention or assessment, and deciding when the athlete may return to sport activity
10. D; History, observation, palpation, special test, active/passive range of motion, strength tests, and functional tests

Chapter 6

1. C; Supination
2. A; Mechanism of injury
3. B; Resistance
4. A; Primary or secondary
5. A; Maintain neutral, in-line position
6. C; Axial loading
7. D; Apneic
8. B; Hyperextension
9. A; With both on
10. B; Minimize swelling

Chapter 7

1. B; Hypertrophic cardiomyopathy
2. C; Ventricles
3. D; Blunt chest trauma
4. A; Volleyball

5. D; All of the above

6. A; Asthma

7. D; All of the above

8. D; Difficulty breathing

9. B; Hypoglycemia

10. C; Spleen rupture

Chapter 8

1. C; Pale and wet skin

2. D; All of the above

3. D; Both A and B

4. A; The athlete loses the ability to shiver

5. B; Remove athlete from outdoors

6. D; All of the above

7. A; Count seconds between lightning and thunder and divide by 5

8. C; Survey the scene for safety

9. B; 5000–11,500 ft

10. D; All of the above

Chapter 9

1. D; Central

2. B; Rotational

3. D; Shoulder

4. C; Scapular circumflex artery

5. A; Air

6. D; Type IV: superior

7. C; Femur

8. D; Tibia

9. A; Hand and wrist

10. C; Shoulder

Chapter 10

1. C; Kidney

2. D; All of the above

3. B; Cullen's sign

4. A; Left upper quadrant

5. B; Hematuria

6. D; Rare

7. C; Clinical picture

8. A; An ectopic pregnancy

9. D; A contusion

10. B; Pain to the shoulder

Chapter 11

1. D; A and B

2. B; Asthma

3. D; Both B and C

4. D. Jugular vein distension

5. D; Air

6. C. Hemathorax

7. A; A life-threatening injury

8. C; Pulmonary embolism

9. D; Flail chest segment

10. B; Occlusive

Chapter 12

1. B; Potentially catastrophic cervical spine injury

2. C; Offer a soft landing surface for gymnasts to fall into while learning new skills

3. C; Placing a mat or other firm landing mat on top of the foam blocks to provide a more stable surface to move on

4. A; The head

5. D; A potentially catastrophic head and/or neck injury from the athlete landing headfirst into the box

6. D; All of the above

7. B; The waveless water entry, which is designed to minimize the movement of the head of neck of the injured athlete

8. A; First rolling the athlete's face out of the water using a head-splint turnover technique

9. D; All of the above

10. C; An axial load resulting from collision with the boards

Chapter 13

1. D; The subjective experience of fear, horror, or helplessness

2. C; 10%

3. D; Lack of social support after the event

4. A; Psycho-educational

5. D; A normal and expected response

6. B; Processing the events and reactions of a potentially traumatic event shortly after it occurs can promote adjustment and prevent the development of long-term psychological problems

7. A; Develop a clear trauma response protocol before events occur

8. B; Ensure physical safety and help reestablish a level of independence

9. D; Cognitive-behavioral therapy

10. C; The empathy they feel and the emotional connection they make with clients

Index

Note: Page numbers followed by "b," "f," and "t" indicate boxes, figures, and tables, respectively.